Concise Medical Textbooks

BIOCHEMISTRY
S. P. Datta and J. H. Ottaway
CARDIOLOGY
D. G. Julian
COMMUNITY HEALTH, PREVENTIVE MEDICINE AND SOCIAL SERVICES
J. B. Meredith Davies
DERMATOLOGY
J. S. Pegum and Harvey Baker
EMBRYOLOGY
M. B. L. Craigmyle and R. Presley
GASTROENTEROLOGY
I. A. D. Bouchier
INTRODUCTION TO GENERAL PRACTICE
Michael Drury and Robin Hull
MEDICAL MICROBIOLOGY
C. G. A. Thomas
OBSTETRICS AND GYNAECOLOGY
R. W. Taylor and M. G. Brush
OPHTHALMOLOGY
Kenneth Wybar
PAEDIATRICS
John Apley
PATHOLOGY
J. R. Tighe
PHARMACOLOGY
R. G. Penn
PSYCHIATRY
W. H. Trethowan
RENAL MEDICINE
Roger Gabriel

Community Health, Preventive Medicine and Social Services

J. B. MEREDITH DAVIES
MD(London), FFCM, DPH

Director of Social Services, City of Liverpool
Lecturer in (Preventive) Paediatrics and in Public Health, University of Liverpool
Formerly Director of Personal Health and Social Services, University of Liverpool

FOURTH EDITION

BAILLIÈRE TINDALL · LONDON

A BAILLIÈRE TINDALL book published by
Cassell Ltd,
35 Red Lion Square, London WC1R 4SG
and at Sydney, Auckland, Toronto, Johannesburg
an affiliate of
Macmillan Publishing Co. Inc.
New York

First published as *Preventive Medicine, Community Health and Social Services* 1966
Third edition 1975
Reprinted 1977
Fourth edition 1979

ISBN 0 7020 0746 3

Set, printed and bound in Great Britain by
Fakenham Press Ltd
Fakenham, Norfolk

British Library Cataloguing in Publication Data

Davies, James Brian Meredith
Community health, preventive medicine and social services. – 4th ed. – (Concise medical textbooks).
1. Medicine, Preventive – Great Britain
2. Medical care – Great Britain 3. Public welfare – Great Britain
I. Title II. Series
614.4'4'0941 RA485

ISBN 0–7020–0746–3

Preface

The last edition was published early in 1975, a few months after the reorganization of the health services and local government. The intervening years have been characterized by many difficulties some of which are related to the introduction of new systems, and others to the financial cut-backs forced upon all public services by the recession.

The uncertainty within the health services was emphasized by the establishment of the Royal Commission in 1976 to examine the 'best use and management of the financial and manpower resources of the National Health Service'. Its report due out in 1979, is awaited with very real interest.

In addition, the last three years have seen the publication of two important reports dealing with children: the report of the Court Committee published late in 1976 dealing with health services for children and the report of the Warnock Committee (on which I had the honour to serve) in May, 1978 on the education of handicapped children. Both reports introduced new concepts of care which will eventually alter the health care of all children and the education of up to 20% of the children attending school who have some substantial special educational need due to some disability or significant learning difficulty. This edition has consequently been changed to describe these features and to set the scene for what are likely to be further evolutionary developments in the next few years.

The format of the book remains the same but many chapters have been extensively rewritten. The first two chapters have been extended to describe Joint Financing and Joint Care Planning.

These are two new features which emphasize the close relationship between the health and social services. In Joint Financing, monies are made available from health authority sources on a short-term basis to enable important community social services to be developed which are essential to the smooth running and development of the health services. The establishment of Joint Care Planning is a clear indication that it is wrong to plan either health or social services separately. Many criticisms of the new management structures within the National Health Service have been made in the last four years and Chapter 2 has been rewritten to include these.

Chapter 3 on the measurement of health has been further extended to include greater emphasis on social class differences in all epidemiological studies. Examples include general morbidity and mortality, perinatal mortality and especially occupational mortality. The year 1978 saw the publication of the analysis of occupational mortality, based upon the 1971 census. Widespread reference has been made in Chapter 3 and in Chapter 14 to this analysis and to the standardized mortality ratios based upon different occupations. An innovation in this edition is that the exact origin of each quoted table has been indicated to enable further statistical studies to be made.

The chapter on Child Health Services has been completely rewritten to include reference to the Court Committee Report and to the government's reaction to it. Greater emphasis is given to care within the neonatal period and more information is given about congenital malformations. The general health surveillance of infants is discussed and the problem of sudden infant deaths (cot deaths) is described in some detail.

The chapter on the health of the schoolchild has likewise been rewritten to include many of the more important points raised in the Warnock Committee's report. The government's reaction to this is awaited and likely to be known shortly after publication of this edition. The report extends special educational help from the 1·8% of handicapped children at present identified to approximately 20% of children known either to have disabilities or significant difficulties. The reasons for doing away with the present system of classification of handicapped children are explained as well as the importance of ensuring greater involvement and support of the parents. The concept of appointing a *named person* to help parents and children is dealt with, as well as the methods of discovery and the importance of multi-professional assessment. The integration of handicapped children into ordinary schools has become a central issue and the types of integration are analysed and described. Many special problems accompany the transitional period from school into adult life for handicapped school children and the role of Employment Rehabilitation Centres, specialist careers officers and further and higher education are briefly discussed. References are included in this edition to the problems of dyslexia which is now becoming more widely recognized and understood.

The changes in family planning introduced in 1975 which included free family planning advice, treatment and supplies (relating to female methods of contraception) are described in Chapter 5.

In the section of the book dealing with communicable diseases, Chapter 13 has been extended to include a full description of the symptoms and epidemiology of the viral haemorrhagic diseases, Lassa fever, Marburg disease and Ebola virus infection, and their prevention is fully discussed. The greatest risks of infection from these serious diseases in the UK certainly occurs in laboratory personnel and health staff who handle patients. A knowledge of how to decrease these risks when dealing with patients or material from Central and West Africa is essential. Rabies has continued to be an increasing danger in this country and the section on this disease has been enlarged.

Chapter 14 on the epidemiology of non-communicable diseases now includes a number of histograms taken from the publication 'Occupational Mortality' (published by the Office of Population Censuses and Surveys) illustrating the effect of social class on mortality.

Parts of Chapter 18 on International Health Control have been rewritten to include a short description of the increasing role the European Health Committee of the Council of Europe and the European Economic Community play in international health developments.

Part III of this book describes the developing social services, many of which have continued to grow at a faster rate than the health services. The new method of 'Partnership' whereby special financial help has been provided by government in an attempt to improve the deprivation of inner city areas is described.

Chapter 22 on the measurement of social problems has been rewritten and revised and now includes the projected changes in the population expected during the next 15 years which are bound to have a marked effect on the educational and social services for children and elderly people. Birth rates for ethnic minorities are now included so that valid comparisons can be made between the percentage of live births in this group and the European population. A new extra section on educational opportunity has been introduced because the extent to which educational opportunity in any country is available is an important factor which influences social problems. The improved educational attainment of girls compared to boys is emphasized.

Chapter 23 includes the changes introduced by the Children Act 1975. Reference is also made to the present disquiet being voiced by magistrates to the Juvenile Courts regarding the Children and Young Persons Act, 1969. Details are given of the codes of guidance now agreed for parts of this Act. The continuing importance of non-accidental injury and child abuse in children is emphasized with special reference to registers and the role of specialist consultant social workers.

The chapter on the disabled now includes an extra section dealing with employment and training of the disabled. The complicated roles of the Manpower Services Commission and its two executive arms, the Training Services Division and the Employment Services Division are described.

The development of more community-based social services for the mentally disordered has become a top national priority and Chapter 25 describes the developments in this field and the current review of the Mental Health Act, 1959. The section on day care for both the mentally ill and handicapped has been extended.

Chapter 26 on the elderly includes a review of the important demographic trends in the elderly with special reference to the likely substantial increases expected during the next 15 years in the proportion of very old persons within the country (over 75 and 85 years of age). Detailed reference is also made to the survey among the elderly published in 1978 by the Office of Population Censuses and Surveys which emphasized the growing proportion of disabled among old people and the various social problems which follow. The growing number of the elderly mentally infirm is rapidly becoming one of the major difficulties facing the health and social services and this problem is discussed in Chapters 25 and 26.

In Chapter 27 a completely new section has been added describing in detail the Housing (Homeless Persons) Act, 1977, which changed the law relating to various types of homeless people. Full details are given of these priority groups for which local authorities now have a clear duty to provide permanent, self-contained accommodation as soon as possible. A code of practice has been issued indicating how various sections of this Act should be implemented and this has been described.

Throughout this book there are many references to the 'primary health care team' which undoubtedly has already developed into a powerful local force in the prevention and treatment of illness and in influencing health and social problems. Approximately 22% of family doctors now work from health centres and the teams centred there include health visitors, home nurses and midwives and there is usually a close link maintained with the local social services.

This book aims mainly at providing doctors, medical students, health visitors and all other members of the primary health care team with a brief up-to-date description of the health and social services as well as explaining the many existing and developing preventive medical services.

The extensive index has been maintained and extended as it is felt that the value of any text book can be measured by the ease and speed of finding information.

Once again my thanks are due to my wife for all her support and help in correcting the proofs, analysing data and for the completion of the index. Without her constant encouragement and help it would have been impossible to have completed this edition.

March 1979 Brian Meredith Davies

Contents

	Preface	v
	Part I Community Health and Preventive Medicine	
1	The Health Services in the UK	3
2	Management within the New Health Services	41
3	Measurement of Health	52
4	Maternity Services	91
5	Child Health Services	106
6	Health of the Schoolchild	126
7	Health Education	153
8	Other Community Health Services	162
9	Epidemiology of Communicable Diseases	171
10	Prevention of Disease by Immunization	180
11	Epidemiology of Air-borne and Droplet Infections	189
12	Epidemiology of Faecal-borne and Food-borne Infections	205
13	Epidemiology of Other Communicable Diseases	222
14	Epidemiology and the Prevention of Non-Communicable Diseases	238

15 Preventive Medicine in Primary Health Care 262

16 Food and Nutrition 276

17 Environmental Health Control 290

18 International Health Control 320

Part II Community Health and Social Services

19 History of Community Health, Preventive Medicine and Social Services 335

20 Management Techniques, Measurement of Need and Determination of Priorities 361

Part III Social Services

21 Administration of the Social Services 383

22 Measurement of Social Problems 396

23 Care of Children in Need 413

24 Care and Rehabilitation of the Disabled 440

25 Care of the Mentally Disordered 464

26 Care of the Elderly 489

27 Other Community Social Services 508

28 Hospital Social Workers 524

Index 541

PART I

Community Health and Preventive Medicine

1 The Health Services in the UK

The National Health Service in the UK which was introduced in 1948 (see p. 350) was completely reorganized with effect from 1st April, 1974. The main object was to improve the health care by providing a unified structure to administer all the health services. This meant that all direct responsibilities concerned with the administration of the national health services were removed from local government.

At the same time local government services outside London were reorganized so that the community supporting social and educational services are provided by new authorities (County Councils or Metropolitan District Councils) which, in the majority of instances, cover exactly the same geographic areas as the new Area Health Authorities (AHAs). In this way, it is hoped to improve coordination between the various services.

Functions of the Secretary of State for Social Services

The Secretary of State for Social Services retains full responsibility for the health services and for the social services and is responsible to Parliament. The Secretary of State who is a member of the Cabinet is also responsible for the system of social security benefits totalling £11 527 million in 1977.

The annual cost of the health services is approximately £6000 million (1978) and represents approximately 10·9% of the total public expenditure and about 4·5% of the gross national product.

The functions of the Secretary of State are to provide throughout England to an extent which he considers necessary:

1. accommodation for the purpose of any service under the National Health Service Acts (health centres, clinics, etc.)
2. hospital accommodation
3. medical, dental, nursing and ambulance services
4. facilities for the care of expectant and nursing mothers and young children
5. facilities for the prevention of illness and aftercare of persons suffering from illness (vaccination and immunization)
6. such other services as are required for the diagnosis and treatment of illness (examples include the blood transfusion and the mass radiography services)
7. school health services (by arrangement with Local Education Authorities)
8. family planning services

At national level, these functions are exercised by the Department of Health and Social Security which both at its headquarters in London and various regional offices throughout the country maintains large teams of civil servants and administrators as well as numerous types of professional staff including doctors, nurses, lawyers, architects, social workers to advise the Secretary of State. Many expert committees are set up from time to time to study special problems within the health services.

The most important of these expert committees is the *Central Health Services Council*, a large body of 31 professional persons drawn from all the major medical, dental, nursing and pharmaceutical organizations as well as 10 other persons with special experience in hospital management or community health services. The Central Health Services Council advises the Secretary of State on all important matters concerning the National Health Service and reports annually.

There are other Standing Advisory Committees each dealing with special aspects. In the community health field, these include those concerned with maternity services and midwifery, with child health, mental health and with the prevention of disease by immunization. In addition, the Secretary of State appoints from time to time special *ad hoc* committees to study special subjects and collect and consider evidence from many sources and to make recommendations in their reports. It then becomes the responsibility of the Secretary of State to decide whether to recommend Parliament to implement any changes necessary.

If the subject is of great public importance, the Secretary of State, through Parliament, may appoint a Royal Commission to study all aspects of the problem. In 1976, such a Royal Commission was set up to examine 'the best use and management of the financial and manpower resources of the National Health Service'. Eventually its report will be presented to the Secretary of State and Parliament who will then decide whether or not to implement its various recommendations. In this way, a Royal Commission can play an important role in suggesting new legislation.

Method of Control exercised by the Department of Health and Social Security

Although the health services are administered peripherally through Regional Health Authorities (RHAs) and Area Health Authorities (AHAs) (see below), the Department of Health and Social Security (DHSS) exercises control over these services through its Regional and Headquarters office in the following way:

Financial

This is now the most important method. The Department supplies all funds, both revenue (for running costs) and capital (for constructing buildings), and therefore is in a powerful position to control development. Each RHA is given its budget and it then allocates to each AHA its financial resources. Both retain independent financial action.

As regards capital, the Department of Health and Social Security provides capital for hospital building or health centres on a 'once and for all' basis and not on any loan basis.

Advisory

This is a most useful function of the DHSS for it acts in an advisory manner issuing important memoranda on many aspects of the health services. Many of these give advice on developments of the service and priorities usually cover aspects both within the community supporting social services and health services. Advice on the development of services for the mentally ill or for the care of the elderly obviously should cover both aspects if it is to be comprehensive.

Advice is also given regarding the planning of new capital—hospital, health centres, etc. Individual plans are examined by the regional and headquarters officers to ensure that each new building can meet the latest requirements and can reach a satisfactory standard. A special National Development Group for the Mentally Handicapped has been set up to review existing policies in this field. The Group issues bulletins and pamphlets advising on the development of both health and social services for the mentally handicapped.

Planning and policy

Another important function of the DHSS is in the planning field. It is hoped that, in the future, long-range planning will play a larger part than in the past. This is because it is now realized that full comprehensive planning of the health services can only be properly achieved by a continuous process of analysis and review in which not only the health service plans are considered but also those of the supporting social services which are provided by the parallel new local authority. Special *Health-Care Planning Teams* have been set up (see p. 22) and include those concerned with all aspects of care. Also *Joint Care Planning* between health and social services has been started locally to ensure that the health and social services prepare jointly an annual strategic plan of development of both their services. In this way it is hoped that the DHSS will be able to ensure a balanced development of services and will, through its financial control, encourage those parts of the health service which need to develop at a faster rate.

The Joint Financing arrangement (see p. 24) helps to balance social service and health service development locally.

This planning aspect will also consider the *effectiveness of any services* provided, i.e. the results these services have upon the health of the people they serve. In this way, it is hoped to discover the most effective health and social service developments so that scarce financial resources can be channelled into fields where the results are most profitable.

Parliamentary Control

Because the Secretary of State is answerable to Parliament for the conduct of the health services, it is open to any member of Parliament to raise any question, however detailed, and this must be answered by the Secretary of State either verbally at question time or in writing.

In very serious instances, the Secretary of State can set up an Inquiry which then considers all aspects of the question and reports to the Secretary of State who then presents that report to Parliament. Recent examples have included fires in hospitals and allegations about the maltreatment of patients in mental hospitals.

These various procedures in Parliament and the continuous individual questioning by members of Parliament ensure that an ever watchful eye is kept on the detailed functions of the health services and does much to prevent bureaucracy.

A further method of control has been the setting up of a Health Service Commissioner for England and a separate one for Wales. Full details of these new services are given below (see p. 37).

General Outline of the National Health Service

The simplest way to understand the functioning of the National Health Service is to look at the plan of its administration (Fig. 1).

It will be seen that:

1. in England the Secretary of State and the DHSS are responsible nationally;
2. peripherally, a three tier system of control is maintained by 14 RHAs and 90 AHAs and 155 Districts.

Officers at Regional, Area and District Levels

Each RHA has its own officers controlled by the Regional Team of Officers (RTO).

Each AHA (unless it only has one district general hospital) has two tiers of officers—at Area level (controlled by the Area Team of Officers) and at District level (District Management Team). In the 28 single district AHAs, there is no separate District Management Team but the Area Team of Officers is strengthened by the addition of the Chairman and Deputy Chairman of

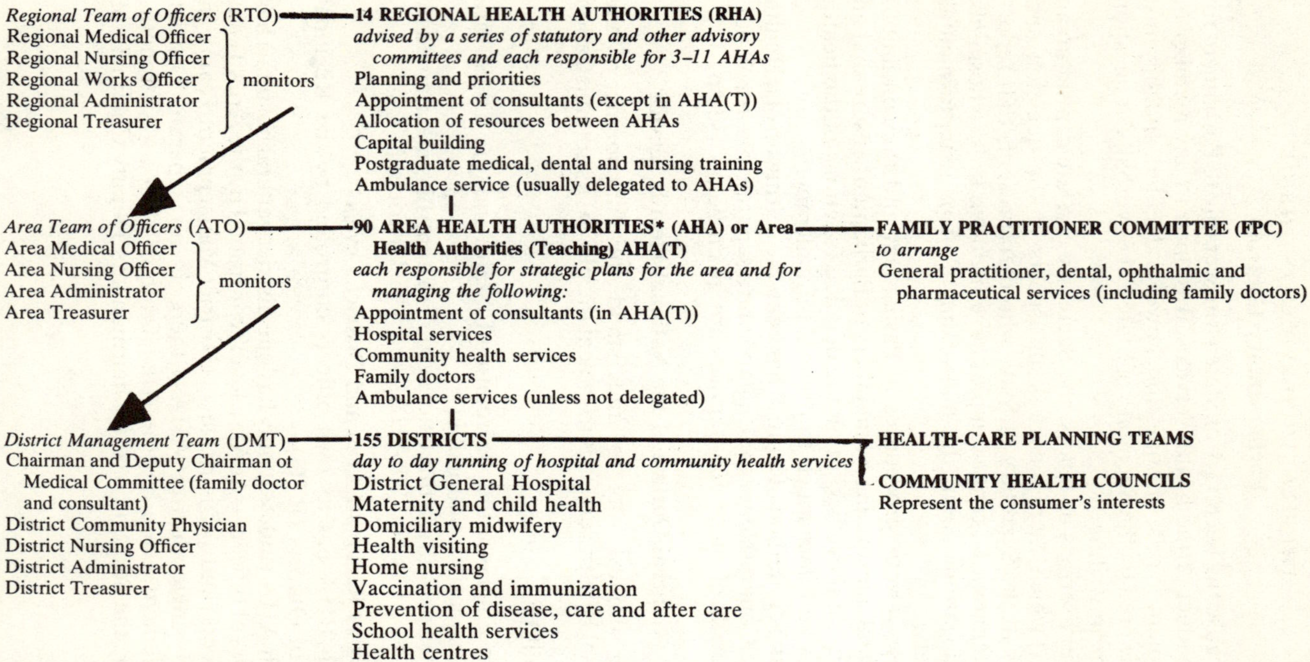

Fig. 1. National Health Service Reorganization Act, 1973, England. In 28 AHAs, there is one district only. In these cases, the ATO can be extended to include the chairman and deputy chairman of the Medical Committee to form an Area Management Team. Each district (or single district AHA) covers a population of between 100 000 and 400 000.

the Medical Committee (family doctor and consultant) to form an Area Management Team.

The diagram shows exactly which officers make up these teams. There are other professional officers at Region—architects and engineers—and at Region and Area—personnel officer, ambulance officer, supplies officer, etc.—who are not in the various 'Teams of Officers'.

Functions of Health Authorities

Regional Health Authorities (RHAs)

Generally the RHA is responsible for the main planning of health services, for capital building programmes, for postgraduate medical, dental and nursing training and for the allocation of financial resources between its constituent AHAs. In all but the AHAs (Teaching), the RHA also appoints all consultants and Senior Registrars. The one point to remember is that the RHA is *not* involved with the ordinary day to day running of the health services (full details, see p. 15).

Area Health Authorities (AHAs)

AHAs generally are responsible for the day to day management of the health services but as regards the general practitioner services, contracts of service are handled by the Family Practitioner Committee (to ensure the independence of general practitioners). Note that general practitioners remain independent contractors.

All hospital services and all the community health services are the responsibility of the AHA which is therefore in charge of:

- District General Hospitals
- Maternity and child health services
- Domiciliary midwifery
- Health visiting
- Home nursing
- Vaccination and immunization
- Prevention of disease care and after-care (health education, chiropody, tuberculosis after-care, occupational therapy and some types of convalescence)
- School health services (in conjunction with the corresponding local education authority)

Health Centres
Ambulances (in large conurbations one AHA is responsible).

AHAs which are also the centres for medical teaching (in conjunction with the medical schools of the corresponding University) are specially designated *Area Health Authorities* (*Teaching*). One interesting additional responsibility which all such authorities have is that they appoint consultants and senior registrars. (In the rest of the service, the appointment of consultants and senior registrars is undertaken by the RHA.)

Within AHAs there is a further division of responsibility. There is a group of officers at Area level responsible for the health services generally for the Area as a whole and at District level for the day-to-day management of the hospital and community health services. There is usually one District for the geographical area served by each District General Hospital. An AHA which therefore includes three District General Hospitals, will normally have three Districts, each controlled by a District Management Team of Officers. These are *directly* responsible to the AHA and *not* through the Area Team of Officers which advises the AHA independently.

LOCAL STRUCTURE AND ADMINISTRATION OF THE HEALTH SERVICES IN ENGLAND

Now follows a more detailed description of the structure and function of the local parts of the health service including:

1. Regional Health Authorities and Regional Team of Officers (see pp. 15 and 17)
2. Area Health Authorities and Area Team of Officers (see pp. 17 and 18)
3. Area Medical Officer (see p. 19)
4. Specialists in Community Medicine (see p. 19)
5. Area Nursing Officer (see p. 20)
6. Area Nurse (Child Health) (see p. 20)
7. Family Practitioner Committee (see p. 20)
8. District Management Team (see p. 21)
9. District Community Physician (see p. 22)
10. Health Care Planning Teams and Joint Care Planning Teams (see p. 22)

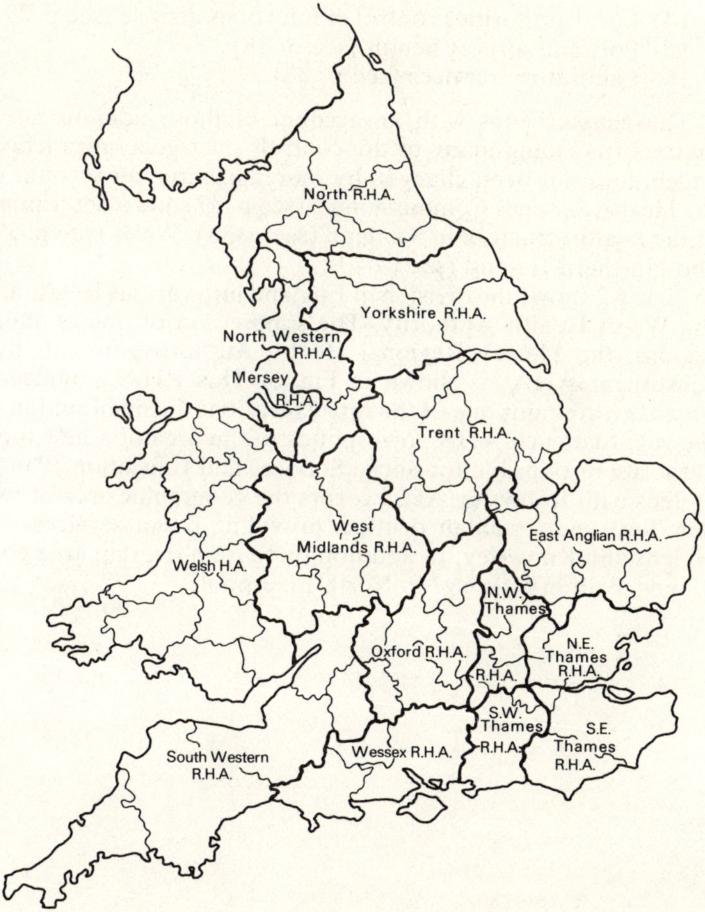

FIG. 2. Regional Health Authorities in England.

11. Joint Consultative Committee (see p. 23)
12. Joint Financing (see p. 24)
13. Community Health Councils (see p. 25)
14. Local authorities control of infectious disease (see p. 27)
15. Port and airport health (see p. 28)
16. Laboratory services (see p. 28)

The chapter ends with an account of those administrative matters (including many of the controls over general practice) which have not been changed by reorganization, an account of the Health Services Commissioners (see p. 37) and a description of the health structure in Scotland (see p. 38), Wales (see p. 39) and Northern Ireland (see p. 40).

Figure 2 shows the division of England into various RHAs and the Welsh Health Authority. The subdivision of one of those regions, the Mersey Regional Health Authority, into its five constituent AHAs is shown in Fig. 3. This RHA is unusual, because it contains one of the rare exceptions outside London to the rule that each AHA corresponds to the area of a new local authority responsible for Social Services and Education. The St Helens with Knowsley AHA covers the geographic area of two new local metropolitan districts providing social services—St Helens and Knowsley. In addition there is an overlap area containing Walton Hospital in North Liverpool.

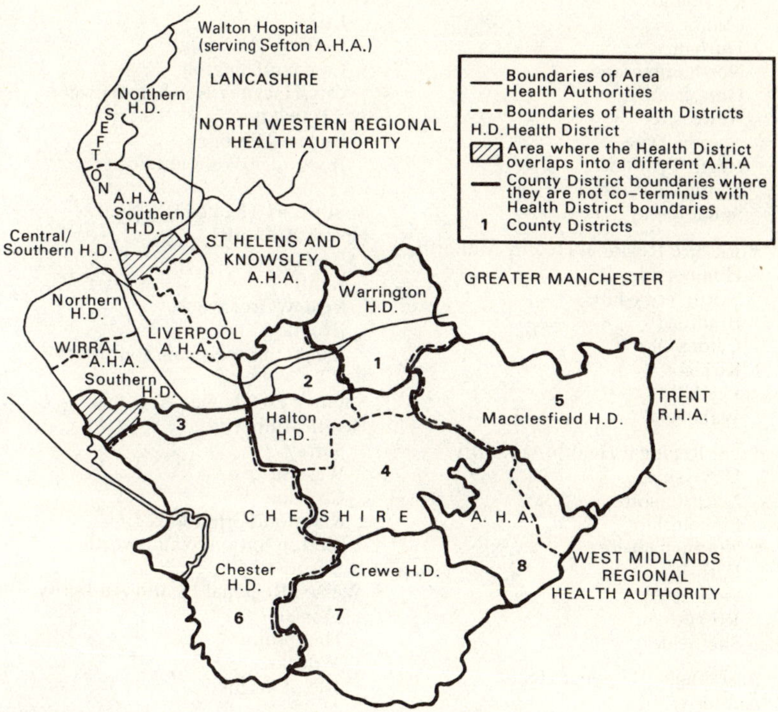

FIG. 3. Mersey Regional Health Authority. Council Districts of Cheshire are marked: (1) Warrington; (2) Halton; (3) Ellesmere Port; (4) Vale Royal; (5) Macclesfield; (6) Chester; (7) Crewe; (8) Congleton. Note that Liverpool AHA(T) is a single health district authority but that Cheshire has five health districts (Warrington, Halton, Chester, Crewe and Macclesfield) covering eight local authority district council councils, but only one county council, Cheshire.

List of RHAs and AHAs with matching local authorities responsible for social services and education services

North Regional Health Authority
- Cleveland
- Cumbria
- Durham
- Northumberland
- Gateshead
- Newcastle upon Tyne
- North Tyneside
- South Tyneside
- Sunderland

Yorkshire Regional Health Authority
- Humberside
- North Yorkshire
- Bradford
- Calderdale
- Kirklees
- Leeds
- Wakefield

Trent Regional Health Authority
- Derbyshire
- Leicestershire
- Lincolnshire
- Nottinghamshire
- Barnsley
- Doncaster
- Rotherham
- Sheffield

East Anglia Regional Health Authority
- Cambridgeshire
- Norfolk
- Suffolk

North-West Thames Regional Health Authority
- Bedfordshire
- Hertfordshire
- Barnet
- Brent/Harrow
- Ealing/Hammersmith/Hounslow
- Hillingdon
- Kensington and Chelsea/Westminster

North-East Thames Regional Health Authority
- Essex
- Barking/Havering
- Camden/Islington
- City/Hackney/Newham/Tower Hamlets
- Enfield/Haringey
- Redbridge/Waltham Forest

South-East Thames Regional Health Authority
- East Sussex
- Kent
- Bexley/Greenwich
- Bromley
- Lambeth/Lewisham/Southwark

South-West Thames Regional Health Authority
- Surrey
- West Sussex
- Croydon
- Kingston/Richmond
- Merton/Sutton/Wandsworth

Wessex Regional Health Authority
- Dorset
- Hampshire
- Wiltshire
- Isle of Wight

Oxford Regional Health Authority
- Berkshire
- Buckinghamshire
- Northamptonshire
- Oxfordshire

South Western Regional Health Authority
- Avon
- Cornwall and Isles of Scilly
- Devon
- Gloucestershire
- Somerset

West Midlands Regional Health Authority
- Hereford and Worcester
- Salop
- Staffordshire
- Warwickshire
- Birmingham
- Coventry
- Dudley
- Sandwell
- Solihull
- Walsall
- Wolverhampton

Mersey Regional Health Authority
- Cheshire
- Liverpool
- St Helens/Knowsley
- Sefton
- Wirral

North Western Regional Health Authority
- Lancashire
- Bolton
- Bury
- Manchester
- Oldham
- Rochdale
- Salford
- Stockport
- Tameside
- Trafford
- Wigan

In London many exceptions to this rule occur. There are 32 London boroughs responsible for social services plus the City of London, but only 16 AHAs. Due to the various boundary problems some London boroughs do cover the whole of an AHA (Hillingdon, Croydon) but in most other cases two or three London boroughs represent an AHA while one AHA is covered by four authorities in the City of London and the London boroughs of Hackney, Newham and Tower Hamlets.

Regional Health Authorities (RHA)

Each of the 14 RHAs will have at least one University providing medical education within its boundaries.

The RHA forms part of the chain of responsibility from the Secretary of State to the AHA.

The main functions of the RHA include:

1. development of strategic plans and priorities based on the needs identified by the relevant AHA
2. allocation of financial resources between the AHAs
3. monitoring the performance and policies of each AHA to ensure that they are consistent and complementary to the needs of the whole region
4. special responsibility for ensuring (with the relevant Uni-

versity and AHA) that adequate medical and dental teaching and research facilities are available

5. appointment of all consultant and senior registrar staff (except in the case of an AHA(T))
6. provision of an ambulance service—day-to-day control is usually delegated to AHAs, with the exception of the large urban conurbations—London, Birmingham, Liverpool, etc.
7. the design and construction of new buildings and works. It will itself undertake the largest capital developments but other new building works will be undertaken by the AHA (subject to approval and guidance of the RHA)
8. development of an overall regional plan for specialist services including deciding the location and degree of provision of the rarer specialities such as chest surgery, radiotherapy, neurosurgery, etc.
9. blood transfusion service

The chairman and members of each RHA are appointed by the Secretary of State after consultation with universities, the large local authorities (those responsible for social services and education) and the main health professions. Members will eventually serve for four years although the first appointments will be made in alternate years with one-half retiring every two years. Members are eligible for reappointment. The chairman is paid on a part time basis but members will be unpaid but entitled to travelling and other expenses. Doctors and nurses will usually be members but there will always be a majority of non-medical members. Membership cannot include any current member of any Area Team of Officers of an AHA within that RHA.

Standing committees will not be appointed as it is intended that all members of the RHA should be concerned with all planning developments and resources allocations. Special committees for specific tasks (i.e. to select AHA members) may be appointed.

Delegation of certain functions of the RHA may be made to the officers.

Officers of the Regional Health Authority

Five senior officers form the Regional Team of Officers (RTO):

Regional Medical Officer
Regional Nursing Officer
Regional Works Officer
Regional Administrator
Regional Treasurer.

The Regional Team of Officers is responsible for recommending regional policies to the RHA. This will be done by the preparation of a *Regional Development Plan* which will deal with:

1. distribution of medical specialities
2. development of medical manpower
3. scheduling of major capital building projects

In addition the Regional Team of Officers will be very much concerned with monitoring its AHA programmes and will subsequently review each AHA planning and budget proposal.

The Regional Team of Officers will act as a body of five officers of equal standing and will elect its chairman who will change from time to time. One of the most important roles is to advise about the performance of each AHA within the region.

Although the Regional Team of Officers will monitor the performance of their counterparts in the various AHAs, they will not be managers of the professional staff making up the Area Team of Officers (the Area Team of Officers are professionally independent).

Area Health Authorities (AHA)

There are 90 AHAs in England (see list, p. 14) and each AHA is the main operational authority for most health services, although, in 62 AHAs with two or more districts, day-to-day administration is delegated to a district organization and a District Team of Officers (DMT) (see p. 21). In the remaining 28 smaller AHAs, there is one district general hospital only and, the Area Team of Officers (with a family doctor and consultant elected from the Medical Committee) acts as an Area Management Team (see p. 9).

The relationship of each AHA to the main structure of the reorganized health service is clearly shown in the list on p. 8. In England each AHA is responsible through the RHA to the Secretary of State for Social Services.

There are two types of AHAs—those with substantial teaching facilities called Area Health Authorities (Teaching) (AHA(T)) and those without called AHAs. The main functional difference is that the AHA(T) make consultant appointments in the area while, in the ordinary AHA the RHA is responsible for such appointments. The chairman of each AHA is appointed by the Secretary of State after consultation with the chairman of the RHA. There are about 15 members in each AHA, four of whom will be appointed by the corresponding local authority and in any AHA(T) by the relevant university. The remaining members are appointed by the RHA after consultations with the main health professions and other organizations. In the largest AHAs which contain many districts, additional members of the AHA are appointed.

Each AHA contains doctors and nurses as members but there is no fixed number of professional members and never a majority of doctors. The chairman is paid on a part time basis but other members are not paid but are entitled to travelling and other expenses.

Area Team of Officers

Each AHA will be serviced by an *Area Team of Officers* (ATO) consisting of:

Area Medical Officer
Area Nursing Officer
Area Administrator
Area Treasurer

This team will act as the planning and evaluation team for the AHA. Plans for developing services are drawn up in conjunction with the corresponding local authority (responsible for social services and education) through joint committees called *Joint Consultative Committees* (see below) and Joint Care Planning Teams (see p. 22). The Area Team of Officers will draw up planning guide lines for each District, will review and monitor district performance and will advise the AHA on the development of health services in the area.

Area Medical Officer

The Area Medical Officer has on his staff subordinate medical officers who are employed in each AHA in clinical work for infants and preschool children, the school health services and other forms of screening (see Chapters 5 and 6). They are members of the staff of the Area Medical Officer. Health education and chiropody are likewise managed by each Area Medical Officer.

Other functions of the Area Medical Officer include:

1. reviewing the health care needs of the area
2. recommending to the AHA health care policies after review of both national and regional policies
3. reviewing the various district plans
4. provision of specialized planning assistance to the District Community Physician (DCP)
5. monitoring and coordinating the District Community Physicians in the area.

Specialists in Community Medicine

In addition three separate Specialists in Community Medicine are appointed to the staff of the Area Medical Officer and are responsible for:

1. giving medical advice to the relevant local authority on *environmental health matters*—Specialist in Community Medicine (Environmental Health)
2. giving medical advice to the relevant local authority on *social services*—Specialist in Community Medicine (Social Services)
3. giving medical advice to the relevant local authority on

child health and school health matters—Specialist in Community Medicine (Child Health)

This individual has dual responsibilities to and is appointed with the agreement of both the AHA and the local education authority. His responsibilities include the organization of the school health service.

Area Nursing Officer

The Area Nursing Officer provides nursing advice to the AHA, to the ATO and to individual officers at area level. She monitors and coordinates the work of District Nursing Officers. On her own staff at area level, she has a specialist nurse, the:

Area Nurse (Child Health)

The Area Nurse is appointed in agreement with the local education authority and is responsible for the provision of nursing services in schools, and for nursing advice on child health. She works closely with the Specialist in Community Medicine (Child Health) to provide a comprehensive school service.

Family Practitioner Committee (FPC)

Each AHA is also responsible for the family doctor services. However the status of the general and dental practitioners, ophthalmic medical practitioners, opticians and pharmacists as independent contractors has remained unchanged. Each AHA has to set up a special committee called the *Family Practitioner Committee* which deals directly with the DHSS on all contractual matters.

The FPC contains 30 members made up in the same way as the former Local Executive Committee it replaces—half of them are appointed by the professions. Of the remaining 15, 11 are appointed by the AHA including at least one AHA member and four by the corresponding local authority. The chairman of the Family Practitioner Committee is appointed by the committee from its own members.

The secretary and staff serving the FPC are employed by the

AHA and are appointed by them after consultation with the committee.

District Management Team

In 62 AHAs, the majority of the day-to-day running of the health services are organized on a district basis within each AHA. The number of districts in such AHAs varies from two to seven. Each district is integrated by a *District Management Team* (DMT) composed of six officers: two clinicians, one a consultant and one a family practitioner, with a District Community Physician (DCP), a District Nursing Officer (DNO), a District Administrator and a District Treasurer. There are no appointed members in the District Management Team which is entirely an officer structure but there is a *District Medical Committee* to represent clinicians. The consultant and family practitioner serving on the District Management Team represent the District Medical Committee as chairman and deputy chairman. It is intended that either a consultant or family doctor will be appointed as chairman of the District Medical Committee. Where a consultant is appointed as chairman, a family practitioner is appointed as vice-chairman and vice versa.

The District Management Team is jointly responsible for the services and is a group of equals (no member is the managerial superior of another). The function of the District Management Team is to manage and coordinate all the main functions of the health services locally. This will include the integration of the various professional skills needed to ensure the best possible patient care. Each District will have working in it all types of clinicians in consultant or general practice; there will be a specialist in community medicine (District Community Physician), and a unified hospital and community nursing service covering all aspects—general nursing, midwifery in hospitals and the community, psychiatric nursing, health visiting and home nursing services—under the control of the District Nursing Officer. In addition the District Management Team will integrate a unified administrative structure for the whole district and administer a District budget following advice from the District Treasurer.

In the remaining 28 single district AHAs, the Area Team of Officers plus a consultant and family practitioner from the Medical Committee act as an Area Management Team (see p. 9).

District Community Physician

Apart from his responsibility as a member of the District Management Team, the tasks of the District Community Physician include:

1. continual assessment of the needs of the community for health care
2. review of the provision of medical services and identification of gaps
3. improvement of medical services so as to provide the best patient care with the resources available
4. coordination of the work of the health-care planning teams
5. organization of special studies for the District Management Team
6. control of work of clinical medical officers attached to him by the Area Medical Officer (including school health services)
7. coordination of health education programmes with the general preventive medical services in the District
8. in certain districts, to act as the 'proper officer' to the local authority (see p. 27)

Health-Care Planning Teams and Joint Care Planning Teams

An important function of the DMT and ATO is concerned with the identification of gaps within the health services and development of ways of improving them. Two types of multidisciplinary teams have evolved to assist in the analysis—Health-Care Planning Teams and Joint Care Planning Teams. Both analyse and assess needs and priorities but the former mainly operates at District level while the Joint Care Planning Team is concerned to ensure that the development of the local health services are complemented by social service changes developed by the matching local authority.

Both teams should be widely multidisciplinary and the actual composition of each health-care planning team will vary with the subject matter but, in most instances, each team will contain general practitioners, consultants, hospital and community nursing staff (midwives, health visitors, home nurses), relevant paramedical staff (including physiotherapists, occupational therapists, chiropodists, radiographers, etc.), hospital social workers and social workers from the local authority social services.

The health-care planning teams provide an opportunity for views on special subjects within each district to be studied in detail and to be presented to the District Management Team and from there to the AHA and RHA and to the DHSS. In this way, the establishment of such teams will enable new developments and policies to be suggested by numerous ordinary professional, medical, nursing and other staff. By allowing social services staff from the relevant local authority which is responsible for many of the community supporting services to take part, it is hoped each team will make a significant contribution towards effective local collaboration.

Joint Consultative Committee (JCC)

Every AHA and the matching local authority must set up a *Joint Consultative Committee* which has the responsibility of advising on the planning and operation of the health services and the social, environmental and education services run by the local authority. The aim of such a committee is to improve cooperation.

In all metropolitan districts, a single Joint Consultative Committee has been set up to deal with all aspects. In non-metropolitan counties there are two Joint Consultative Committees, one for social services and education set up with the county council and one for environmental health matters set up with the local district councils in their area which are responsible for environmental health matters.

Working groups of officers from the health authorities and the local authorities will also be available to help and support the Joint Consultative Committee.

JCCs receive reports from the health and local authority services and in particular considers reports from the Joint Care Planning Team set up by both. Although the JCC has no executive power, it is now considered to be very important for it is the main advisory committee in each area responsible for ensuring joint development between both services. With the growing trend for all health care to be concentrated in the community rather than in hospitals, the quality of that care depends very much on the level of support services provided by local authorities and especially by social service departments.

Joint Financing

A novel system of central funding called *Joint Financing* was introduced in 1975 to encourage the development of local authority social services in the matching local authority. Finance is made available centrally to each AHA who then fund agreed projects in the social service field for a limited period (at present for a maximum of seven years). Finance is provided on a diminishing basis and at an agreed proportion. Thus a project may initially be financed by say 60% or 80% or 100% from the AHA for the first year (and 40%, 20% or nil respectively from the local authority) but gradually the proportion from the AHA is reduced so that, by the end of the agreed period, the local authority is completely funding the project.

Many different types of community schemes have been developed in this way but especially in the field of the elderly and mentally disabled. *The criterion which must always be satisfied is that the scheme must benefit the development of the local health services.*

The JCC has an important role to play in Joint Financing schemes as it debates and *determines which projects should be given priority* and recommends them to the AHA and local authority for implementation.

The Secretary of State provides Joint Financing funds direct to AHAs who can only use these resources for that purpose. The Rate Support Grant is likewise increased annually to enable local authorities to take up their share of the costs.

Community Health Councils

Community Health Councils have been introduced into the health services following the National Health Service Reorganization Act, 1973. There is one Community Health Council for each district or single district AHA. Their main function is to represent the local consumers' interests and to ensure that the development of local health services do take regard of local opinion. Each community health council will contain between 18 and 30 members.

Not less than one-half the total membership of the Community Health Council is appointed by the relevant local authority or authorities. Members appointed in this way may be either councillors or non-councillors. *At least one-third of the members* are appointed by voluntary organizations active locally in relevant fields such as Councils of Social Service, Age Concern and the various organizations associated with the physically and mentally disabled. In the selection of the voluntary bodies to be represented, the RHA (but not the AHA) has a part to play. The remaining members (approximately one-sixth) are appointed by the RHA after consultation with local authorities and such other organizations as it seems fit. Persons should be selected from individuals who already have a special knowledge of the health service (such as representatives of women's organizations, trades unions, the Churches, youth and immigrant bodies who might not otherwise be appointed).

Members of RHAs, AHAs or Family Practitioner Committees are not eligible to serve on any Community Health Council. Nor can members of Community Health Councils be chosen from family doctors, consultants or any other National Health Service employee. People over 70 cannot normally be appointed.

Any permanent staff to service Community Health Councils are provided by the RHA.

Functions of Community Health Councils

The main function of Community Health Councils is to make sure that the public has a full say in the local health services; it also should help the managing authorities (AHA and DMT) by making them better informed on local priorities, needs and deficiencies.

Each AHA and District Management Team has a duty to supply promptly to each Community Health Council health information of all sorts (except confidential information about individual patients). Statistics and minutes of AHA meetings should be provided. The Community Health Council is expected to provide the DMT with local views on the needs and problems of the community served by the health district. The AHA has discretion to withhold any information which it may regard as confidential but the Community Health Council has the right of appeal to the RHA if the relevant AHA refuses to supply particular information requested.

There should be friendly consultation between the AHA and each Community Health Council and the AHA (or not less than one-third of the members of it) should meet each Community Health Council each year.

Members of each Community Health Council are allowed to visit or inspect premises under the control of the AHA such as hospitals, offices, clinics, health centres, staff residential accommodation. The clinician and nursing officer in charge should be informed beforehand of any proposed visit.

Each Community Health Council may publish at any time reports or statements and must produce an annual report which must then be sent to the relevant RHA and AHA.

Each Community Health Council must admit the public to its meetings and ensure that the public is aware of the names of the chairman and members.

Matters which Community Health Councils are concerned with include:

1. general effectiveness of the health services in the district
2. planning of health services
3. variation in local health services—closure of hospitals or hospital departments
4. collaboration between the health services and local authority social and education services
5. standards of service, i.e. number of hospital beds in the district, the average number of patients on family doctor's lists

6. patient facilities including hospital outpatients, open visiting of children, waiting times, amenities for hospital patients and arrangements for rehabilitation of patients
7. waiting periods for in-patients and out-patients treatment and for domiciliary services
8. quality of catering in hospitals and in other health service institutions
9. complaints—not individual patient complaints (see below, p. 33) but the general type of complaint
10. advising individual members of the public how and where they should lodge a complaint and the facts that should be provided

Local Authority Control of Notifiable Disease and Food Poisoning

Local authorities (metropolitan district councils or district councils) have many responsibilities in relation to environmental health including the investigation of notifiable disease and food poisoning. The public health inspector staff (usually now under a Chief Officer named 'Environmental Health Officer') are responsible for much of this work but require the advice and guidance of experienced community physicians. To ensure that such help is readily available, every local authority must designate a '*proper officer*' for functions relating to notifiable disease and food poisoning, and this must be a doctor who is a community physician of the AHA. Usually this will be the Specialist in Community Health (Environmental Health) in the case of a metropolitan district or a single London borough or a non-metropolitan county with one health district only. Where, in a non-metropolitan county, there are two or more health districts, this function is undertaken by the District Community Physician of each district.

Notifications of infectious diseases are reported by the patient's doctor to the 'proper officer' (the community physician as above) and then by him to the AHA (see p. 33).

In the case of an outbreak of infectious disease, the 'proper officer' has, for the purpose of carrying out an epidemiological investigation, executive control over the appropriate staff of both the local authority and the National Health Service in any part of his district. This means that the investigating community physician (the 'proper officer') would have control over public health inspectors, port health inspectors and health visitors as regards that investigation.

Port and Airport Health

Similar arrangements apply, and local authorities which are concerned with port or airport health must appoint a 'proper officer'—a community physician responsible for medical epidemiological investigation.

Laboratory Services

Each large District General Hospital has its own bacteriological and pathological laboratories. In addition, there is a regional system of specialized laboratories organized outside AHAs' control called the *Public Health Laboratory Service*, whose function is to provide a network of bacteriological and virological laboratories to assist in the investigation of infectious diseases. They are maintained by the Secretary of State through the Public Health Laboratory Board and are quite separate from the hospital laboratories. The headquarters of this service is at Colindale, London, where there is also provided: (*a*) the central enteric reference laboratory for typing salmonella organisms; (*b*) standard laboratory of serological reagents; (*c*) national collection of type cultures.

Regional laboratories are in the main in University towns with smaller laboratories elsewhere. Wherever possible, general practitioners should send specimens to their local Public Health Laboratory, which will always be ready to help.

Every month, the Public Health Laboratory Service publishes a bulletin on bacteriological and virological subjects and this contains all unusual bacteriological and virological findings which are likely to be of significance to doctors.

Administration of General Practice

The Family Practitioner Committee (FPC) (see p. 20) administers the contracts of service of general practitioners and controls the number practising in its area. The buying and selling of goodwill was abolished by the National Health Service Act, 1946, and doctors wishing to join the service as principals must apply to the FPC.

There is, however, special machinery set up to assist in the more equal distribution of doctors throughout the country. This is done by an important national committee set up by the Secretary of State—called the *Medical Practices Committee*—which constantly assesses the number of general practitioners practising in any area and its population. It then classifies each area into one of four types.

1. *Designated area*—this is a district in which there is an inadequate number of doctors. It is defined as an area where the average number of patients per doctor exceeds 2500. No difficulty is ever experienced by a doctor wishing to practise in such an area and a special inducement payment of £960+ a year is payable to a doctor whose main surgery is situated in an area that has been 'designated' for a continuous period of three years up to the date of payment. This allowance is one of the ways in which doctors are encouraged to move to 'underdoctored' areas. In 1976, 15·2% of general practitioners worked in such practices.

2. *Open area*—an area with an adequate number of doctors and where the doctor/patient ratio is between 1/2200 and 1/2500. Admission to the medical list (i.e. permission to practise in such an area) is usually automatic. In 1976, 30% of general practitioners were in such practices.

3. *Intermediate area*—an area where the doctor/patient ratio is between 1/1800 and 1/2200. Applications to practise in such areas are never automatically granted and each application is considered separately with special reference to the trends in the area. Generally in areas where the ratio of patients to doctors is falling, it is unlikely that permission will be given to start a new practice and vice versa. In 1976, 38·8% of general practitioners worked in such practices.

4. *Restricted area*—an area where the number of doctors is adequate (where the average number of patients per doctor is below 1800) and all new applications to practise in such areas will be refused. Entry into practice can only be obtained by applying for a vacancy (on death, retirement or through a partnership). In 1976, 16% of general practitioners were working in restricted areas.

All applications for entry are first made to the FPC which has to forward the request to the Medical Practices Committee. If there is more than one application for the vacancy, the Medical Practices Committee has the responsibility of making the appointment.

There are provisions for any practitioner who is aggrieved by the selection to lodge an appeal with the Secretary of State who then decides whether the appeal should be heard orally. If so, the Secretary of State appoints the persons to hear the appeal.

Drugs and medicines. In the majority of practices, prescriptions for medicines and drugs are issued by the doctor and dispensed by the pharmacist. However approximately 10% of general practitioners (situated in the more rural areas) carry out the dispensing themselves.

Size of practice. A limit of 3500 is fixed on the total number of patients any single-handed doctor may have on his list. If a doctor employs an assistant (he must have the permission of the FPC to do this), the limit of his list is raised by a further 2000 patients.

Choice of doctor. The public have a completely free choice of doctor and the doctor also is free to decide whether or not to accept the patient on to his list.

The FPC is required to keep a list of doctors practising in the area, called the Medical List, which must indicate separately the general practitioners who undertake maternity medical services. This list is available at the local FPC headquarters and main Post Offices, where it may be examined by any member of the public to help in his choice of a doctor.

If a patient has difficulty in finding a doctor to accept him, he can apply to the Allocation Committee (another sub-committee of the FPC) which will then allocate the patient to a convenient doctor.

Local Medical Committee

One of the most important committees of any FPC is the Local Medical Committee which acts as the local medical advisory committee to the FPC. It mainly consists of doctors practising in the area and the chairman is invariably a general practitioner. There are representatives of the consultant services and it is usual for the Area Medical Officer to be a member of this Committee. The Local Medical Committee has many functions to perform;

any difficulties connected with particular practices or with local policies are usually referred to this committee which then advises the FPC. The Local Medical Committee has to carry out an investigation if the Secretary of State considers there has been excessive prescribing by a practitioner (see p. 34). In the same way, the Secretary of State may ask the Local Medical Committee to investigate a complaint that a general practitioner has not exercised sufficient care in certification. Other similar expert committees help with the administration of the dental services (the Dental Services Committee), the pharmaceutical services (the Area Chemists Contractors Committee), and the ophthalmic services (Optical Committee).

Terms of service of general practitioners

Once a doctor has accepted a patient on his list, he is required to render to him all proper and necessary treatment.

Under his terms of service, a doctor may contract out of night and weekend work if alternative arrangements can be made. A separate form of payment is added to the basic practice allowance for doctors agreeing to cover these periods. If the doctor has also agreed to give maternity medical services, he must render all necessary maternity care for which he will receive additional payment. In 1976, approximately 75% of general practitioners provided such services.

In addition, the doctor must arrange further treatment for his patients such as admission to hospital or attendance at out-patient departments. Every general practitioner is responsible for ensuring adequate medical cover in his absence on holiday or for sickness.

Every doctor must provide proper and sufficient surgery premises, including waiting room facilities for his patients. Rent which is accepted by the District Valuer plus full rates and up to 70% of expenditure on ancillary help are directly reimbursed (this latter allowance does not apply to wives, or other dependents, who assist the general practitioner in his practice).

The doctor must provide free of charge certificates needed under the National Insurance Acts and many other statutes. Records of the illnesses of his patients must be kept by each doctor.

Fees are paid to doctors carrying out particular services which are specially recommended by the Secretary of State. At present, these cover: (*a*) cervical smears £2·90 and (*b*) vaccinations and immunizations £1·00 to £1·45. These can be divided into three groups:

1. *General*—including those immunizations and vaccinations carried out in children on Government recommendation and other special groups.

These include:

Poliomyelitis: Groups at special risk, e.g. general practitioners; ambulance staff; medical students; practising dental surgeons and others who come into contact with dental patients; practising nurses in hospitals and elsewhere; hospital staff who come into contact with poliomyelitis cases; families of the above groups.

Anthrax: those at special risk, e.g. workers in establishments such as tanneries, glue, gelatine, soap and bone-meal factories and woollen mills, who are regularly handling certain raw materials.

Typhoid and paratyphoid: hospital staff likely to come into contact with cases.

Changes in the list of diseases and of the categories of people for whom vaccination is recommended, may need to be made from time to time.

2. *Travellers abroad* as follows:

Diseases	*Groups affected*
Smallpox	Those travelling from UK to any country where smallpox may be encountered.
Typhoid, paratyphoid	Those travelling out of UK.
Cholera	Those travelling to countries where cholera is likely to occur.

Vaccinations required by the Government of the country to which the patient is travelling.

3. *Vaccination in local outbreaks*—this covers emergency programmes of vaccination, but only if the person vaccinated is a member of a group for which vaccination is recommended, or, if the patient vaccinated is a close contact of a person diagnosed by the general practitioner and the vaccination is subsequently approved by the District Community Physicians or Specialist in Community Medicine (Environmental Health), i.e. vaccination is in the public interest.

To qualify for such fees the doctor must submit special forms signed by the patient.

Methods of controlling practice

There is a central Tribunal which is set up by the Secretary of State with a chairman who must be a barrister or solicitor of at least 10 years' standing, to which the FPC may refer cases of doctors, dentists, chemists and opticians, if they consider that such persons should no longer be employed within the National Health Service because of inefficient practice. The Tribunal then holds an inquiry and, if it is satisfied that the report is serious enough, can order the removal of the offender from the National Health Service. In such a case, there is always a right of appeal to the Secretary of State.

Informal procedure for complaints

A proportion of complaints should be investigated informally and each FPC must now appoint one of its lay members to assist the Administrator to the FPC to do this. This informal stage should not normally take longer than a week or two. If the complaint cannot be satisfactorily cleared up informally, the formal procedure described below must be used. Some cases of complaint may, from the first, appear to indicate so serious a state of affairs that an informal enquiry would be inappropriate.

Formal procedure for complaints

Each FPC must also appoint a Medical Services Committee which consists of a lay chairman of the FPC acceptable to both sides, plus six other members, of whom three must be from the Local Medical Committee. The Medical Services Committee has the responsibility of investigating any complaints raised by a patient about the service given to him by his doctor.

There is a set procedure laid down for the investigation of such complaints. The hearing is always in private and the doctor's name is never made public. This method may seem unfair, but unless the doctor's name is kept secret, great damage would be done to his reputation even if he was completely innocent and the complaint frivolous.

After the hearing, the Medical Services Committee reports its finding to the FPC which then sends its decision to the Secretary of State. The doctor has the right of appeal to the Secretary of State. In the case of the proved complaint, one of the following actions can be recommended to the Secretary of State who then decides:

1. a sum be deducted from the doctor's remuneration to cover the expenses of the complainant only, and the doctor may be warned
2. a sum be withheld from the doctor's remuneration
3. a special limit, as to the number of patients on the doctor's list, be imposed (this is rarely done)
4. reference to the Tribunal that in the opinion of the FPC the doctor should not be permitted to continue in the National Health Service. The Tribunal then decides on the facts

The doctor may appeal to the Secretary of State against 1, 2 and 3 but not against 4.

It is important to stress that the Medical Services Committee is only empowered to inquire into an alleged failure of a general practitioner to comply with the terms of service under the National Health Service Acts. It has no power to deal with matters of civil or criminal law or with professional disciplinary matters dealt with by the General Medical Council.

The Local Medical Committee also has certain duties in connection with *alleged excessive prescribing by doctors*. If a doctor is considered by the Secretary of State to have prescribed excessive quantities of drugs or appliances for his patients, the Local Medical Committee has the task of carrying out an investigation. If as a result of their inquiry the Local Medical Committee come to the conclusion that there has been excessive prescribing, then they must report the case to the FPC, who may then recommend the Secretary of State to withhold a certain sum from the remuneration of the doctor as a penalty. In practice, such action is rarely taken without a warning first being given to the doctor.

Financial provisions

All forms of hospital treatment are free, and if a single room is necessary, this is also provided free. If the patient requires additional privacy, he may be given an amenity bed, usually in a double room, at a cost of £1·50 to £3·00 per day, but treatment for such patients is free. A certain number of private beds are provided in many hospitals, the charge for which varies. In the case of private patients only, consultants may charge a fee on an agreed scale.

The general practitioner may only demand a fee in certain circumstances—from schools or employers for medical examination of pupils or employees, from patients not on his list or that of his partner or assistant, for treatment in private nursing homes and from a dental practitioner in respect of an anaesthetic given to a patient receiving dental treatment or for any treatment given to stop the bleeding of such a patient.

There is no additional cost to the individual patient in obtaining all the medical services provided by general medical practitioners. Small charges are levied for prescriptions, for spectacles and certain appliances (elastic hosiery, etc.). Prescriptions for the following people can be obtained without charges by completing the declaration on the back of the prescription form, children aged 15 and under, women aged 60 years and over and men aged 65 years and over, and people holding exemption certificates. These are issued to expectant and nursing mothers, people suffering from certain medical conditions, persons and their dependents receiving supplementary benefit and family income supplement. A part charge is made for dental treatment, but such treatment is free for young persons and expectant and nursing mothers.

The method of remunerating doctors in general practice is as follows (1978 figures):

1. *A basic practice allowance* of £3030 per year payable to all doctors with at least 1000 patients on their lists (with proportionate payment if lower than 1000 patients on the list).
2. *A standard capitation fee* for every patient on the doctor's list which is £2·70 per year for each patient aged under 65 years, £3·50 per year for each patient aged 65–74 years and £4·30 per year for each patient aged 75 and over.
3. *Special payments for out of hours services* (nightly from 7 p.m. to 8 a.m., and from 1 p.m. Saturdays to 8 a.m. Mondays):
   a. supplementary practice allowance of £595 per year

b. supplementary capitation fee for each patient in excess of 1000 on the list—£0·54 per year
c. a fee of £5·75 for each visit requested and made between 11 p.m. and 7 a.m.

4. Additional payments are added to the basic practice allowance as follows:
a. to a doctor in an area that has been designated for a continuous period of three years—£940 per year or £1440 (with over 3000 patients)
b. to a doctor practising in a group practice—£525 per year
c. seniority payments (subject to attendance at a prescribed number of sessions of postgraduate training), as detailed below
d. allowances for vocational training (not payable to a doctor who qualifies for any of the seniority payments)—£725 per year
c. postgraduate training allowance—£270 per year for five years

Seniority payments

(*a*) to a doctor whose name has been continuously included in the Medical Register for 15 years and who has been a principal providing unrestricted general medical services under the National Health Service for at least the last five years—£725 per year. (*b*) to such a principal, after 10 years more of practice in the general medical services, £1235 per year. (*c*) to such a principal, after a further 10 years of practice in the general medical services, £1965 per year.

Miscellaneous payments

A doctor is paid £41·60 if on the obstetric list (£24·25 if not on the list), for providing complete maternity services for each patient confined.

For every temporary resident the doctor is paid £2·70 if the visitor is staying not more than 15 days and £3·30 if the stay is longer than 15 days.

Trainee practitioners are paid a varying annual sum depending upon their post in the hospital service before becoming a trainee. The sum varies from £4869 to £7156. The principal providing the training receives £1625 annually.

Initial practice allowances are paid at varying rates where a general practitioner provides a service for the first time in a new developing area (housing estate or new town). Such payments are graduated so that they fall off as more and more potential patients move into the new area.

Special payments are made to doctors practising in rural areas and remote island communities.

Reference has already been made to the extra fees for cervical cytology and immunization.

Health Service Commissioners

Separate Health Service Commissioners for England and Wales have been set up by the National Health Service Reorganization Act, 1973, to investigate complaints against the relevant health bodies.

Both these Commissioners are only removable on an address from both Houses of Parliament and their salaries are paid directly out of the Consolidated Fund. They are therefore in the same independent position as High Court Judges.

The main functions of the Health Services Commissioners are to investigate:

1. an alleged failure in a service provided by a relevant body—RHA, AHA, FPC, Public Health Laboratory Service Board or any special body appointed before and after 1 April 1974
2. an alleged failure of a relevant body to provide a service which it was a function of that body to provide
3. any other act taken by or on behalf of a relevant body in a case where it is alleged any person has sustained injustice or hardship in consequence of the failure or of maladministration

It is important to note that the Health Services Commissioner is specifically excluded from dealing with:

1. professional complaints against decisions of individual doctors or nurses in regard to individual patients
2. any action which is dealt with by the Tribunal set up to deal with serious complaints (see p. 34)

3. any complaint which is subject to action in a court of law

Complaints may be made to the Health Service Commissioners by the patient, his relatives or a friend or by a member of any hospital staff. The Health Service Commissioners will only investigate a complaint when the complainant remains dissatisfied *after the health authority has had an opportunity to investigate the complaint and reply to it*.

SCOTLAND

The reform of the health services in Scotland followed separate legislation, the National Health Services (Scotland) Act, 1972. General principles are the same—the removal of all community health functions from local authorities and the establishment of a unified health service, under 14 *single health boards*.

The Secretary of State for Scotland remains responsible to Parliament and the *Scottish Health Services Planning Council* advises the Secretary of State and reviews the development of health services in Scotland. National consultative committees advise the Scottish Health Services Council and are formed from members representing the professions providing health care and treatment.

A new body called a *Common Services Agency* provide the Scottish Health Services Council, the Scottish Health and Housing Department and the 14 Health Boards with certain executive and advisory services including:

1. major building project control
2. complex management service provision
3. health service staffing and training
4. secretarial services for the Scottish Health Services Council

In the Scottish health services reorganization much emphasis has been laid on integration of services at the patient level and not only at senior management level. The need to plan health services to meet the needs of patients and to make the best possible use of the staff, money and physical resources available is also emphasized. Team work in all aspects of the health services in Scotland is stressed as well as the involvement of doctors and clinical workers fully in managerial matters.

Two important advisory committees have been introduced:

1. *University Liaison Committee* to advise on the provision of facilities for undergraduate and postgraduate teaching and research.

2. *Area Consultative Committee* representing doctors, dentists, nurses, midwives, pharmacists and ophthalmic and dispensary opticians to advise on professional matters.

WALES

The reorganization was introduced by the same legislation as in England—The *National Health Services (Reorganization) Act, 1973*.

No regional tier of authorities has been set up. The Secretary of State for Wales has overall responsibility to Parliament for the health services in Wales and particularly to:

1. determine health policies in Wales
2. allocate resources between the eight AHAs
3. ensure that objectives are achieved
4. ensure the standards of health services are satisfactory

A new body, the *Welsh Health Technical Services Organization*, has been set up and is directly accountable to the Secretary of State. Its function includes:

1. designing and building all major hospital and other capital works
2. running a central computer service for the health services in Wales
3. negotiating central supply contracts

There are eight AHAs in Wales, each consisting of 15 part-time members who will be responsible to the Secretary of State for planning and providing health services and for ensuring that the plans are implemented.

There is a District organization similar to the English pattern (see p. 21). A senior member of each health profession is appointed adviser to give advice to the Area Team of Officers and to the AHA about matters which are relevant to his/her profession. This is in addition to any advice which comes from any formal advisory structures set up by each health profession.

NORTHERN IRELAND

The reorganization in Northern Ireland was carried out in 1973 and covered both the health and social services. A unified structure was then created outside local political control dealing with the hospital, family practitioner, community health and social services. The probation and education services were *not* included. At provincial level the DHSS acts as government agency and also like an English Regional Health Authority, being responsible for policies and the allocation of resources. There are four Boards, each consisting of 30 members all appointed by the Secretary of State. Approximately one-third are drawn from the local government District Councils, one-third from the professions and one-third from industrialists, trades unions, voluntary bodies and the universities. Each Board is responsible for planning, delivering and monitoring the health and social services. Each Board has an Area Executive Team consisting of four chief officers of equal status, a Chief Administrative Officer, a Chief Administrative Medical Officer, a Chief Administrative Nursing Officer and a Director of Social Services. Each Board has from three to six Districts dealing with the day-to-day delivery of health and social services. District Committees consist of local members of the public and are non-executive, but act as a focus for local opinion. Various district professional officers make up the District Executive Team and are individual subordinates to the corresponding Chief Officer at Board Level.

This combined structure has attracted much attention and has resulted in more positive moves towards multidisciplinary assessment and more flexible use of all the various facilities in each Board such as hospitals, homes, hostels, day care units, day nurseries. It has also resulted in better understanding between all those working in the health and social services.

2 Management within the New Health Services

The aim of any health service must be to improve the health care of the population and this includes three main functions: *prevention of disease, early diagnosis of illness*, and *effective treatment of disease including if possible, rehabilitation of the patient* so that he no longer needs any supporting help.

Many complicated factors influence these three functions including the habit and attitudes of people, environmental and occupational features, the very nature of certain diseases, the availability of medical, nursing and other professional staff, financial resources, the capital available, etc. But the *quality of health care* can also depend upon how effectively all these available parts integrate to form a smooth uninterrupted service to the patient. The art of doing just this is loosely termed 'the management of the health services'. Many consultants and general practitioners have criticized the reorganized health service on the grounds that management seems to have become too important. Some of this criticism stems from a misunderstanding of the part management should play within any health service but some of the criticism is justified because some management seems unproductive: it fails to help the deliverers of health to provide the best possible service.

Good management should always be concerned with ensuring that, once an individual comes into the ambit of the health service, the delivery of the right kind of medical and other professional care is prompt and effective and readily accepted and understood by the patient. Even the simplest examples call for a great deal of integration and sharing by many different parts of the health service. The failure of even one small section to deliver health care may effectively reduce the chance of helping a patient.

Many clinicians (and others) have seen at first hand the ill-effects on their patients of these failures and have naturally been sceptical when it has been pointed out that improvements will follow only if the management of the health services is improved.

Any health service must always be largely dependent on the individual clinical work of doctors (consultants and general practitioners). Nothing can replace sound individual clinical practice and the reorganized health services have stressed the importance of ensuring that the management of all parts of the service should be designed to support and encourage it. But good individual clinical practice can be wrecked if the necessary supporting health or social services either in hospital or in the community are not readily available. In particular, the reorganized health services aim to achieve:

1. complete integration of all health services
2. a satisfactory balance of services between hospital and the community
3. the development of adequate services for every type of patient and especially for chronic patients (the elderly, the mentally ill) as well as for acute patients
4. the development of balanced general practitioner services and primary health-care teams to tackle problems early in disease and within the community
5. the prevention of disease

Health services are already widely decentralized, individual clinicians see individual patients and make important decisions without any reference to any others in the service. Management must also be decentralized to groups which are small enough so that each clinician feels part of the team and can understand the main local problems. This means that doctors must be prepared to play their part in managing and planning the local services.

There must also be clear lines of responsibility and it is important that those managing the services can take quick effective action to respond to obvious urgent patient needs. There is now some evidence that the establishment of three tiers in the health service in England—District, Area and Region—has not encouraged sensible quick and efficient decisions. Much of the present management at Area and Regional level seems to have become too remote from the day-to-day problems of patients. This leads to decisions being taken in isolation or even not being taken at all; this has naturally caused resentment among doctors, nurses and all other care staff at field level. These are indications of poor management and not of the need for no management.

MONITORING OF HEALTH SERVICES

It is important that local developments of the services fit into the pattern of other developments both regionally and nationally, and equally essential that national policy is decided by analysis of reliable information collected locally and that national policies are always initiated locally from the experience of individual clinicians. As there are over 22 000 family doctors in England and Wales this means developing information systems which will enable local problems and the results of local medical practice to be accurately assessed so that the effect of different alternatives can be analysed, assessed and a constructive national policy finally determined. This process is often referred to as 'a monitoring of health services' and the various techniques used are still in an early stage of development and need much research.

A further complication is that the environmental circumstances in different parts of the country vary so much that different patterns of local health care are obviously necessary. A service which works well in a town of 10 000 may need much modification in a city of half a million or in a scattered rural community.

A further problem is that, in the past, the level of health services and especially the number of hospital beds available, has been unequal. This means that certain parts of the country already have more than their fair share of beds. But the process of readjusting this is difficult for many of these areas are now experiencing a reduction in their population (which, of course, aggravates the problem) and have high unemployment rates. Organized labour naturally resents any efforts made to reduce the number of hospital beds available (and so staff employed) and rational management decisions which would eventually lead to more health services where they are urgently needed are foiled.

Essentials for Good Health Service Management

To summarize, management of the reorganized health services requires:

1. integration of services at local level. This entails active participation by clinicians who must help in the development of health services
2. acceptance of multidisciplinary teams. The services can only function effectively if there is team work between doctors, nurses, administrators, technical officers, paramedical staff, community supporting staff, architects, engineers, supplies officers, ambulance officers, etc.
3. clear lines of responsibility to be established so that if a defect in any service develops, it is obvious where the responsibility lies
4. flexible methods of managing the health services to meet the different needs of all types of communities

Practical examples are now given of how the new health reorganization will assist in reaching these four requirements.

Integration of services at local level

The general practitioner represents the basic unit within the health service. In most instances the patient seeks help and advice first from his general practitioner working in a Primary Health Care Team. Integration therefore must be effective at this level between other general practitioners in the same neighbourhood (whether in partnership or not), between general practitioners and the consultant services, and between general practitioners and the supporting services (i.e. social services). Many patterns of general practice organization exist but increasingly it is accepted that better integration will result from the development of larger groups. The primary health care team, consisting of a number of doctors practising from a health centre or from the general practitioners' own purpose built premises, is an ideal way to assist integration. Such a unit is small enough to enable individual general practitioners to feel a complete part of the team and large enough to arrange a very effective attachment of health visitors, home nurses, and social workers. Such a team would probably be responsible for approximately 10 000 to 20 000 persons and therefore a typical social services area would usually have at least three to five primary health care teams within its neighbourhood.

The size of the district (managed by the District Management Team) must also be flexible but most will contain a population of 200 000 to 250 000. This means that each district might have 80 to 100 general practitioners, four to five social service areas plus one District General Hospital (with 22 to 25 consultants covering various specialities including psychiatry).

A glance at these figures makes it clear that the number of doctors involved, about 125, should be small enough to make personal integration a very real feature.

There is increasing evidence that integration at local level is improving especially with the development of multidisciplinary teams; it is in the relationship between this local level and the District and Area that integration at present seems uncertain.

Multidisciplinary team development

Primary health care

The primary health care team particularly when operating from a health centre or group practice is multidisciplinary; each team is still small and this helps local integration between the general practitioner, health visitors, home nurses and midwives and social workers. The better integration of these services which follows has improved the efficiency and management of health care to any patient.

District and Area Management

Much more complicated issues occur when the development and management of all the various health and social services in a district or area are concerned.

The various formal groups—District Management Teams (DMT) and Area Team of Officers (ATO)—are also multidisciplinary but involve very few clinicians and this has tended to make both bodies rather remote from day-to-day problems. This criticism is greater in those 62 AHAs where the ATO has a number of districts to deal with. The operation of consensus management in the ATO has also tended to make for greater delays and less individual commitment on the part of individual members to develop and change services to meet present day needs.

Health-Care Planning Teams and Joint Care Planning Teams

In theory both these multidisciplinary teams should improve local management because they encourage clinicians and other health and social care professionals to become involved on a more practical basis. The way such teams have concentrated on patient groups, children, mentally ill, mentally handicapped, physically disabled and elderly has helped to emphasize demographic local changes and local deficiencies. The greatest problems of both types of teams has been that they have, so far, been operating in a 'no growth' situation and the changes they have been able to effect have been minimal or non-existent. In such a case, not unnaturally, doubt has been cast by many individuals about the efficiency of such teams.

However, there has already been ample evidence that such multidisciplinary teams can be most effective. Perhaps the best examples are in the case of children—the setting up of new integrated services—the *District Handicap Teams* following the Court Reports recommendations (see p. 124) and the better local coordination and understanding which has followed the *Area Review Committees in non-accidental injury* (see p. 435).

Clear lines of responsibility

The line of responsibility from Parliament to RHA to AHA to DMT or to the FPC and to the individual doctor, nurse or other health care worker is usually clear. The National Health Service is a very complicated body and every one in it must understand his/her responsibility and to whom he/she is accountable.

Policy

Members of RHAs and AHAs are responsible for major issues of policy and allocation of resources. Officers of RHAs, AHAs and DMTs should advise the members so that the major issues requiring decision are clearly defined.

Executive action

Officers must have executive authority to implement policies and plans and work towards agreed targets. Senior Officers can then check how effective the performance has been; this is called *monitoring the services*. Note that the Regional Medical Officer coordinates and monitors the work of the Area Medical Officer in the region without being in charge of the Area Medical Officer. The Area Medical Officer monitors the work of the District Community Physicians in the same way.

In practice, this monitoring works in a very uncertain way. This is mainly because the new management system in the health service is a complicated mixture of consensus and line management. In this, many officers have more freedom of action (which is desirable) but no chance to make and carry out effective executive action. A perfect example is that the DMTs are *not* accountable to the ATOs in a management sense but the ATO has very considerable power to determine the budget the DMT controls. In such a situation, it is not surprising that so far *the best and most effective forms of management have emerged in single district AHAs*, where the one team (ATO) has had to tackle both tasks. Criticism has also increased regarding the role of the RHA which is certainly very remote and separated from day-to-day problems of patient care. There is considerable evidence that the Welsh, Scottish and Northern Ireland systems which do not have a regional tier are cheaper and more effective. Obviously the smaller size of these three countries makes it easier to dispense with a regional tier but a slightly extended regional structure of the DHSS itself could take on such a task.

None of this interferes with the individual clinical responsibility of the clinician. However, professional advisory committees and representative professional committees set up by the RHA and AHA will obviously be needed to advise on the best possible balance of clinical resources to achieve the highest standards of care.

The need for flexibility

The sizes of the various RHAs and AHAs vary widely. The largest RHA outside London is West Midlands with eleven districts and a population of 5·1 million. The smallest is East Anglia with three districts and a population of 1·7 million. The populations covered by AHAs also differ widely, from approximately 200 000 to over 1 million. Flexibility will obviously be necessary.

Some of the current problems of management of the health services seem to be connected with the degree of variation in the size of the AHAs. The comments above about how the single district AHA has seemed to be the most effective has suggested that less flexibility of organization size might help. There was much criticism in the past that the administration of hospital and community health services have been too hierarchical and inflexible and few would wish to see a return to rigid systems of control. But the present systems suffer from the defect that they are too indefinite and executive action often very difficult especially if the personality of one officer clashes with another. Simpler systems of management with one person eventually responsible have much to recommend them provided that delegation is used to a large extent in the control and management of local services.

Clinical decisions have always been made on an entirely different basis, with every clinician making his own clinical decisions although, if he wishes, he can seek advice and help from senior colleagues and consultants. It was hoped that the management of the health services would involve clinicians to a greater extent. The inclusion of two clinicians (one specialist and one general practitioner) in the DMT was a step in that direction. This, together with the influence of the specialist advisory committees has helped, but so far has resulted in little real change of emphasis in the management of the health services. This is partly due to the very small new developments which have been possible since 1974 but also is connected with the unsatisfactory financial control exercised locally on health service development.

Any new development will obviously depend on a satisfactory system developing to ensure that financial resources are deployed sensibly to meet the most urgent needs. So far the weakest part of the management of the health services seems to be in the methods used to control finances. This is clearly being considered by the Royal Commission at present looking at changes needed in the health service. The DHSS eventually decides the size of the finances available, to various RHAs. The most frustrating elements are:

1. *a lack of local political control* in deciding the finances made available (the action of Community Health Councils is very marginal)
2. the cumbersome management structure introduced between the DHSS and those delivering patient care. The chain DHSS → RHA → AHA → DMT is expensive, relatively ineffective and has produced much irritation in those professionals delivering patient care who, for instance, find it often very difficult to keep their hospital equipment up to date, but see a great deal of resources being spent on petty administrative features—to many professionals there seems little justification in the need to have such a system

Management within the health services

As indicated above, the new management structure introduced into the health services in 1974 has been widely criticized. The type of management was chosen in an attempt to overcome the rigid hierarchical structure of the past. Many parts of the present management have excellent theoretical features. For instance, it should be an advantage that there is a greater likelihood of relatively junior members in the service being able to influence developments than in a hierarchical management system. This is valuable as it is totally wrong to suggest that only those in the higher management positions are fit to suggest new developments. Many senior staff are necessarily somewhat remote from everyday problems and unless field work staff are encouraged to play a part, the chances of developments being even abreast of professional trends become less likely.

The reorganized health service management was so designed that the disadvantages of the old-fashioned hierarchical system have been largely done away with. Many unusual features have been included, and it is certain that conflicting opinions will be advanced by doctors, nurses or others especially when the reports of different health-care planning teams are considered.

Many may believe that such conflicting or different opinions could magnify difficulties of management. This is certainly *not* true of the forward planning processes in management *for here conflict and controversy are not only unavoidable, but actually helpful* if the development of any service is to remain up to date and dynamic. Often it is only by a process of discussion, analysis and argument in which two or three conflicting views are studied that all aspects of any subject can be fully and properly considered.

Continued conflict can, however, become counter-productive when *it comes to executive action.* It is in this respect, that the present management in the health services is most suspect; consensus management does not always overcome controversy but may only increase it in a negative way and lack of agreement within an executive team soon leads to no effective action at all.

Curiously the traditional or hierarchical systems of management can be more effective in an executive capacity, for in such a system one very senior officer, after full consultation, finally decides which executive action should be followed and then takes responsibility for its problems or deficiencies. In such systems minor adjustments to ensure relative success are quickly made by the most senior officer who has a very obvious personal interest in the success of the scheme for he is clearly responsible. Of course hierarchical management is only effective where there is complete professional consultation and plenty of delegation of smaller decisions, otherwise it can equally lead to stagnation as the most senior struggle to deal with far too much. Many professionals are suspicious of hierarchical management because they believe it encourages a dictatorial approach. A further difficulty is that many professional groups in the health service, i.e. doctors and nurses, demand that their service must always have at its head that type of professional.

Consensus management has been developed in the health services in an attempt to overcome these difficulties and its success will only be able to be judged when the other controversial features are sorted out and, especially, the relationship between the RHA, AHA, and DMT (see p. 8).

Consumer participation

The introduction for the first time in the health service management structure of a body who will watch the consumer interest, the *Community Health Council*, has added to the constructive criticism and to the controversy. Community Health Councils have been specially designed (see p. 26) to ensure that no member of an AHA nor an officer or employee of the local national health service can be a member. Community Health Councils, therefore, must always be completely independent and their very terms of reference encourage constructive criticism. Their introduction into the management structure of the health service emphasizes that the value of controversy has been clearly recognized. It could prove one of the most valuable changes in the control of the health services for it accepts completely that possible developments in the health services will only take place if many different viewpoints are constantly considered.

3 Measurement of Health

The assessment of the health of a nation or community can best be measured by an intelligent use of vital statistics. These can be defined as the study of various numerical data connected with the life and health of man within the community. This includes information concerning births, marriages, deaths and population and the collection of data about the incidence of disease (*morbidity*) as well as the number of persons dying from disease (*mortality*).

SOURCES OF VITAL STATISTICS

In 1970, there was an amalgamation between the General Registrar's Office for England and Wales and the Government Social Survey to form the Office of Population Censuses and Surveys (OPCS). This is an independent department headed by a director and is responsible for the registration of births, marriages and deaths and for some medical statistics. It is also responsible for the Census (tasks formerly undertaken by the General Register Office). The Government Social Survey carries out many of the larger statistical surveys for the Government.

The Central Statistical Office is the main central government department dealing with all types of statistical information including vital statistics. It is now closely linked with the office of Population Censuses and Surveys by a policy committee chaired by the Director of the Central Statistical Office with the Director of OPCS as its deputy chairman and with members drawn from many government departments who have a major interest in statistics (the Home Office, Department of Education and Science, Department of Environment, and DHSS).

There are many publications which act as the main sources of vital statistics. Two of the most useful are *Population Trends* (published by the OPCS quarterly) and *Social Trends* published annually by the Central Statistical Office.

Population Trends

This gives the latest population and vital statistics for England, Wales and Scotland and the various regions. In addition, each publication contains four or five specialist articles on population and medical statistical topics. Each issue contains a valuable idea of the present and past publications and the topics dealt with.

Social Trends

This deals with many types of information about population, leisure activities, personal income and wealth, health and social services, education, housing, environment, justice and law and public expenditure. It contains many statistical tables and diagrams which are all designed to present the subject in an easily understood way and, in particular, to illustrate the trends which the various figures demonstrate. This publication also contains important articles on specific topics of current interest, useful definitions of many terms used and a bibliography.

The following annual publications give more details:

1. *Health and Personal Social Services Statistics for England* (with summary tables for Great Britain) (DHSS). A collection of the most useful information including vital statistics, population projections, costs of health and personal social services, manpower details, community health services, personal social services, maternity and child health services, psychiatric services, preventive medicine, morbidity statistics, abortions and blood transfusion services.

   Much of these data come from the annual surveys and enquiries detailed below:
2. *Annual Report of the Chief Medical Officer to DHSS*
3. *General Household Survey* (OPCS). Multipurpose survey giving information on a large number of topics about

private households in UK. Useful to pick up trend data in the years between censuses

4. *Family Expenditure Survey* (OPCS). Continuous enquiry into the expenditure pattern in approximately 11 000 households
5. *National Food Survey* (Ministry of Agriculture, Fisheries and Food). Continuous enquiry into domestic food consumed and good budgets of 7000–8000 households
6. *Local Authority Vital Statistics* (OPCS). Replaces Registrar General's Statistical Review of England and Wales, gives following information for each local authority area and for each RHA and AHA: population, live births, stillbirths, deaths, infant and perinatal mortality (published two years in arrears)
7. *Hospital In-Patient Enquiry* (jointly by DHSS and OPCS). Covers a 1 in 10 sample in England and Wales and all records in Scotland for non-psychiatric patients in NHS hospitals
8. *Mental Health Enquiry* (DHSS)—analysis of individual in-patient records of admission to and discharge from (or death in) psychiatric hospitals or units
9. *Annual Returns from NHS Hospitals* (DHSS), covering in-patients, out-patients and day patients
10. *Annual Report of Health Advisory Service* (DHSS)

Additional information is available from:

a. Census returns, full censuses every 10 years (last 1971) and usually 10% census held every five years. There was no 10% census in England, Wales and Scotland in 1976, but there was one in Northern Ireland

b. Special surveys such as the *Reports on Confidential Enquiries into Maternal Deaths* usually published every three years

c. *Health Bulletin* (Public Health Laboratory Service) published quarterly giving up to date epidemiological data

d. Special *ad hoc* enquiries such as the *Survey into Handicapped and Impaired in Great Britain* (OPCS) 1971 and the National Development Group for Mentally Handicapped publications *e*. Various DHSS Publications such as *Better Services for the Mentally Ill* (1976); *The Way Ahead* (1977) and *A Happier Old Age* (1978)

f. The reports of various government committees of enquiry such as *Fit for the Future* (1976), Court Report on Child Health Services (DHSS) and the *Special Educational Needs*, report of the Committee of Enquiry into the Education of Handicapped Children and Young People (The Warnock Committee) (1978) (Department of Education and Science)

g. *Health Trends* published by DHSS and Welsh Office quarterly. Articles of topical value on national and international health topics

h. World Health Organization (WHO) publications. This organization publishes a weekly *Epidemiological Bulletin* giving world-wide information on very serious communicable diseases. WHO also publishes many specialist reports and an annual report

Local Statistical Information

Many planning departments of major local authorities have specialized statistical sections which analyse the local OPCS population figures and various local statistics.

In addition the following can provide useful local information on health:

1. notifications of communicable diseases (see p. 176)
2. notification of births and deaths to Area Medical Officer
3. local hospital records
4. first medical certificates issued for social insurance purposes to the local officer of the DHSS
5. school medical records
6. cancer registration schemes

Collection of Statistical Information

Registration of birth

The parent has a duty to register the birth of every child to the local Registrar of Births, Marriages and Deaths within 42 days.

Notification of birth

This is for a different purpose and is mainly to ensure that the local preventive health services of the Area Medical Officer and District Nursing Officer learn rapidly of the occurrence of each birth. This allows the infant health services to assist the mother without delay (i.e. to allow the health visitor to call, see p. 115). Every birth or stillbirth must be notified to the Area Medical Officer within 36 hours. It is usual for this notification to be carried out by the midwife or doctor attending the birth.

Registration of stillbirth

Every stillbirth must be registered with the local Registrar of Births, Marriages and Death. A special certificate from the midwife or doctor attending the birth must record that the child was stillborn. The legal definition of stillbirth is 'any child which has issued forth from its mother after the twenty-eighth week of pregnancy and which did not at any time after being completely expelled from the mother breathe or show any other sign of life'.

Registration of death

Any death must be registered by the nearest relative (or other person in charge) within five days of the death. The doctor who has attended the patient during the last illness must provide a certificate as to the cause of death. The cause of death on the death certificate provides the Registrar General with his records of mortality and accurate certification is important.

Statistical rates

It is obviously desirable to refer to all statistics in terms of the same unit of population and this is usually per 1000 persons. This is used for births and for mortality rates.

Enumeration of the Population

The population of the UK is counted in the census and is estimated by the Registrar General during the intervening years. A combination of methods are used for this purpose.

The Census

The first census was taken in 1801. The census is usually carried out every 10 years although there is authority to take it in a modified form every five years. A 10% sample census was held in 1966 but for reasons of economy no such census was held in 1976 (except in Northern Ireland). The last full census was in April 1971. In the census the responsibility for collecting the information is that of the Registrar General although he is assisted by local authorities. The Census Act gives specific directions as to how the census must be carried out and it is usual to undertake it on the first Sunday in April provided this is not Easter Sunday. This is because the population is most static at this period of the year. An 'enumerator' (usually a member of the staff of the local authority) visits each home and leaves the census form. This has to be completed by the head of the house in respect of everyone resident in that house on census day. The enumerator then calls to collect the form and is able to give any advice as to its final completion.

The details collected at the 1971 census were outlined in the Census Regulations, 1970, and included: name, sex, age; relationship to head of family; marital condition; place of birth; country of birth of mother and father; present address, address one and five years ago; qualifications obtained including certificates of education; name and business of individual's employer; classification of occupation as employee, employing large or small number; apprenticeship, trainee or full-time student; number of hours worked per week; means of transport to work. For women only, details of any births, date of marriage and any divorce.

Details of accommodation occupied were also recorded including whether owner-occupier or tenant (with type of renting); whether house is shared; number of rooms; how many cars or vans normally used by members of household; whether there is a cooker or cooker with oven, a fixed bath and shower, hot water supply, flush toilet with entrance inside or outside.

SOCIAL CLASS

To compare many vital statistics and especially mortality, the Registrar General classifies the census population into six different *Social Classes*, based upon the occupation of the chief wage earner of the family:

Non-manual

Class I	Professional occupations (i.e. lawyers and doctors) (5·5%)
Class II	Managerial and lower professional occupations (i.e. sales managers, teachers and nurses) (18·5%)
Class IIIN	Non-manual skilled occupations (e.g. clerks and shop assistants) (12·0%)

Manual

Class IIIM	Skilled manual occupations (i.e. bricklayers and underground coal miners) (37·5%)
Class IV	Partly skilled occupations (i.e. bus conductors and postmen) (18·0%)
Class V	Unskilled occupations (i.e. porters, ticket collectors and general labourers) (8·5%)

N.B. The percentages in each social class in the 1971 census are shown in brackets.

Population

In 1977, in England and Wales the total mid-year population was 49 247 000 consisting of 24 014 600 males and 25 232 000 females.

The distribution of the various age groups throughout the population is of interest to all doctors as the medical problems of different age groups are so varied.

TABLE 1 Age and sex structure of population of England and Wales mid-1976

	Males		*Females*		*Total*	
Age groups	Thousands	%	Thousands	%	Thousands	%
0–14	5601·2	23·4	5301·6	21·0	10 902·8	22·2
15–44	10 001·2	41·9	9697·6	38·4	19 698·8	40·1
45–64	5533·6	23·1	5859·5	23·2	11 373·1	23·2
65–74	1962·5	8·3	2577·3	10·3	4539·8	9·3
75–84	706·9	2·9	1419·4	5·6	2126·3	4·3
85+	117·2	0·4	361·5	1·4	478·5	0·9

The proportion of the various age groups as shown in Table 1 varies because of an increasing incidence of mortality in men with age and also because of the varied birth rates in the past. It is important to realize that 14·0% of the population of England and Wales are now aged 65 years and over. The difference between the sexes rises sharply after age 65 and *by the age group 85 + there are more than three times the number of women than men*—a very significant fact when planning social services for the very old. The proportion of elderly people in the population has risen steadily in the last 60 years—in 1901 there were 4·67% of persons aged 65 years and over compared with the present-day figure. It will clearly be seen how there are many more elderly women in the community compared with elderly men.

BIRTH RATE

The birth rate is the number of children born per year per 1000 of the population. Another way of expressing this is:

$$\text{Birth rate} = \frac{\text{number of births in the year} \times 1000}{\text{mid-year population}}$$

The birth rate has varied considerably in England and Wales in the last 80 years (Fig. 4).

It will be seen that in 1900 the birth rate was 28·2. The rate then fell steadily to the low figure of 14·4 in 1933, except for the sharp increase for the years immediately after the 1914–18 war. It fell again during the early part of the 1939–45 war, but rose steeply in 1946, immediately after the war, as many families became reunited. The rate then fell steadily for several years and by 1955 was 15·0. For reasons still imperfectly understood, it then began to rise and reached 18·5 in 1964. This sudden change in the trend produced exceptional pressure on maternity accommodation. In the period 1951–5 there was an average of 675 420 births annually, but by 1964 the number of births had risen to 865 000.

Since 1965, the birth rate has been steadily falling until in 1977 it had reached 11·6 (the lowest recorded rate since the 1930s) and the number of births fell to 567 000 (Table 2). There is no certainty that this trend will continue and it is most important for anyone concerned with the planning of obstetric and child health services to watch for future changes.

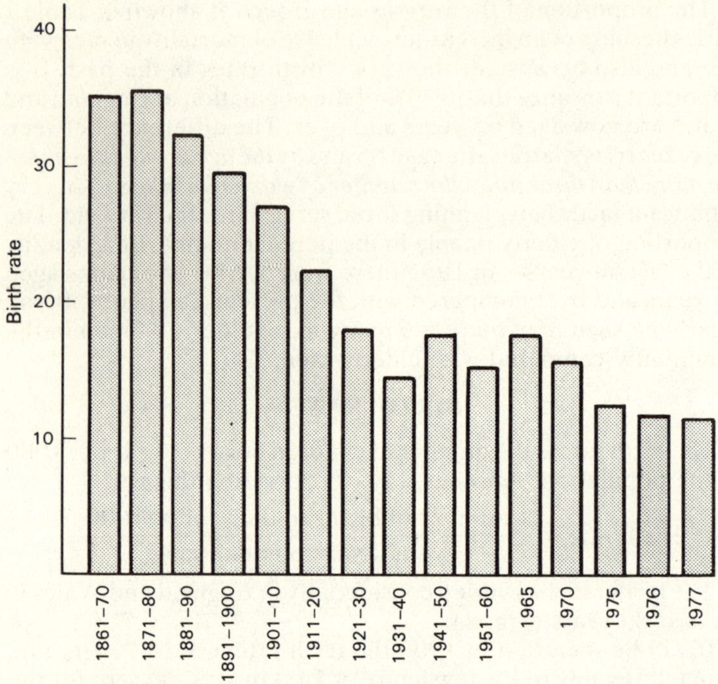

FIG. 4. Birth rate, England and Wales, 1861–77.

TABLE 2 Birth rate, England and Wales, 1955–77

Year	*Birth rate*	*Year*	*Birth rate*
1955	15·0	1965	18·1
1956	15·6	1966	17·7
1957	16·1	1967	17·2
1958	16·4	1968	16·9
1959	16·5	1969	16·3
1960	17·2	1970	16·1
1961	17·4	1972	14·8
1962	18·0	1974	13·0
1963	18·2	1976	11·9
1964	18·5	1977	11·6

Social factors in a community cause changes in the birth rate, and, in the past, poorer sections of the community have tended to show higher birth rates than the wealthier sections.

This is, however, changing in the UK. Tables 3 and 4 show this. In both social classes I and II have been amalgamated, and also social classes IV and V.

TABLE 3 Social class and births—England and Wales 1975

Social class	% of population	% of live births
I and II	24	26
IIIN	12	14
IIIM	37·5	39
IV and V	23·5	20

(from *Population Trends*, 1977, OPCS)

This has been a recent trend as shown by Table 4 in which the 1970 births are indexed at 100. The rate of fall recorded is greatest in social class IV and V (67) and least in social classes I and II (96).

TABLE 4 Social class and Births—1970–1975 (Index 1970-100)

	All classes	*I and II*	*IIIN*	*IIIM*	*IV and V*
1970	100	100	100	100	100
1972	92	102	94	90	84
1974	81	99	78	77	72
1975	76	96	75	71	67

(from *Population Trends*, 1977, OPCS)

These figures suggest that families in social classes IV–V are now limiting the size of their family to a much greater extent than in the past. The explanation is probably connected with much more effective contraception available and the high unemployment rates in social classes IV and V.

The age of the mother having her first child falls with the social class as shown in a survey in England and Wales in 1970–2, illustrated in Table 5.

TABLE 5 Average age of mother at first live birth within marriage

Social class of husband	*Average age of mother*
I	26·3
II	25·8
IIIN	24·9
IIIM	23·4
IV	22·9
V	21·9

(from *Population Trends*, 1977, OPCS)

The birth rate is high in underdeveloped countries: many African countries have birth rates between 34 and 52 and Pakistan had an average rate of 50·0 for the period 1965–70. The rate for India in 1971 was 42·8 and in the middle east, Jordan has the highest rate, 47·8. Rapidly developing countries often show high birth rates. Israel had a rate of 28·3 in 1975. Most European countries have rates well below 20, but Albania still has a very high rate, 35·3. Religion may have a marked effect, the rate in Eire (a Roman Catholic country) was 21·6 in 1975.

It is interesting to note that *male births always exceed female births in the ratio of 105 to 100*, but the male death rate exceeds the female death rate so that after age 50 there are more women than men.

In 1976 of all live births, 9·1% were illegitimate but *nearly twice that number (17%) were pre-maritally conceived* (birth occurring within eight months of first marriage). In mothers aged under 20 years, approximately 65% of all births are pre-maritally conceived but the figure falls to 15% for ages 20–24 and 6% for age 25 and over.

DEATH RATE

The crude death rate is the number of deaths per year per 1000 of the population. Another way of expressing this is:

$$\text{Death rate} = \frac{\text{number of deaths in the year} \times 1000}{\text{mid-year population}}$$

The crude death rate is of little value, as the relative age of populations in districts and towns is never known accurately. Where there is a large proportion of elderly persons, the number of deaths in the community is bound to be higher, irrespective of the living conditions. For this reason, it is not possible to deduce from a high crude death rate that the area is unhealthy. The deaths of strangers in a locality are deducted and allocated to the districts in which they permanently reside. Such deaths are known as 'transferable deaths'. The Registrar General notifies each Area Medical Officer of such deaths so that corrections may be made locally.

In 1977, 570 000 deaths occurred in England and Wales. The crude death rate was 11·7.

Because of the extreme difficulty in correcting the death rate for age and sex distribution locally, it has never been possible to produce a perfect method by which death rates may be compared. For this reason, it is better to use other mortality rates (such as infant mortality rate—see below) to compare the health problems of different districts.

If crude death rates are used, an approximation to standardization can be obtained by using the Registrar General's Area Comparability Factor. The crude death rate is multiplied by the area comparability factor to give the adjusted rate. An example is given in Table 6 by comparing the crude death rates of seven local authorities.

It will be seen that Hastings and Torbay have the highest crude death rates (20·6 and 17·2), but that the adjusted rates are 11·74 and 9·80. This is due to the large number of elderly people living in these places and this produces proportionately many more

TABLE 6 Crude death rates of seven local authorities, 1975

	Population	*Crude death rate*	*Area comparability factor*	*Adjusted death rate**	*Adjusted death rate order*
Hastings	75 000	20·6	0·57	11·74	3
Torbay	110 000	17·2	0·57	9·80	6
Bath	84 000	12·9	0·80	10·32	5
Worcester	74 000	11·4	1·01	11·5	4
Cambridge	103 000	9·3	1·01	9·4	7
Knowsley	191 400	8·4	1·58	13·37	1
Harlow	80 000	5·6	2·20	12·32	2

* Crude Death Rate × Area Comparability Factor
(from *Local Authority Vital Statistics*, 1975, OPCS)

deaths. On the other hand, Knowsley, which contains Kirkby in its area, and Harlow, a new town, have a very high proportion of young people and their crude death rates are very low, 8·4 and 5·6. But when these are multiplied by the area comparability factors this gives an adjusted rate of 13·37 and 12·32, and instead of seeming to be the best authorities in the table actually are the worst. Also included in the table are two cities, Cambridge and Worcester, whose populations are very typical in age range of the whole country, having therefore an area comparability factor of 1·01 and their crude and adjusted death rates are very similar.

Expectation of Life

Very accurate estimations of the expectation of life are made by insurance companies, as they base their premiums for life assurance on the estimated expectation of life. Life tables are constructed from a knowledge of the make-up of the population at individual ages and from the deaths at such ages. The way the expectation of life has improved since 1838 is seen from Table 7.

It is interesting to note the difference between the two sexes: *women on an average live six years longer than men* (an important difference when planning services for the elderly).

TABLE 7 Expectation of life (in years), England and Wales

Years	*Males*	*Females*
1838–44	40	42
1871–80	41	45
1910–12	52	55
1930–2	59	63
1942	62	67
1955	68	73
1965	68·5	74·7
1971	69·0	75·3
1973–5	69·5	75·7

However, the improvement in the expectation of life slows down the older the person (Table 8).

TABLE 8 Improvement in expectation of life comparing 1901 with 1973–5, England and Wales

	Males		*Females*	
Expectation of life	*1901*	*1973–5*	*1901*	*1973–5*
at birth	48·1	69·5	51·8	75·7
at age 10 years	51·4	61·1	54·0	67·1
at age 20 years	42·7	51·7	45·4	57·2
at age 30 years	34·5	41·8	37·1	47·5
at age 40 years	26·8	32·3	29·2	37·9
at age 50 years	19·7	23·4	21·7	28·7
at age 60 years	13·4	15·7	14·9	20·3
at age 70 years	8·4	9·6	9·2	12·9
at age 80 years	4·9	5·8	5·3	7·3
at age 85 years	—	4·6	—	5·6

It will be seen that whereas the expectation of life has improved 21·4 years at birth for men (an improvement of 44%) the expectation of life of a man of 70 has improved 0·8 years only (an improvement of 10·5%).

At all ages the life expectancy of women is greater than men. After the age of 70 years, this difference falls and at age 85 the life expectation of women is one year greater than men.

Specialized Death Rates

The crude death rate is rarely used to indicate the preventive medical problems of an area. But there are a number of specialized death rates which are of much greater value.

The infant mortality rate

This is the number of infants under one year of age who die per year per 1000 live related births.

$$\text{Infant mortality rate (IMR)} = \frac{\text{Deaths of infants under one year of age during the year} \times 1000}{\text{Number of live births during the year}}$$

In 1977 in England and Wales the rate was 14·0 which means that 1·40% of babies born alive died in their first year of life. The infant mortality rate is one of the most widely used death rates; it gives an excellent indication of the living conditions in an area because the main factors influencing a baby's progress are closely connected with his home. If the living conditions in the home are poor, the child is much more likely to fall ill and the results of that illness to be more serious, and this is reflected in the number of deaths recorded in children under one year of age in the area.

A deterioration in the social circumstances of an area, such as a sudden change in the level of unemployment, will be rapidly reflected in the infant mortality rate. In the depressed areas in the 1930s the rate was very high. The infant mortality rate can be used to compare the living conditions of towns as shown in Table 9. A casual visitor to, say, the London Borough of Havering or Reading would probably have little idea that living conditions were considerably worse in Chester, Rugby or Neath.

It is interesting to note that the differences between boys and girls in each country are roughly similar (Table 10).

There is also a marked difference between the infant mortality rate for legitimate and illegitimate births (1971 England and Wales legitimate IMR = 17·5; illegitimate IMR = 25·4), but the degree of difference has narrowed over the last 60 years (Table 11).

TABLE 9 Infant mortality rate per 1000 live births, England, 1975 (England and Wales IMR = 16)

Havering (London)	9	Bolton	18
Reading	9	Manchester	21
Oxford	10	Hackney (London)	23
Exeter	11	Chester	24
Cardiff	13	Rugby	25
Liverpool	16	Neath	31

(from *Local Authority Vital Statistics*, 1975, OPCS)

There is a significant difference between the infant mortality rate of boys and girls in England and Wales, Scotland and Northern Ireland (Table 10).

TABLE 10 Infant mortality rate per 1000 live births, England and Wales, Scotland and Northern Ireland, 1971

	Males	*Females*
England and Wales	19·8	15·1
Scotland	22·2	17·4
Northern Ireland	24·5	20·8

TABLE 11 Infant mortality rate, legitimate and illegitimate births, England and Wales, 1911 to 1976

Year	*Legitimate*	*Illegitimate*
1911–20	95	194
1921–30	69	130
1931–40	57	94
1941–50	42	61
1951–60	24	31
1961–70	19	26
1976	12·5	19

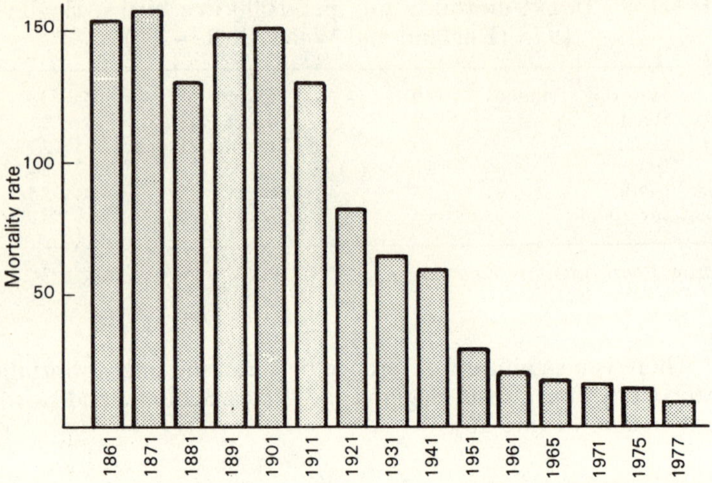

FIG. 5. Infant mortality rate, England and Wales, 1861–77.

TABLE 12 Infant mortality rate per 1000 live births, England and Wales

Year	*Rate*	*Year*	*Rate*
1841	147	1941	60
1851	154	1951	30
1861	153	1960	21·8
1871	158	1965	19·0
1881	130	1970	18·2
1891	149	1971	17·3
1901	151	1975	15·7
1911	130	1976	14·3
1921	83	1977	13·8
1931	66		

The changes in infant mortality during the last 130 years in England and Wales are given in Table 12 and are illustrated in Fig. 5. There is a markedly higher infant mortality in boys than in girls. There is also a marked social class differential in infant mortality. The *lowest rates are in social class I (9·6) and the highest in social class V (26·5).*

TABLE 13 Infant Mortality Rate (IMR) per 1000 live births, England and Wales

Years	*Males*	*Females*
1966	21·4	16·5
1971	19·8	15·1
1973	18·9	14·7
1976	16·2	12·2

(from *Population Trends*, 1978, OPCS)

Causes of infant mortality

The principal causes of infant mortality in boys and girls in 1974 in England and Wales are given in Table 14.

It is important to note that one-fifth are caused by congenital abnormalities and that this is the single largest cause. Complications of pregnancy and labour are responsible for one-eighth and immaturity, infections and pneumonia are the next commonest causes.

TABLE 14. Principal causes of infant mortality per 1000 live births, England and Wales, 1974

	Males	*Females*
Certain causes of perinatal morbidity and mortality	3·59	3·72
Congenital anomalies	3·89	3·85
Diseases of respiratory system	2·63	1·74
Pneumonia	1·48	1·05
Acute respiratory infections in influenza	0·86	0·52
Accidents	0·45	0·34
Infectious diseases	0·66	0·47
Enteritis and diarrhoea diseases	0·32	0·21
All other causes	4·72	2·00
Total	18·60	13·90

(from *Fit for the Future*, the Court Report)

Many doctors find it difficult to understand why the level of paediatric services are not the determining factor in infant mortality. They do, of course, play their part in keeping death rates lower than they might otherwise be, but they are not a major factor in determining the level of infant mortality. This is confirmed by the fact that the infant mortality rate is lower in rural areas with good living conditions, but where there are no specialized paediatric services on the scale of those in large cities.

International comparisons in Infant Mortality Rate

There are still wide variations between the infant mortality rates of different countries of the world (Table 15). Sweden is clearly the lowest, with Japan and the Netherlands also with low figures. Many other results may seem surprising. England and Wales at 15·7 is above USA and Germany, but below France. Portugal has a high rate in comparison to her neighbour Spain. The Eastern European countries have high rates similar to many African and Asian countries.

TABLE 15 Infant mortality rates in different countries, 1975

Sweden	8·3	New Zealand	16·0
Netherlands	10·6	USA	16·1
Denmark	10·7	Germany (Federal)	19·7
Japan	10·8	Israel	21·8
France	13·6	USSR	27·8
Spain	13·8	Hungary	32·6
Canada	15·0*	Romania	35·0*
England and Wales	15·7	Portugal	37·9*
Germany (East)	15·7	Yugoslavia	40·5

* 1974
(from *On the State of the Public Health*, 1976, DHSS)

Neonatal mortality rate

This figure is the number of infants who die in the first four weeks of life per year per 1000 live related births.

$$\text{Neonatal mortality rate} = \frac{\text{infant deaths in first four weeks of life during the year} \times 1000}{\text{number of live births during the year.}}$$

The neonatal mortality rate is, of course, contained within the infant mortality rate. Because of the exceptional hazards to very young infants, the neonatal rate is responsible for approximately two-thirds of the total infant mortality in the first year of life. In 1977 the neonatal mortality rate was 9·3 per 1000 live births in England and Wales. Of these, 7·6 occurred in the first week and 1·7 in the period 7–28 days. It is interesting to note that the rate is much higher in boys.

Perinatal mortality rate

This is the combined total of the number of stillbirths and deaths within the first week of life per year per 1000 total births.

$$\text{Perinatal mortality rate} = \frac{\text{still births plus deaths in first week of life during the year} \times 1000}{\text{number of total births during the year}}$$

The value of the perinatal mortality rate is that it gives a good indication of the hazards to a baby immediately before and after birth. The perinatal mortality rate overcomes the disadvantage of separating stillbirths from those infant deaths which occur a short time after birth. The child might have little chance of survival, but exceptionally skilful midwifery could convert a likely stillbirth to a first week death; in either event the death will be shown in the perinatal mortality rate.

In 1977, the perinatal mortality rate in England and Wales was 17·0 per 1000 total births. The improvement in the perinatal mortality rate in the last 23 years is shown in Table 16:

TABLE 16 Perinatal mortality rate and stillbirth rate, England and Wales, 1950 to 1977

	Perinatal Mortality	*Stillbirth*		*Perinatal Mortality*	*Stillbirth*
1950	37·4	22·6	1968	24·7	14·3
1953	36·9	22·4	1971	22·3	12·5
1956	36·7	22·9	1973	21·0	11·5
1959	34·1	20·8	1976	17·7	9·7
1962	30·8	18·1	1977	17·0	9·4
1965	26·9	15·8			

(from *Population Trends*, 1978, OPCS)

There are three important factors which affect perinatal mortality, *maternal age*, *parity* and *social class*. Table 17 illustrates

TABLE 17 Perinatal mortality by maternal age, parity and social class, England and Wales 1973

Maternal age	*Rate*	*Parity*	*Rate*	*Social class*	*Rate*
Less than 20	23·0	0	20·1	I	13·9
20–24	17·5	1	15·3	II	15·6
25–29	16·6	2	19·0	III	19·2
30–34	20·4	3	24·6	IV	21·8
35–39	27·1	4	28·2	V	26·8
40–44	41·8	5	37·2		

(from *Population Trends*, 1977, OPCS

the way these three influence the rate. Note that the older classification of Social Class into five groups is used and that the lowest rates are found in mothers in social classes I and II having a second child, while in her twenties and the highest rates are seen in a mother having her fifth or later child. The perinatal mortality rate is higher in illegitimate births (in 1972 the total rate was 21·7, but 21·0 in legitimate births and 28·2 in illegitimate births).

International comparisons

Examination of the perinatal mortality rates of different countries (Table 18) shows a marked variation which, however,

TABLE 18 Perinatal mortality in different countries, 1974

Sweden	13·2	Romania	20·0
Denmark	14·5	England and Wales	20·4
Netherlands	15·4	USA	21·9
Japan	16·7	Germany (Federal)	23·0
Canada	17·6	Italy	29·2
Germany (East)	18·0	Portugal	32·2
France	18·6	Hungary	34·1
New Zealand	19·2*		

* 1971
(from *On the State of Public Health*, 1976, DHSS)

is not quite so great as in the case of the infant mortality rate (see p. 66). Sweden, Netherlands and Denmark still head the table and the position of England and Wales is disappointingly low.

Stillbirth rate

This is the number of stillbirths per year per 1000 total births. A stillbirth is a late fetal death at or over 28 weeks gestation. Table 16 shows that in the last 20 years the stillbirth rate has improved faster than first week deaths (a 58% improvement compared with 52%). In 1977 the rate was 9·4.

The stillbirth rate shows the same proportional variations in respect of age of mother, parity and social class as does the perinatal mortality rate.

A history of previous stillbirths also adds considerably to the chances of a further stillbirth.

Maternal mortality rate

The maternal mortality rate is the number of women who die from causes associated with childbirth per year per 1000 total births:

$$\text{Maternal mortality rate} = \frac{\text{deaths during the year in women associated with childbirth} \times 1000}{\text{number of total births during the year.}}$$

The maternal mortality rate is a measure of the risk to the mother connected with childbirth. Deaths are only counted if they are directly related to pregnancy. For example, death from renal failure which had commenced with a severe toxaemia of pregnancy and pyelonephritis would be counted as a maternal death even if the woman died years later. But death from a completely unrelated cause (such as a road accident or medical or surgical emergency) would not be counted as a maternal death even if it took place during pregnancy.

Maternal mortality rates have fallen dramatically since 1935. The rate was then 4·33 while in 1976 it was 0·13 (including abortions)—an improvement of 33 times (Fig. 6).

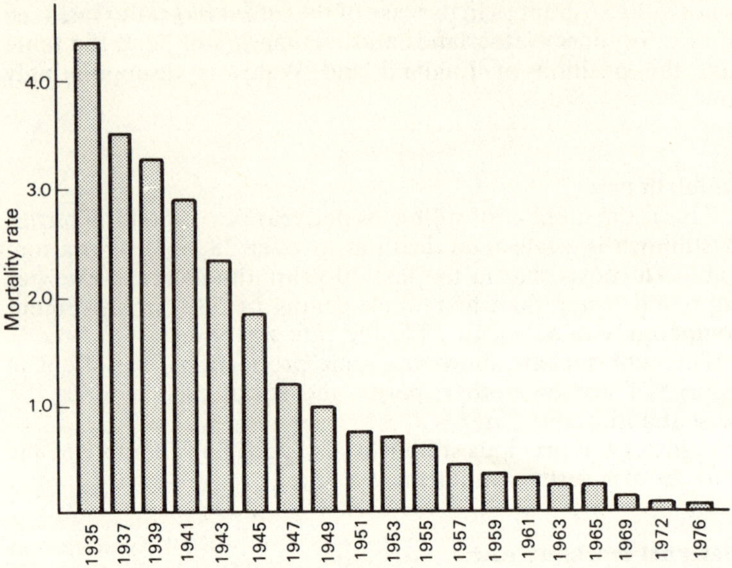

FIG. 6. Maternal mortality rate (including abortion), England and Wales, 1935–76.

Examination of Table 19 shows that the maternal mortality rate improved in quite a different manner compared with the infant mortality rate. The infant mortality rate has improved steadily throughout the last 60 years, whereas the maternal mortality rate hardly altered between 1900 and 1930. At the beginning of the 1930s it had actually risen to 4·24. After 1937 it fell rapidly and has continued to fall steadily until the early 1970s (it has risen slightly in the last five years). The reason for these different trends in infant mortality and maternal mortality is that they are affected by entirely different factors—whereas infant mortality is mainly connected with living conditions, the maternal mortality rate is related to the standard of obstetric practice. The introduction in 1937 of chemotherapy and then antibiotics produced a rapid fall as the dangers of death from puerperal infection were dramatically reduced. Further advances in treatment have lessened the hazards of pre-eclamptic toxaemia and haemorrhage, thus reducing further the maternal mortality rate.

TABLE 19 Maternal mortality rate (including abortion), England and Wales, 1870–1976

Year	MMR	Year	MMR	Year	MMR
1870–2	4·81	1941	2·90	1961	0·34
1880–2	4·61	1943	2·37	1963	0·28
1890–2	5·31	1945	1·85	1965	0·25
1900–2	4·67	1947	1·20	1967	0·24
1910–12	3·67	1949	1·00	1969	0·19
1920–2	4·03	1951	0·78	1971	0·17
1930–2	4·24	1953	0·72	1973	0·12
1935	4·33	1955	0·61	1975	0·11
1937	3·51	1957	0·46	1976	0·13
1939	3·25	1959	0·39		

Causes of maternal mortality

Maternal mortality is rare today and consequently extreme care must be taken in quoting this rate for populations under 8–10 million. The principal causes of maternal mortality in England in 1976 are given in Table 20.

TABLE 20 Principal causes of maternal mortality, England, 1975–6

Causes	*Deaths*
Other deaths from delivery	17
Toxaemias of pregnancy	15
Puerperal phlebitis and pulmonary embolism	10
Other complications of puerperium	9
Abortion	6
Other complications of pregnancy	6
Ectopic pregnancy	5
Postpartum haemorrhage	5
Haemorrhage of pregnancy	1

(from *On the State of the Public Health*, 1976, DHSS)

Note that *toxaemias of pregnancy still represent the largest single identifiable cause.* There has been an improvement in deaths from haemorrhage and 1975–6 was the first two years without any maternal deaths from placenta praevia or antepartum haemorrhage.

See p. 100 for confidential returns into maternal deaths.

MORBIDITY

Much research is now proceeding to perfect methods of measuring disease incidence (*morbidity*). Certain infectious diseases are notifiable, but for most diseases indirect methods have to be used. These include the various sources of statistics mentioned on pp. 52–55. The General Household Survey reported the incidence of long standing illnesses in 1974–5 classified by age and social class (see Table 21).

TABLE 21 Long-standing illness by social class, age and sex, 1974–5, Great Britain (as rate per 1000)

Social class	*Age*				
	0–14	*15–44*	*45–64*	*65+*	*All*
Males					
I	36	66	161	239	88
II	50	74	162	336	122
IIIN	40	83	274	363	148
IIIM	45	85	237	397	138
IV	47	84	265	373	155
V	56	112	390	377	226
Total	46	83	234	366	140
Females					
I	28	79	134	286	84
II	26	72	161	412	119
IIIN	20	66	200	417	148
IIIM	35	93	202	419	132
IV	25	95	260	437	197
V	44	115	264	419	246
Total	29	84	209	424	155

(from *Social Trends*, 1977, OPCS)

It is interesting to note the usual pattern of increased illness in social classes IV and V compared with I and II is seen; also there is more chronic illness in boys than girls in the 0–14 age group, but much more in women than in men in the 65 years and over age group.

HOSPITAL STATISTICS

The Hospital In-patient Enquiry and Hospital Activity Analysis published annually gives many interesting morbidity returns.

TABLE 22 Discharges and deaths in all hospitals, excluding mental hospitals, in Great Britain, 1974 (numbers per 100 000)

Cause	*No.*
Males	
1. Diseases of digestive system	1138
2. Diseases of respiratory system	1006
3. Symptoms and ill-defined conditions	930
4. Other injuries and reactions	836
5. Rheumatic fever, hypertensive disease and heart disease	670
6. Cancer	588
7. Diseases of peripheral circulatory system	486
8. Fractures, dislocations and sprains	418
9. Male genital disorders	335
10. Mental illness	333
11. Infective and parasitic diseases	213
12. Congenital anomalies	208
13. Disease of the eye	206
14. Diseases of the skin	186
Females	
1. Diseases of breast and female genital system	1020
2. Diseases of digestive system	902
3. Symptoms and ill-defined conditions	893
4. Diseases of respiratory system	728
5. Other injuries and reactions	615
6. Cancer	560
7. Diseases of peripheral circulatory system	489
8. Rheumatic fever, hypertensive diseases and heart disease	470
9. Mental illness	445
10. Other neoplasms	341
11. Fractures, dislocations and sprains	338
12. Diseases of the eye	228
13. Endocrine, nutritional and metabolic diseases	217
14. Diseases of the nervous system	180
15. Infective and parasitic diseases	176

Note: Had pregnancy, childbirth and puerperium discharges been included, they would have formed the largest group in women.
(from *Hospital In-patient Enquiry*, 1974)

There are broad similarities in the discharge pattern of both sexes. The number of women exceed men but this excess is greater in mental illness (37%) than in physical illness (13%). Digestive system, respiratory and heart disease are all greater in men, but disease of the breast and female genital system are the largest cause in women and represent at 1020 admissions a much larger figure than male genital disorders (335). Note also that 'other neoplasms' and 'endocrine, nutritional and metabolic disease' figure among the 15 commonest causes in women but not in men.

Table 23 gives an analysis of all admissions to mental hospitals and units. There are fundamental differences in the sexes: in both schizophrenia, depressive psychosis and psychoneuroses head

TABLE 23 Mental Illness: All admissions to mental hospitals and psychiatric units, England, 1975

Cause	*No.*
Males	
1. Schizophrenia	14 650
2. Personality and behavioural disorders	8305
3. Psychoneurosis	7385
4. Alcoholism	7102
5. Depressive psychosis	6808
6. Other psychoses	5018
7. Senile and presenile dementia	2917
8. Other psychiatric conditions	2419
9. Drug dependence	1087
Total	55 691
Females	
1. Schizophrenia	15 716
2. Depressive psychosis	15 461
3. Psychoneurosis	15 046
4. Personality and behavioural disorders	9428
5. Other psychoses	8256
6. Senile and presenile dementia	6744
7. Other psychiatric conditions	3360
8. Alcoholism	2509
9. Drug dependence	570
Total	66 892

(from *Mental Health Enquiry*, 1975, DHSS)

the list in that order but the incidence of depressive psychoses in women is nearly double that in men, a factor which is certainly influenced by the larger proportion of women in the older age groups. Many of the other causes are very similar in incidence, but alcoholism is nearly three times commoner in men than women.

Number of beds occupied daily

Because of the great variation in length of stay in hospitals, the figures given above do not represent the daily usage of hospital beds. This is best shown as in Fig. 7, which shows clearly, for

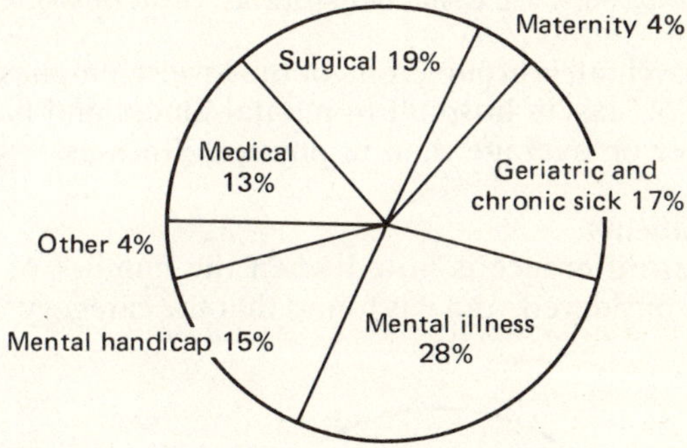

FIG. 7. Percentage of hospital beds occupied daily by different disease categories, Great Britain, 1975.

example, the large number of hospital beds occupied by mental disability—43% (mental illness 28% and mental handicap 15%). It is particularly interesting to note that although pregnancy is the largest single cause of hospital discharge in women, it accounts for only 4% of hospital bed usage due to the very short stay in hospital of such women.

Discharges and deaths of in-patients

An entirely different picture is given if the proportion of discharges and deaths of in-patients are compared (see Fig. 8).

Here the three largest groups are surgical, medical and mater-

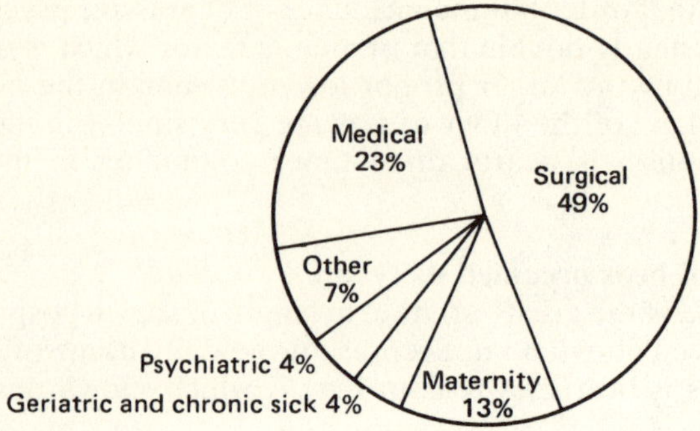

FIG. 8. Discharges and deaths of in-patients, Great Britain, 1975.

nity. The psychiatric group is one of the lowest, emphasizing that the length of stay in hospital in mental illness and handicap is much longer on average than in physical illnesses.

New out-patients

A further difference is noted when the number of new out-patients is considered, and it is found that the category 'accidents

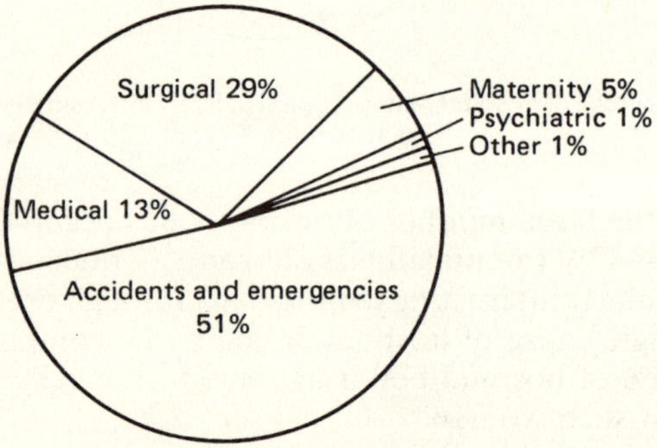

FIG. 9. New out-patients in hospitals, Great Britain, 1974.

and emergency' becomes the largest single group. The other interesting feature is that psychiatric figures fall to a very low level—1% of all new out-patient attendances.

Sickness Benefit Returns

There are two main ways of presenting such returns:

1. new spells of sickness (rate per 1000 at risk, Table 24)
2. days of sickness per 1000 persons at risk (Table 25)

The first certainly represents the initial call on general practitioners and the second the total loss of productive power due to disease.

TABLE 24 The 12 commonest causes of new spells of certified incapacity (rate per 1000 persons at risk, Great Britain, 1975)

Cause	*No.*
Males	
1. Other diseases of respiratory system	79·4
2. Influenza	47·8
3. Symptoms and ill-defined	44·9
4. Infections and parasitic diseases	38·5
5. Accidents	34·1
6. Disease of digestive system, Bronchitis	33·7
8. Sprains and strains (joints)	23·5
9. Arthritis	23·3
10. Other diseases of musculoskeletal system	19·1
11. Mental illness	13.9
12. Skin diseases	11·5
Females	
1. Other diseases of respiratory system	125·1
2. Symptoms and ill-defined	70·5
3. Influenza	49·9
4. Infections and parasitic diseases	48·8
5. Complications of pregnancy	26·8
6. Diseases of digestive system	25·8
7. Bronchitis, Mental illness	25·4
9. Accidents	21·8
10. Diseases of urinary system	15·0
11. Arthritis	14·7
12. Other diseases of musculoskeletal system	12·9

(from *Health and Personal Social Services Statistics*, DHSS, 1977)

TABLE 25 The 12 commonest causes of working days lost 1975 (rate per 1000 persons at risk), Great Britain

Cause	Days lost
Males	
1. Bronchitis	1844
2. Symptoms and ill-defined	1745
3. Ischaemic heart disease	1728
4. Mental illness	1374
5. Other diseases of respiratory system	1185
6. Arthritis	1167
7. Other diseases of circulatory system	1052
8. Diseases of digestive system	1026
9. Accidents	896
10. Diseases of nervous system	859
11. Other diseases of musculoskeletal system	713
12. Influenza	494
Females	
1. Mental illness	2460
2. Symptoms and ill-defined	2234
3. Other diseases of respiratory system	1451
4. Arthritis	1276
5. Complications of pregnancy	1261
6. Diseases of nervous system	904
7. Bronchitis	811
8. Other diseases of circulatory system	798
9. Ischaemic heart disease	709
10. Diseases of digestive system	701
11. Infections and parasitic diseases	601
12. Other diseases of musculoskeletal system	532

(from *Health and Personal Social Services Statistics*, DHSS, 1977)

It is most interesting to compare these tables both for differences between the sexes and to see how, in some diseases, although the number of spells of sickness is smaller, the days lost are very large. Ischaemic heart disease is not among the 12 commonest causes of new spells of sickness, but is third in importance in days lost in males and ninth in females. The importance of mental illness in women is once more emphasized, being first in days lost in women (fourth in men) and seventh in spells of sickness in women (eleventh in men). Bronchitis causes more than twice the number of days lost in men (1844) compared with women (811). Diseases of the digestive system, influenza, unspecified (symptoms and ill-defined) are very similar in both sexes. Disease of the urinary system and of the breast and genital systems do not appear in either sex (are fourteenth in women).

Communicable diseases

The main figures for 1976 in Great Britain are given in Table 26. Most of these figures are fairly typical with the exception of measles (1976 saw a very low incidence). Typhoid fever for the second year in succession exceeds 200 cases and the number of paralytic poliomyelitis cases were higher than any year since 1968.

TABLE 26 Communicable diseases notified—Great Britain, 1976

Disease	*No. of cases*
1. Measles	68 112
2. Food poisoning	11 119
3. Scarlet fever	10 442
4. Tuberculosis (pulmonary)	8959
5. Dysentery	7239
6. Infective hepatitis	6823
7. Whooping cough	4289
8. Acute meningitis	2179
9. Ophthalmia neonatorum	282
10. Typhoid fever	215
11. Tuberculosis (of meninges and central nervous system)	114*
12. Paratyphoid fever	78
13. Acute poliomyelitis (paralytic)	13
14. Anthrax	4
15. Acute poliomyelitis (non-paralytic)	3
16. Diphtheria	2

* 1975

(from *Health and Personal Social Services Statistics*, DHSS, 1977)

Cancer registration

Most of these statistics originate in hospital figures, and these are collected together and analysed by the DHSS. The 12 commonest malignant cancers recorded in this way in England and Wales in 1970 are given in Table 27. In this year there were a total of 154 352 cases registered (1263 in age groups under 15 years, 71 941 in ages 15–64 and 81 147 in ages 65 and over). It is interesting to note there are marked differences in the incidence in men and women in some cancers (lung, bladder and kidney, and stomach). While breast cancer in women is the commonest cancer seen, it is rare in men. In others the incidence is very similar (skin, pancreas).

TABLE 27 Cancer registrations (malignant neoplasms only), England and Wales, 1970, the 12 commonest specified causes

Cancer	*Male*	*Female*	*Total*
1. Lung, bronchus	23 962	5269	29 231
2. Breast	168	18 156	18 324
3. Skin	8555	7637	15 192
4. Intestine (except rectum)	4863	6499	11 362
5. Stomach	6538	4556	11 094
6. Bladder and kidney	6546	2576	9122
7. Total lymphatic and haemopoietic tissues	4532	3665	8197
8. Prostate	5247	—	5247
9. Pancreas	2412	2002	4414
10. Cervix uteri	—	4099	4099
11. Ovary	—	3975	3975
12. Uterus (other than cervix)	—	3364	3364

(from *Health and Personal Social Services Statistics*, DHSS, 1977)

Maximum age incidence of cancers

An interesting feature of the incidence of different cancers is that some are much commoner under 65 years of age, some have a similar incidence in ages 15 to 65 and 65 years and over and some have a greater incidence over 65 (Table 28).

Sexually transmitted (venereal) diseases

Statistics are collected at hospital clinics treating these diseases and are given in Chapter 13 (p. 228).

TABLE 28 Varying age incidences of certain cancers, England and Wales, 1970

Site	*15–64*	*65 and over*
Greater incidence in ages 15 to 64		
Breast (women)	11 198	6958
Cervix uteri	3084	1015
Ovary	2427	1540
Lymphatic and haematopoietic tissue (men)	2536	1715
Eye, brain and nervous system	2051	571
Similar incidence at 15–64 and 65 years and over		
Lung	15 278	15 834
Skin	7367	8800
Greater incidence over age 65 years		
Stomach	3780	7313
Intestine (except rectum)	4000	7357
Rectum	2776	4770
Bladder	3645	5293
Prostate	889	4357

(from *Health and Personal Social Service Statistics*, DHSS, 1977)

MORTALITY RATES

The causes of death are grouped together as mortality rates. Most of these are very reliable as there is an obvious need for doctors to be very accurate when certifying death, even in the more primitive countries, so that mortality statistics are widely used to compare international statistics of disease. The WHO collects and publishes a comprehensive yearly report in which mortality statistics are given by death rates per 100 000 population.

To ensure that every country and every statistician is using the same basis for description of any disease, an *International Statistical Classification of Diseases, Injuries and Causes of Death* is used and each disease is given a ICD number. The last review of this list internationally occurred in 1965.

It is possible to compare different mortality rates by giving the death per 1000, 10 000, or 100 000 but for deaths in England and Wales a better way is to use the *Standardized Mortality Ratio (SMR)*.

Standardized Mortality Ratio (SMR)

By definition the Standardized Mortality Ratio (SMR) is the percentage ratio of the number of deaths observed in the group studied to the number expected from the age-specific death rates for England and Wales. The SMR is used in two ways:

1. To compare mortality from one year to another:

First an adjustment is made for changes in sex/age of the population of different years and a base year is selected. Then the SMR is expressed as the percentage of deaths in the year in question compared with the base year.

At present, by convention, the base year is 1968 and a year with a SMR of 200 has a mortality of 200/100 or twice as great as 1968. If the SMR was 75, it would mean that the mortality for that year was 75/100 or three-quarters that of the base year.

Table 29 shows the SMR for a number of causes of death for the four years 1961, 1966, 1970, 1975 for Great Britain, all expressed in terms of the base year 1968 (i.e. for all those diseases the 1968 figure was 100). The table shows the marked way in which mortality has altered even in this 17 year period. For example, the deaths from tuberculosis have declined from 171 to 56 in men (165 to 64 in women)—an improvement in the order of three times. Deaths from hypertensive disease show an improvement in both sexes which is almost as great. But the table shows that there are diseases which are increasing: cancer of the lung in women accounted in 1975 for almost twice as many deaths as in 1961. The trend in men is also upwards but the increase is flattening out during the last four years. Yet many cancers are showing a slow decline—cancer of digestive system and cancer of the cervix uteri.

It is curious to note that deaths from pneumonia show a steady increase from 1961to 1975. It is difficult to determine the reason (these are age-standardized figures) but clearly calls for great vigilance on the part of doctors to diagnose and to treat pneumonia promptly and effectively.

It is interesting to realize that had this table covered a longer period of time, some of the changes that would have been demonstrated would have been even more dramatic. For instance, the SMR for all forms of tuberculosis would have been in the region of 1100 for 1901–10, 600 for 1921–30, 350 for 1940–9 and 190 for 1950–2. This means that mortality in 1901–10 was eleven times greater than in 1968 and as the mortality has nearly halved since then (SMR in 1971 = 56), a straight comparison between 1901–10 and 1975 would show a reduction of mortality for all forms of tuberculosis in the region of twenty times.

TABLE 29 Standardized Mortality Ratio. Deaths by selected causes, Great Britain, 1961–75 (base year 1968 = 100)

	Males				*Females*			
Cause of death	*1961*	*1966*	*1970*	*1975*	*1961*	*1966*	*1970*	*1975*
Tuberculosis (all forms)	171	115	76	56	165	109	114	64
Cancer								
Lung	88	97	102	102	72	90	108	131
Digestive system	102	100	98	98	105	100	95	94
Cervix uteri	—	—	—	—	105	100	95	87
Ischaemic heart disease	90	97	100	103	97	97	97	100
Hypertensive disease	156	108	92	69	170	112	85	63
Pneumonia (except newborn)	84	91	105	106	76	88	100	107
Suicide	117	106	86	81	115	113	88	82
All causes	103	101	95	94	105	102	95	87

(From *Social Trends*, 1977, OPCS)

2. To compare group mortality with total mortality. The standardized ratio can also be used to express the mortality of a section of the community compared with the whole population. The average mortality of the whole country is called 100 and the mortality of the group is given as a ratio of this figure.

To compare the impact of mortality on different groups, the social class classification already discussed on p. 58 is used. The decennial supplement 'Occupational Mortality' published in 1978 gives full details of SMRs of different occupations for the years 1970–2 and is based upon the population distribution of the 1971 census. Table 30 shows the wide variation in the mortal-

TABLE 30 Standardized mortality ratio by cause and social class, England and Wales, 1970–2

	Social Class					
Cause of death	*I*	*II*	*IIIN*	*IIIM*	*IV*	*V*
All causes (men)	77	81	99	106	114	137
All causes (women)	82	87	92	115	119	135
Carcinoma of lung, trachea and bronchus (men)	53	68	84	118	123	143
Carcinoma of lung, trachea and bronchus (women)	73	82	89	118	125	134
Carcinoma of breast (women)	117	112	110	109	103	92
Ischaemic heart disease (men)	88	91	114	107	108	111
Ischaemic heart disease (women)	58	77	81	125	123	146
Suicide (women)	124	110	118	83	87	94
Pneumonia (men)	41	53	78	92	115	195
Carcinoma of cervix uteri	44	66	69	120	140	161

(from *Occupational Mortality*, 1970–2, OPCS)

ity between the social classes. It is interesting to note that social classes I and II enjoy a greatly reduced mortality compared with social class V. The disadvantage is marked in carcinoma of the lung (men) ($2\frac{3}{4}$ times the mortality in social class V compared with social class I) and pneumonia (men) ($4\frac{1}{2}$ times the mortality in social class V). The well known greater hazard in women of carcinoma of the cervix uteri is well illustrated (SMR 44 in social class I compared with 161 in social class V). But there are diseases where the opposite occurs, i.e. a higher mortality is observed in social classes I and II than in V. Carcinoma of the breast in women shows a steady increased incidence in the higher social classes. Suicide in married women is another example: SMR 124 in social class I and 87 and 94 in social classes IV and V.

Occupational mortality

If the mortality of members of different individual occupations is compared (rather than social class), it will be seen that quite wide variations occur. Table 31 lists the SMRs for men aged 15–64 by occupation for the year 1970–2. It will be seen that the

TABLE 31 Standardized Mortality Ratios (SMRs) for men aged 15–64 years, England and Wales, 1970–2

Occupation	*SMR*	*Occupation*	*SMR*
Teachers	70	Dock labourers	106
Postmen	72	Furnacemen	111
Porters (railway)	83	Police officers	113
Radiographers	86	Judges, barristers, solicitors	120
Agricultural workers	90	Coal miners (underground)	132
Electricians	92	Steelworkers (rolling mills)	137
Shop assistants	93	Nurses	138
Clergy	96	Pharmacists	147
Fire brigade officers and men	100	Fishermen	151
Painters and decorators	105	Stage managers, actors	154
Car assembly workers	105	Publicans, innkeepers	190
Medical practitioners	105	Bricklayers, labourers	240

(from *Occupational Mortality*, 1970–2, OPCS)

mortality in teachers (70) is almost half that of nurses (138). Even in the health services, there are wide variations: radiographers (86), medical practitioners (105), nurses (138) and pharmacists (147). These mortality rates do not only indicate particular hazards of different occupations, they are also influenced by the type of individual employed or who chooses such an occupation.

There are full details in the OPCS publication *Occupational Mortality* of the reasons why certain occupations show a high mortality rate. For instance, suicide is a high mortality risk of pharmacists, no doubt connected with the ease with which this profession can obtain lethal drugs. Publicans and innkeepers have very high rates from cirrhosis of the liver and also showed high death rates from cancer of the lung. Cirrhosis of the liver was also high in medical practitioners, as were suicide and accidents. It is interesting to note that cancer of the lung is now relatively rare in doctors, this no doubt being connected with the low number of cigarette-smokers in that profession.

Possible aetiological connections between diseases and occupations are further considered in Chapter 13.

Value of Vital Statistics

It is important to realize that vital statistics can make fascinating study. The way diseases occur unequally throughout different social classes and occupations emphasizes that there are many social aspects of disease and many of these are as yet imperfectly understood. No doctor in hospital or general practice need become an expert in vital statistics, but a simple knowledge and understanding of the potentials of statistics will make their work more interesting. There are many opportunities for morbidity studies related to occupation and social class which could yield much useful research in everyday hospital and general practice.

4 Maternity Services

In 1977, 568 000 births occurred in England and Wales and the care of the mother is an important part of the preventive and curative health services. Pregnancy is a physiological process and this has helped to produce strong preventive features in all maternity services. The main emphasis in obstetrics is how to avoid and prevent abnormalities occurring, and how to recognize and diagnose them early, so that their effects can be minimized.

The maternity services are more closely coordinated than any other health service in the UK and this is essential for efficiency as the service is shared between hospitals and domiciliary services.

HOSPITAL CONFINEMENTS

In 1976 in *England and Wales 97·5% of mothers were delivered in hospital and 2·5% at home.*

It is now clear that the trend noticeable during the last 20 years for more and more mothers to be delivered in hospital is almost complete. There are still variations throughout the country but the following groups of mothers should always be delivered in hospital:

1. mothers with some abnormality (such as toxaemia of pregnancy or any malpresentation) or a 'small for dates' baby
2. mothers with three or more children. Perinatal mortality is high in this group (see p. 72) and the risks to the mother greater

3. mothers over the age of 35 years—the incidence of certain abnormalities of labour is higher in this group
4. all primigravida
5. mothers living in poor home conditions where a home delivery might be very difficult or dangerous

Recently it has been emphasized that *the 'small for dates' baby is at particular risk around the time of delivery* and all such cases should be delivered in a maternity hospital unit.

Ideally each mother should spend 7–10 days in hospital after delivery. Earlier discharge has become more popular during the last 15 years but there is now a tendency for less very early discharges (under five days) to occur; this may well be due to less pressure on maternity beds due to the falling birth rate. In England in 1977, 57% of women delivered in hospital, returned home six days or less after confinement (64% in 1972). The mean postnatal stay in hospital of all women delivered then was 5·9 days (England and Wales).

Many social and domiciliary care problems can be created by very early discharge for no mother is fit to look after her home so early in the puerperium and must have special help. Arrangements must be made for the domiciliary midwife to call and see all women discharged home early to continue the postnatal care of the mother and child. Towards the end of the puerperium, the midwife should ideally meet the health visitor in the home (see p. 115).

MATERNITY SERVICES

The Midwives' Acts prohibit, except in a sudden emergency, any unqualified person who is not either a doctor or midwife (or students in training) from attending any woman in childbirth except under the personal direction of a doctor or midwife.

The Central Midwives Board maintains a strict control over all the midwifery services. Their rules are supervised locally by officers of AHAs and include:

1. supervision over all certified midwives practising in the area. This includes midwives in maternity hospitals as well as those in nursing homes or employed as domiciliary midwives. In practice, the detailed supervision of midwives in

hospitals is left to their senior staff, but the DNO and her staff supervise carefully midwives in nursing homes and in domiciliary practice. No midwife may practice until she has given her notice to do so to the AHA

2. power to suspend a midwife from practice if it is necessary to do so. This may have to be done to reduce the likelihood of the spread of infection if the midwife is found to be a nasal carrier of pathogenic streptococci

The Central Midwives Board lays down a code of practice and rules for all midwives. These specify the records she must keep, the standards she must follow in her midwifery practice, the drugs and the anaesthetics she can use, as well as defining the medical emergencies in which she has a duty to call in medical aid. The Central Midwives Board also insists that every practising midwife shall attend a refresher course once every five years.

Role of General Medical Practitioner and Midwife in Domiciliary Midwifery

In the few cases where the mother is delivered at home, there are three possibilities open to her:

1. in a minority of cases, her own general practitioner carries out the antenatal care, delivers the patient and the midwife acts as a maternity nurse. Postnatal care also is undertaken by the general practitioner.
2. in most cases, the general practitioner does the antenatal care but the midwife delivers the patient calling him only in case of need. The midwife reports delivery to the general practitioner who then completes the postnatal care.
3. the patient may choose to be delivered solely by a midwife who, in this instance, accepts full responsibility for looking after the patient in the antenatal period and in her confinement

General practitioners who have had special experience in midwifery and who undertake regular domiciliary midwifery are placed on the 'obstetric list'.

Midwives to carry out both hospital and community services are provided by every AHA through its district services and are supervised by the DNO. At present there are very few private midwives practising.

A midwife employed in domiciliary practice is usually provided with a house or flat in her district from which to practise and it is usual for a midwife to have a car for her use. This is important as often she has to reach her patients quickly at any hour of the day or night, and to carry heavy mobile gas and oxygen or Trilene analgesia equipment.

Maternity outfits, which include all the necessary sterile dressings for the confinement and puerperium, are supplied free to each mother. It therefore should not be necessary for the general practitioner to have to supply extra dressings for the confinement.

Every midwife is trained in giving Trilene and gas and oxygen analgesia. The patient's own doctor must examine her to certify that she is fit for analgesia. Modern analgesia apparatus is very reliable and is designed for the anaesthetic to be given either by the midwife or doctor attending, or in the first stage of labour by the patient herself. Tuition by the midwife is always given in the self-administration of analgesia. The patient lies on her side, presses the mask to her face, releasing a pressure valve, and breathes the anaesthetic; as she loses consciousness, her grip relaxes, the mask falls away, shutting off the valve and anaesthetic, and she regains consciousness to repeat the cycle when necessary.

ANTENATAL CARE

The prevention of many of the complications of pregnancy rests with careful antenatal care. It is the responsibility of the general practitioner and/or midwife to ensure that adequate antenatal care is carried out on all women being delivered in domiciliary practice.

A mother who is to be delivered in hospital usually receives her antenatal care from that hospital. Occasionally, where this is difficult, arrangement may be made for her to attend her own doctor for this care. The pressure on most hospital antenatal clinics is so great that it is not possible to carry out health education or mothercraft clinics in the hospital. Usually the mother attends a special health education mothercraft clinic.

First Antenatal Examination

The first antenatal examination is most important and usually takes place at the time of confirmation of the pregnancy, at about the third month of pregnancy. A complete *general medical examination* is undertaken to check that the woman has no undetected illness. At this time, a complete record should be obtained of the past medical history with particular attention paid to any past history of tuberculosis, diabetes, heart disease and any virus infections from which the patient may have suffered. The chest may be X-rayed either by mass miniature radiography if available or by using large films at a hospital radiography unit.

Next, a complete *obstetric history* is taken of any previous pregnancies. Special note is made of any difficulties or abnormalities which may have occurred either in the mother's or baby's health. In addition, blood samples are collected and tests should always include:

1. A *Wassermann* or *Kahn* test to make certain that the mother has no hidden infection of syphilis. This test is of the greatest importance, for if the woman has latent syphilis a possible congenital syphilitic infection in the infant can be prevented if treatment is immediately started at the third month of pregnancy.
2. *Haemogloblin* estimation. If this is below normal, immediate treatment is started. Haemorrhage may occur later unexpectedly and anaemic women are more prone to bleed. Obviously haemorrhage will be more serious in cases where the haemogloblin level is lower than normal.
3. *Blood group* is estimated and recorded. In any subsequent emergency, such information will be invaluable to enable a blood transfusion to be given quickly.
4. *Rhesus factor* estimation is carried out. If the mother is Rhesus positive then no problems will arise. If, however, the mother is Rhesus negative, difficulties may occur later affecting the health of the child. If the father is also Rhesus negative then all will be well. If, however, the father is Rhesus positive, which is more likely, problems may occur shortly after the birth of the child especially in a second and subsequent pregnancy. *In all such cases, the expectant*

mother should be immunized with anti-D immunoglobulin (see below)

In first pregnancies *a further blood examination* must be undertaken at the thirty-fourth week of pregnancy to check whether antibodies are present in the mother's blood. If these are present, it is likely that the baby will develop serious haemolytic jaundice after birth and may need an exchange transfusion. In such a case, the delivery must be undertaken in hospital and the neighbouring paediatric unit alerted before birth. As a further precaution, even if antibodies are absent at the thirty-fourth week, cord blood from the baby should be collected at birth and tested for antibodies.

Prevention of Rhesus incompatibility by immunization

It is now possible to prevent many of the problems of Rhesus incompatibility by immunization with anti-D immunoglobulin of Rhesus negative women immediately after their first confinement or miscarriage. The problem in Rhesus incompatibility is due to red blood cells from a Rhesus positive child crossing the placental barrier and entering the mother's blood stream. Shortly after the birth of the first child, the Rhesus negative mother manufactures antibodies against these Rhesus positive red blood cells of her child which, in this way, are then destroyed. In second and subsequent pregnancies, these antibodies increase and, when they recross the placental barrier and enter the baby's blood stream, they lead to massive destruction of the baby's blood cells usually after birth, but in serious instances, before birth which may lead to a stillbirth.

Immunization with anti-D immunoglobulin should be given *immediately following the first delivery* of a child or after a *first miscarriage or abortion.* An anti-D immunoglobulin then destroys the Rhesus positive red blood cells of the baby within the mother's blood stream and there is not time enough for the mother to develop antibodies. Therefore a consequent pregnancy will be like a first pregnancy and no problems will arise. It is, however, necessary in such cases to *reimmunize the mother after all subsequent pregnancies or miscarriages to prevent antibody formation.*

Recommendations in regard to treatment are as follows:

1. In all cases the anti-D immunoglobulin should be given within 60 hours of delivery or termination of pregnancy (miscarriage or abortion)
2. All Rhesus negative women giving birth to a Rhesus positive baby after the 20th week should be screened for fetal cells so that women who have large transplacental haemorrhages can be given large doses of anti-D immunoglobulin
3. The usual dose of anti-D immunoglobulin for all Rhesus negative women having had Rhesus positive babies regardless of parity or ABO group, should initially be 100 mg. Further doses may be necessary for cases in which large transplacental haemorrhages have occurred
4. A standard dose of 50 mg should be provided for all women known to be Rhesus negative, having therapeutic abortions up to and including the twentieth week of pregnancy, except for those who are sterilized at the same operation. Rhesus negative women whose pregnancy with a Rhesus positive fetus is terminated after the twentieth week, should receive a dose of 100 mg
5. The decision to use anti-D immunoglobulin for Rhesus negative women having spontaneous abortions should be left to the individual clinician

Health education

The first antenatal examination should be completed by giving general health education advice on diet and general management of the pregnancy.

Recent research has emphasized that there is a greater risk to the baby of a mother who smokes during pregnancy. The Health Education Council recently ran a campaign against smoking in pregnancy pointing out that over 1500 babies annually might not have died if their mothers had given up smoking when they had become pregnant.

Prescription charges are waived to expectant mothers and until their babies are one year old. A Family Practitioner Committee Exemption certificate is needed which can be obtained by filling in Form FW8 available from the doctor, midwife or health visitor.

Diet in Pregnancy

A well-balanced diet with a good proportion of high class protein is required. Many mothers have strange ideas about diet in pregnancy and a simple explanation is needed to ensure that the essential ingredients are fully understood. At least a pint of milk should be drunk per day and foodstuffs rich in iron, calcium, phosphorus and vitamins should be eaten. Vitamin preparations either in the form of tablets or orange juice or cod-liver oil may be obtained from the local maternity and child health clinic, or alternatively these may be taken in the diet as fresh fruit and various fats. Good well-balanced meals will reduce the likelihood of unexplained prematurity and pre-eclamptic toxaemia.

Free milk

An expectant mother with two or more children under school age is entitled to free milk, regardless of her family income. The claim should be made on Form FW8 for seven pints of liquid milk or one pack of dried milk per week.

Free milk is also available to expectant mothers and all children under school age where the family income is below a certain level and to all handicapped children aged 5–16 who are not registered at school and to children attending a registered day nursery.

Continued Antenatal Care

Further antenatal examinations are regularly and frequently carried out during pregnancy—once a month until the twenty-eighth week and then more frequently, until the patient is being seen at least every week from the thirty-fourth to fortieth weeks. An abdominal examination is made to check the level of the uterus and, later, the position of the child. During the later weeks of pregnancy, particularly in primipara, the early engagement of the head in the pelvis is checked.

At each visit the blood pressure is examined—the warning signs of toxaemia are a rise above the level of 130 to 140/90. The urine is tested for albumen and the legs palpated for oedema. A careful record is kept of the weight gain during pregnancy, especially between the twentieth and thirtieth weeks. If the weight gain exceeds 3·3 kg (7 lb) during this period, especially in young primipara, this should be regarded as a possible early sign of toxaemia of pregnancy. Such patients should be treated accordingly with rest and observed very carefully. If there are any other signs of impending toxaemia (raised blood pressure, albuminuria or oedema) immediate bed rest and treatment should be started.

Value of antenatal care in the prevention of serious abnormalities of pregnancy

The prevention of serious abnormalities of pregnancy is closely linked with good careful antenatal care. Any abnormal symptom or sign must be completely investigated as it may be an early indication of a more serious condition. A loss of blood per vaginam, even though slight, may indicate such a potentially serious condition as placenta praevia. In the primipara, when the baby's head fails to engage the mother's pelvis, this is usually indicative of an abnormality such as a malpresentation—persistent occipitoposterior or an unusually small pelvis. An immediate full investigation prevents serious complications later.

Towards the end of the pregnancy, it becomes even more important that antenatal examinations take place regularly. If the patient defaults from attending any antenatal visit, it is essential that the doctor or midwife calls on the patient to discover the reason. In many instances, the reason may only be slackness on the part of the patient, but it could be that she has developed some symptom which she does not recognize as serious, but which gives her an excuse to postpone her visit. Many serious cases of toxaemia and eclampsia have been prevented by a midwife or doctor following up a non-attender in this way.

Dental care in pregnancy

Dental care in pregnancy is always very important as any mother's teeth can deteriorate rapidly. Each mother should visit the dentist early in pregnancy for a complete check-up and treatment. All pregnant and nursing women (up to one year after confinement) are entitled to free treatment including, if need be, the provision of dentures, and health authority dental staff provide this treatment at clinics.

Preventive aspects of maternal mortality

At present in the UK, approximately one mother in 7700 loses her life as a result of child bearing. A consultant obstetrician and community physician should investigate fully every maternal death to find the cause. The most recent series of such investigations called *Report on Confidential Enquiries into Maternal Deaths in England and Wales* covered the period 1970–2 and was published by the DHSS. It showed that 53·8% of all maternal deaths were avoidable and would have been prevented if some mistake or omission had not occurred (if abortion and ectopic pregnancy are excluded the figures fall to 33·8%).

The types of 'preventable factors' varied from mistakes and omissions on the part of doctors and midwives to lack of cooperation from the patient herself.

Table 32 gives the main causes of maternal deaths.

TABLE 32 Causes of maternal death, England and Wales, 1970–2* (rates per 100 000 maternities)

Abortion	81	(115)
Pulmonary embolism	61	(75)
Toxaemia	47	(51)
Miscellaneous	39	(30)
Anaesthetic deaths	37	(34)
Ectopic pregnancy	34	(31)
Sepsis (excluding abortion)	32	(33)
Haemorrhage	27	(41)
Amniotic fluid embolism	22	(27)

NB Mean maternal mortality rate for years 1970–2 was 0·129 per 1000 births.
* The 1967–9 rates are in parentheses.

Compared with the 1967–9 investigation, there has been a fall in all causes except sepsis and ectopic pregnancy. The most significant reductions have been in abortion, pulmonary embolism and haemorrhage. Toxaemia of pregnancy still accounts for a rate of 47 deaths per 100 000 maternities and ectopic for 34. Inadequate antenatal care is often an important factor in toxaemia of pregnancy. In particular, it is most important to carry out an immediate follow-up by home visiting of all defaulters from antenatal clinics particularly if they are known to have signs of toxaemia. Every pregnant woman should carry on her person a 'cooperation card' (see below) which describes essential information and which may be a life-saving measure if she collapses away from home.

In the early antenatal programme of any mother, *the possible danger of an ectopic pregnancy must be borne in mind.* Half these deaths occurred at home or in the ambulance during transfer to hospital. A further 22% died in hospital awaiting operation. *Immediate operation is most important* and should be carried out as soon as possible after the diagnosis has been made. Resuscitation should *not* precede the operation, but be coincidental to it.

Cooperation card

Although the majority of women are now delivered in hospital, cooperation is of the greatest importance especially in an emergency and every woman wherever she is booked to have her delivery, in hospital or at home, should always carry a special cooperation card with her. This is a simple record of her antenatal care and contains the results of all the tests carried out including her blood group. In an emergency when a pregnant woman is unexpectedly admitted to hospital, her cooperation card is of great value in arranging prompt treatment.

Management of Labour in Domiciliary Practice

Although only 2·5% of births now occur at home, the following account is still given in detail as all home deliveries may present special hazards for the mother and child.

Whether or not the patient has booked a doctor, usually the midwife is notified when labour starts. She then visits and examines the mother, and, if she confirms that labour has started, arranges for her care. In booked cases, the doctor is notified at this stage, but as most doctors have to carry on their busy practices, it is usual for the midwife to continue to look after the mother, only calling the doctor if some difficulty arises. The midwife brings to the home all the equipment for the labour including analgesic apparatus. As explained earlier, the mother can give herself a whiff of anaesthetic using either gas (nitrous oxide) and oxygen or Trilene. Of the two forms, Trilene is more popular for domiciliary practice today. It has the following advantages: (*a*) a longer period of analgesia is obtained; (*b*) there is less danger to the child from anoxia. (This risk can be reduced by using gas/oxygen rather than gas/air, but this adds considerably to the weight of the equipment.) (*c*) The apparatus is very light when Trilene is used.

A high degree of surgical cleanliness is maintained in domiciliary midwifery by using sterile gowns, gloves, masks, caps and sheets. Increasing use is being made of disposable sterile materials including disposable towels, masks, caps and syringes. Any gown used remains at the patient's home to reduce the risk of carrying infection from patient to patient.

Dependent upon the progress of labour and condition of the patient, midwives may leave the patient for a short time during the first stage of labour. They are allowed pethidine or more commonly pethilorfan which has a less depressant effect upon the child but as labour often progresses rapidly after giving such drugs, no midwife leaves a patient after administering pethilorfan until the patient is delivered.

If, during the delivery, the midwife meets with any abnormality she must send immediately for medical aid whilst staying herself to continue the delivery. Medical aid is provided by the patient's doctor in most cases, but, if no doctor has been booked, the midwife sends for a nearby practitioner who is on the obstetric list. For very urgent and serious problems, the midwife may send directly for the special mobile hospital team, the obstetric 'flying squad'. In some areas, midwives have been issued with light mobile wireless transmitters so that they can summon help in an emergency without having to leave the patient.

Use of the obstetric 'flying squad'

Each maternity hospital provides a mobile team ('flying squad') consisting of an experienced obstetrician (consultant or senior registrar) plus an experienced hospital midwife, who will go to the home of a patient to deal with any emergency in labour or to any general practitioner maternity unit. In a recent survey, it was found that the 'flying squad' was called out to one in 70 domiciliary deliveries. The commonest cause was retained placenta (half the cases) and haemorrhage (a third of the cases) as well as other complications of labour—such as an unexpected breech presentation. It is usual for the 'flying squad' to be taken to the patient's home by ambulance which, after the patient has been resuscitated, can transfer her to hospital. In cases of haemorrhage it is very important to resuscitate the mother with a blood transfusion set up in her home before her removal to hospital. A midwife and doctor should always accompany such a patient so that oxytocic drugs can be given during the journey.

Care of the mother and child during the puerperium

The midwife has full responsibility for the domiciliary care of the newly delivered mother and child during the puerperium. Midwives must visit for a minimum of 10 days and a maximum of 28 days and usually also visit in the evenings for the first three days. Records of pulse and temperature are maintained. If a temperature of 38°C (100·4°F) occurs or a reading of at least 37·5°C (99·4°F) on two successive days, medical aid must be sent for.

Blood for the Guthrie test (to discover phenylketonuria) is collected by the midwife from the baby on the fourth day (see p. 113).

Breast feeding should be started whenever possible and much patience, encouragement and care will be needed to do this. In the puerperium the midwife helps the mother with all aspects of mothercraft which she has learnt in her health education classes—how to bathe the baby and generally care for the new-born child.

POSTNATAL CARE

A careful examination of every mother delivered in hospital should always be undertaken before her discharge home. In addition six weeks after delivery a full postnatal examination should be carried out either at the hospital where the baby was born or at the doctor's surgery or at the clinic. By this time the health visitor should be acting as one of the most important advisors to the mother.

Family Planning and Abortion

Family planning advice should always be available to all women as part of their postnatal care. Full details are given later (see p. 168). Expectant mothers should also be able to receive pregnancy advice services early in pregnancy if they are considering an abortion. The whole object of the Abortion Acts was to reduce the high risks to mothers who had decided to have an abortion by making legal abortion in certain circumstances (see p. 271). All those working with expectant mothers must realize that this *preventive aspect* is of great importance and should give unbiased advice or refer to an official pregnancy advice centre women who seek such help.

THE CARE OF THE UNMARRIED MOTHER

The care of the unmarried mother in pregnancy is a special problem. In 1976 in England and Wales 9·1% of all births occurred in mothers who were unmarried (53 800 births). This proportion is rising (it was 5% in 1960). Illegitimacy produces many difficulties and, from the preventive health point of view, the most serious problem is that the disturbed social circumstances surrounding an unmarried mother produce greater hazards for both mother and child. This is shown by a higher infant mortality rate (IMR) in illegitimate births (see Table 11). The reasons are mainly connected with the fact that antenatal care may not have been carried out because of concealment of the pregnancy or because the mother was forced to leave her home due to the unsympathetic reaction of her parents.

Many social service departments and voluntary bodies make special provision to assist the unmarried mother. Often many cases drift towards the large cities and special arrangements are made there. Wherever possible, the unmarried mother is given help to stay at home, going to hospital for the delivery. If conflict, so often created between the mother-to-be and her parents, can be avoided, problems tend to be reduced.

In some cases, however, the unmarried mother cannot or does not wish to remain at home. In such instances, the best solution is for her to be helped by a social services department who can usually arrange a suitable hostel or similar unit, many of which are run by voluntary or church organizations. After the birth of her child in hospital many unmarried mothers need time to decide whether they wish to care for the child or arrange adoption.

Sheltered Housing for Unmarried Mothers

An increasing number now care for their children and are accommodated in special 'sheltered housing' flats or flatlets run by voluntary bodies and housing associations. Later permanent housing is usually arranged and the unmarried mother can leave her child in the care of a day nursery run by a social service department while she undertakes a full time job (see p. 413).

5 Child Health Services

More has been done during the past 75 years to develop effective medical services for young children than for any other group in the community. Yet there are still many hazards and problems facing the infant and these are unequal in their effects throughout different regions of the country and different social classes.

In December, 1976, an exhaustive review of the child health services in the UK by a Committee set up by the DHSS under the chairmanship of Professor S. D. M. Court, was published (*Fit for the Future*, Comm. 6684). Reference is made at the end of this chapter to its main recommendations and the governments reaction to them, but many of the facts discussed in that report have been emphasized throughout this chapter.

The surveillance (or 'watching over') of the health of all children can only be successfully carried out by the team work of many professionals helped by the parents. All working in the primary health care team play an essential part—general practitioners, health visitors, midwives and district nurses—but a wide range of experts from the paediatric hospital services will be involved in special cases. In addition, in all instances where there is a health or social handicap, those in the educational and social service fields will be concerned from an early age.

Yet, the key community worker in the preventive child health services is the *health visitor* attached to a health centre or large group practice. She works very closely with general practitioners and paediatricians. Her detailed role is discussed later (see p. 115).

Notification of births

All births must be notified within 36 hours to the Area Medical Officer. This is to make absolutely certain that the health visitor and midwife know of every birth.

CARE IN THE NEONATAL PERIOD

The first month of any child's life (and especially the first week) is one of the most critical. Reference has already been made (p. 70) to the neonatal and perinatal mortality rates but Table 33

TABLE 33 Deaths at different ages in childhood and adolescence, England and Wales, 1974

Stillbirths (*a*)	7175
First week (*b*)	5994
Perinatal (*a* + *b*)	13 169
1 week to 1 year (*d*)	4465
First year (*b* + *d*)	10 459
Years 1–4	1922
Years 5–9	1225
Years 10–14	1091
Years 15–19	2212

(from *Fit for the Future*, 1976, Comm. 6684)

emphasizes even better the critical nature of the hazards of pregnancy, birth and first week of any child's life. It will clearly be seen that first year deaths (10 459) easily exceed all those in the next 19 years and first week deaths exceed deaths for one week to one year. The main reasons for these deaths are failure of fetal growth, complications during delivery (especially insufficient oxygen reaching the brain), severe malformations and the immaturity or malnutrition of babies of low birth weight.

The vast majority of babies (97·5%) are now born in hospital, but many of those will be home within a few days (see p. 92). Therefore the care of the child in the neonatal period occurs both in hospital and in the community and both must work closely together.

Every newborn infant should be fully examined between the ages of 6 and 10 days before he leaves hospital by a paediatrician or doctor trained in neonatal paediatrics. This examination should form the first stage of a continual process of health care surveillance of the child. Ideally the parents should be present at this examination and certainly the doctor should always communicate his findings in person to the mother (or other adult responsible). Where any abnormality is found or where there is a social problem, the health visitor should be informed (either directly or through the hospital social worker).

In addition to feeding and general care difficulties, there are five special problems found in the neonatal period: (1) haemolytic disease of the newborn; (2) neonatal cold injury; (3) care of low weight (premature) babies; (4) congenital malformations; (5) screening tests to exclude phenylketonuria and congenital dislocation of the hip.

Haemolytic Disease of the Newborn

Reference has already been made to this disease and its prevention (see p. 96). As a further check a blood estimation of bilirubin should be done routinely on all infants before being discharged home from hospital. For those delivered at home the midwife carries a simple Perspex device (an icterometer) for estimating quickly the depth of jaundice in the newborn child and in cases of doubt will arrange a bilirubin blood test.

Neonatal Cold Injury

All newborn infants may suffer from neonatal cold injury, but the danger is greatest in low weight babies.

If any baby, in the first few weeks of life, becomes seriously chilled, its body temperature may fall dangerously low (to 32·2° (90°F) or lower). The infant then becomes quiet and difficult to rouse or feed. He may have a deceptively florid complexion but the skin surface is much colder than usual and later he becomes oedematous. This is a dangerous condition which can prove fatal.

Prevention depends on ensuring that the temperature of the room in which the baby is sleeping does not fall below 18°C (65°F). Most midwives carry a wall thermometer which is used to record the maximum and minimum temperatures of the room. This check is needed both in winter and in summer when unexpectedly low temperatures may occur at night.

Care of Low Birth Weight (Premature) Babies

Approximately 6·5% of all live births involve a baby of low birth weight, less than 2·5 kg. It is convenient to subdivide such infants into two groups: (1) those under 2·04 kg, who should always be admitted for a period into an intensive care unit, and (2) those whose weight is between 2·04 kg and 2·49 kg, who may need a short period in an intensive care unit (a day or so) but who mainly can be looked after in normal circumstances although some may require a special home care service.

Intensive care units for low birth weight babies (formerly called premature baby units)

About 1–2% of all live births require a period of prolonged care in an intensive care unit until their weight reaches that of the second group (i.e. exceeds 2·04 kg). Approximately 14–15% of other live births are admitted to such units for a short time after birth for observation and resuscitation. The Court Committee advocate that such units where possible should act as a regional centre and where at least 25 cots and preferably 40, would enable them to be expertly staffed and equipped. They also emphasize *how important adequate and special transport arrangements are to enable a very low birth weight baby safely to be transferred to such a unit.*

There are three special aspects in the case of low birth weight babies in intensive care units: (1) incubator care; (2) feeding; and (3) prevention of infection.

Incubator care

This is needed for the very small premature baby. The value of the incubator is that it allows easier control of the atmosphere in which the baby lives. There are three factors which must be carefully balanced: (*a*) The *temperature* of the incubator should be maintained so that the child's temperature is kept constant just below 36·6°C. (*b*) There should be a constancy in the *relative humidity* of the air (level of water vapour) within the incubator. It is best to maintain this at 60%. (*c*) The *supply of oxygen* must be controlled. As many tiny babies have difficulties in pulmonary ventilation, oxygen can be most helpful, but great care must be taken not to increase the level of oxygen too high, for if this happens there is a danger of damaging the retina of the newborn child and producing blindness (retrolental fibroplasia). The level of oxygen should always be the lowest which will give adequate relief to the child.

Feeding

Because of the effort of suckling, breast feeding is rarely possible for very tiny babies. But human breast milk should be used if available. Many large paediatric and maternity centres maintain human breast milk banks. Various forms of artificial feeding are used—usually graduated weaker feeds of dried milks. These are always given more frequently than normal, two or three hourly, and often by nasal catheter, allowing the measured feed to flow by gravity.

Prevention of infection

Infection represents the greatest hazard to all low birth weight babies. The development of a respiratory infection may be so sudden and dramatic that death can occur after a few hours; prevention of infection is one of the most important functions of any intensive care unit. No one should visit the unit unless his presence is essential and parents and other visitors are not allowed in. No staff should enter it suffering from an infection (cold or upper respiratory infection) and all staff must wear a sterile cap, mask and gown. Hand washing must, at all times, be scrupulously carried out. Great care is necessary to avoid carrying infection from one cot to another and very high nursing standards are essential. New admissions from home should be separated from those already being nursed. In some units, air sterilization is practised using ultraviolet light filters.

Domiciliary care of low birthweight babies

Many AHAs run a domiciliary premature baby service to care for the larger premature baby (from 2·04 to 2·49 kg) at home. Specially trained neonatal midwives or nurses undertake this care, and feeding equipment, cots and thermometers can be loaned. The nurse instructs the mother in all the special methods of care and feeding and follows this up with twice-daily visits to ensure that all is continuing properly. In this way, constant advisory help is made available to the mothers of premature babies at home and enables continued supervision of babies who have spent a period in an intensive care unit when they are eventually discharged home. These nurses must do no other type of work and must be careful to avoid introducing infection into the home. Visitors should be as carefully controlled as in hospital intensive care baby units. In practice, the risk of infection within the home is less than in hospital.

Congenital Malformations

About 1 in 50 babies is born with a congenital abnormality. These vary from serious defects such as myelomeningocele (spina bifida), intestinal obstruction or some kind of congenital heart disease to foot defects and cleft lips. In the worst, immediate specialized hospital care is essential but in others a plan of future action needs to be discussed. In all instances, there should be sympathetic and full communication with both parents and a full explanation given. It is also helpful if the health visitor can be involved at an early stage so that the mother may know to whom she can turn for day-to-day advice.

In all cases of the birth of a child with an inherited abnormality whether of an anatomical type (spina bifida, cleft palate) or of a metabolic origin (phenylketonuria) the parents should be offered *genetic counselling*.

In all cases where a permanent disability is likely, the *district handicap team* (see p. 124) should be involved at any early stage and the parents clearly made aware of the wide range of professionals and services ready to help.

Morbidity of congenital malformations

The demonstration that prenatal infections such as rubella, and drugs such as thalidomide, have caused congenital abnormalities makes it essential that some continuous observation is maintained throughout the country on the level of congenital malformations. A scheme of voluntary notification of all abnormalities observable at birth (or found within seven days after birth) was introduced in the United Kingdom in 1964. The doctor or midwife who completes the notification of birth form states on it whether any abnormality was apparent at birth. The Area Medical Officer then finds out from the general practitioner and hospital concerned the precise diagnosis and the completed form is then sent at the end of the month following that in which the birth occurs to the Office of Population Census and Surveys which maintains a national register. Note that this scheme is designed to detect *changes in frequency of reporting* rather than to estimate the absolute incidence of malformation.

In 1974, 12 730 babies in England and Wales were notified with one or more congenital malformations. Approximately 83·5% of children had one, 12·5% two, 3% three and 1% four or more malformations. The age and parity of the mother are also factors in determining the levels of incidence; the lowest rates are in the younger mothers having their second child while the highest rates in mothers over 40 having their fourth child.

Talipes is the commonest malformation followed by spina bifida or hydrocephalus, anencephaly, cleft lip or palate, congenital dislocation of the hip and Down's syndrome. More abnormalities occur in boys than girls, on a 5:4 basis, but this is mainly due to external genital abnormalities.

The incidence of abnormalities grouped on an anatomical basis is given in Table 34.

TABLE 34 Congenital malformation by anatomical site, England and Wales, 1974

Site	*Live birth malformations (rate per 10 000 live births)*		*All babies' malformations (rate per 10 000 live and stillbirths)*
	Male	*Female*	
Limbs	60·4	62·3	67·0
Central nervous system	13·3	16·8	37·9
External genitalia	28·8	1·6	16·3
Cleft lip/cleft palate	15·0	11·2	15·1
Cardiovascular system	7·8	7·7	10·1
Chromosomes	5·8	6·5	7·3
Intestines	5·6	4·0	6·5
Ear	4·6	4·4	5·2
Eye	1·1	1·5	1·7
Total	175·2	146·3	196·7

(from *Fit for the Future*, 1976, Comm. 6684–1)

Screening Tests to Exclude Phenylketonuria and Congenital Dislocation of the Hip

Two important screening tests should be carried out during the first few weeks of a child's life to ensure that neither of the following is present: (*a*) phenylketonuria, (*b*) congenital dislocation of the hip.

Phenylketonuria is a rare inherited metabolic disease in which faulty metabolism results in poisonous phenylalanine metabolites being produced which lead, after a few months, to markedly retarded mental development and severe mental handicap. Only if the disease can be diagnosed within a few weeks of birth and the child given a special diet can mental deterioration be avoided.

To ensure that every case of phenylketonuria is discovered early enough, a Guthrie test is carried out on a specimen of blood taken from the baby between the sixth and the fourteenth day of life. Several spots of blood from the young infant are collected from a heel prick on to specially absorbent filter paper. In the laboratory a small disc is punched out of each of the blood impregnated filter papers and up to one hundred individual discs are placed on a special agar plate containing a spore suspension of *Bacillus subtilis* and an inhibitory substance. Phenylalanine acts as an antagonist to the inhibitor and, after incubation, growth of the organism will be observed around blood discs which contain phenylalanine. The Guthrie test is the best available but some authorities still use the Phenistix test or the Scriver test.

Congenital dislocation of the hip is a condition which, if diagnosed very early, can often be effectively treated. If, however, diagnosis is delayed, it is much more difficult to correct and may lead to permanent disability. It is now known that the main cause of this condition is inadequate development of the acetabulum of the pelvis. There is a simple test (eliciting Ortolani's or von Rosen's sign) which the midwife or health visitor should carry out on all babies at 6–14 days after birth and at monthly intervals until the child is four months old. This test consists of manipulating the hip of the child from the adducted to the abducted position while the thigh is flexed. A positive or abnormal result is indicated by a 'click' or 'snap' being produced during the test and corresponds with the dislocated femoral head moving into the proper position in the acetabulum.

Whenever this test is abnormal, the child should be immediately referred to an orthopaedic surgeon. Treatment is simple and consists of maintaining the hips continuously in abduction by application of a plaster spica or special splint. This produces constant pressure by the head of the femur in the centre of the acetabulum and causes it to deepen and develop normally. After six to nine months of such treatment the danger of permanent congenital dislocation of the hip has passed. Diagnosis within a week or two of birth means that treatment can be completed before the infant would normally have reached the stage of standing.

Health Surveillance in Children

All children, whether normal or presenting any signs of illness and congenital malformations, should have their health carefully watched over (surveillance). For the first four to five years, this is carried out by the community health services but, when the child goes to school, the school medical service usually takes over much of this role (see Chapter 6). There are four main features in this surveillance:

1. oversight of the health, physical growth and developmental progress of the child
2. providing health educational advice and support to parents including training in parenthood
3. linking these preventive health services with treatment sought for illnesses or accidents
4. prevention of infectious diseases by immunizations

All these functions overlap but the first three will be discussed as a group now while immunization is described in Chapter 10 (see p. 182).

The primary health care team should be mainly responsible for this health surveillance but can only undertake this function properly when a health visitor is an integral part of that team. In practice, the health visitor is largely responsible for (1) and (2) above and the general practitioner, paediatrician and health visitor for (3).

Role of health visitor

During the puerperium the midwife is responsible for the care of the newborn infant. At the end of this period the health visitor becomes the main health education adviser and is responsible for helping and instructing the mother in all aspects connected with the upbringing of the child—infant feeding, prevention of accidents, immunization, etc. The general practitioner is usually only consulted in the case of illness, but the health visitor should help in all normal and abnormal cases, maintaining the closest liaison at all times with the general practitioner. The health visitor should always meet the mother during pregnancy at the mothercraft classes and, at the end of the puerperium, takes over from the midwife. This is best carried out by a meeting at the mother's home on the fourteenth day after delivery.

The first important factor upon which the health visitor concentrates is the *feeding of the child*. Wherever possible, breast feeding is recommended and much patience and perseverance are needed to establish it. Usually not more than 25% of mothers are breast feeding their child at the age of four months. Encouragement is often required to allay the fears of mothers that their breast fed babies are not getting enough milk. The increased tendency for mothers to return to work after two months and the ease and convenience of artificial feeding have tended to increase bottle feeding. There is, however, plenty of evidence to show that breast feeding gives a child the best possible start in life and the incidence of all types of infection is lower. In outbreaks of infantile gastroenteritis, which can be a dangerous disease in infants, the breast fed child almost invariably escapes. There is also evidence that the personal bond between mother and the breast-fed child is very close. From the mother's point of view, as mentioned on p. 245, the incidence of carcinoma of the breast is lowest in women who have breast fed their children.

When, for some reason, breast feeding cannot be established the health visitor advises the mother on artificial feeding. Dried and evaporated milks are used, being reconstituted just before the baby's feed.

One of the most valuable aspects of a health visitor's work is that she visits the home regularly where she can give practical health education advice about frequency of feeding, clothing, the temperature of the baby's room and general hygiene. She can make certain that the mother fully understands all the intricacies attached to caring for a small baby.

The health visitor usually works from a health centre or group practice, but may visit a child health clinic set up separately. After her initial home visits, she endeavours to persuade the mother to bring the baby to the appropriate clinic (at approximately six weeks) where the range of child health services can be increased. The majority of mothers attend regularly especially during the first year of the baby's life. The fact that the mother comes to a child health centre does not mean that the health visitor ceases to visit the home although the frequency of visiting may be reduced.

CHILD HEALTH CLINIC

Many general practitioners are now running their own child health clinics in health centres or large group practices. One great advantage of such an arrangement is that the healthy child can see a doctor without mixing with other ill persons, some of whom may have upper respiratory infections. Other mothers attend separate child health clinics run by health visitors at which either general practitioners or clinical medical officers attend on a sessional basis. The services provided include:

Education in Mothercraft

Individual tuition is given by health visitors to mothers or by group tuition with the help of leaflets, posters, lectures and films. Every possible health education topic is discussed including nutrition of children, prevention of accidents in the home, etc.

Sale of Infant Foods

These include: suitable dried milks (full cream and half cream); National cod-liver oil; concentrated orange juice; vitamin A and D tablets; proprietary dried milks (usually sold in specially cheap clinic packs); certain other baby foods.

Routine Health Surveillance

The main function of any child health clinic is to arrange routine health surveillance on a team basis. Each child and mother are always seen by their health visitor and the doctor at the clinic sees both when they first attend (usually when the child is about six weeks old), annually or when there may be a special problem. The purpose of these examinations is to check that the baby is perfectly fit and to discover any abnormalities as soon as possible. Treatment is not carried out at child health clinics and any defects discovered should be referred to the family doctor or through him to hospital for further investigation and treatment.

The function of a child health centre is essentially preventive and not curative. No ill child should ever be brought to a child health clinic because of the risk of spreading infection, but should be seen at the general practitioner's normal surgery. In cases of doubt, the health visitor will make a home visit to advise.

Health Education Advice

Advice is given by health visitors on minor problems as they arise and this is an extension of the work done on home visits. The majority of queries are on feeding problems and difficulties connected with the development of the child.

Immunization of Infants

This can either be undertaken by the general practitioner or, if there is a separate clinic, by the doctor attending. Such immunizations include protection against whooping cough, diphtheria, tetanus and poliomyelitis. Full details and schedules are given on p. 182.

NORMAL PROGRESS IN THE INFANT

Much of the preventive medical services for young children depend on recognizing the normal stages in a child's development. Considerable variation occurs and no reliance should ever be placed on too stereotyped tables of progress, but usually a baby will double his birth weight by five months and treble it by a year. Regular weighing is useful only to indicate generally a change in progress—a sudden loss of weight or a halt in the gain of weight calls for further investigation. Care must always be taken not to overstress the baby's weight, for it should never be a mother's main guide to progress. Some of the fittest babies are those who have been breast fed and these are usually lighter than average although very active and alert.

The healthy infant normally sits with support by the third or fourth month of life. By the eighth or ninth month he can usually stand with support and will probably stand without support between the tenth and fourteenth months, and walk soon after. Crawling and creeping often occur at about the ninth or tenth month but may not always be shown.

Weaning from either the breast or from bottled feeds usually commences between four and six months. With the many specially prepared foods available (including a wide range of tinned foods) weaning is simple. Once it has started, it is wise gradually to extend the range of foods used so that the child becomes accustomed to different tastes. Many weaning foods are sold at child health clinics and the health visitor is always available to advise which to use.

The *development of speech* is a very important stage. During the first two to three months of life, the child will make reflex noises—crying loudly if uncomfortable and gurgling if content. This stage is similar in both normal and deaf children. By the fourth month, the very first attempts at vocalization are made in the normal child and by seven to eight months, he babbles away loudly and tunefully and has a very definite ability to listen. It is at this stage of development that the deaf child's reflex vocalizations begin to diminish and, by the eighth month, he is making fewer and fewer attempts to produce sounds. Because of this change, the *health visitor should be careful to observe all children from seven to eight months of age.*

The normal child learns to speak by imitating what he hears and by $1\frac{1}{2}$ years of age he should be using simple words and sentences. A slow development of speech always calls for investigations to exclude: (*a*) deafness and (*b*) mental handicap.

Careful observation and investigation at frequent intervals usually defines the problem. It is important for the general practitioner to realize that the diagnosis of either condition may be extremely difficult in the very young child. If deafness is suspected, an immediate audiometric test should be carried out at the local specialist unit. Special equipment and sound-proof rooms are essential to define the extent of the deafness. Mentally handicapped children show delay in all stages of development—sitting, standing, walking—as well as a retarded development of speech.

Sphincter control of the bladder of the baby is slow to develop and may not be completely reliable until the child is $2\frac{1}{2}$ to 3 years old. It is important that the mother realizes this fact, for futile attempts to train the baby too early will only cause irritation and tensions, and may produce enuresis later. The health visitor should discuss these problems with the mother.

The general behaviour is an important guide, as every infant should be a happy active child constantly exploring his home in an inquisitive way. It is most important that he should feel secure in his home.

Children in Special Need

All children should have routine health surveillance by the health visitor and primary health care team but there is a need in some infants for more intensive oversight of their health and for monitoring their development progress with special care. Such children represent about 15–20% of all births in whom either the prenatal, family, perinatal or postnatal history are in some way abnormal. The group will also include families known to be living in poor social conditions (problem families). The selection of such a group to receive special care should be flexible but will certainly include those with a history of low birth weight, any congenital malformations, history of rubella in the mother, hyperemesis or toxaemia of pregnancy, difficulties in the neonatal period—anoxia, convulsions—and those infants with any marked illness postnatally. The occurrence in other members of the family of hereditary disorder or markedly abnormal behaviour should also be warning signs.

Such children are known to be *at special risk and their health surveillance should be undertaken by the health visitor and primary health care team to a greater degree than usual.* For instance, extra medical routine examinations should be carried out (to exclude congenital malformations such as congenital heart disease which may only present signs and symptoms later). An extra *careful watch should be kept to exclude deafness*, to deal with special social problems at an early stage (such as non-accidental injury) and to help the mother overcome various small problems of feeding and care.

The concept of 'at risk' registers whereby health surveillance is only or mainly carried out on perhaps 10–15% of selected children is no longer accepted as it is now certain that regular health surveillance is essential for all children. But special additional care is needed for the group of children outlined above who are at special risk and it should always be left to the health visitor and primary health care team to include in this group children and their families for whom special concern is felt.

Particular Hazards of the Post Neonatal Period

Apart from the continual dangers from serious congenital malformations already being treated, there are two main hazards facing the infant in the neonatal period (one month to one year)—*respiratory diseases and cot deaths* (Fig. 10). In some cases, these conditions are connected because cot deaths are more likely to occur in social class V and where there is limited parental understanding and early symptoms are not recognized which results in the parents failing to use the available primary health care services properly.

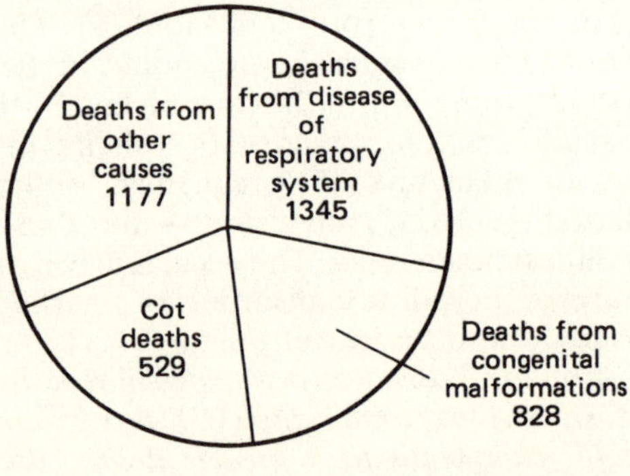

FIG 10. Post-neonatal (one month to one year) mortality, England and Wales, 1973. (From *Fit for the Future*, 1976, DHSS)

Cot deaths (sudden infant death)

The sudden infant death syndrome—often called 'cot death'—is a very distressing event, for such a death occurs very suddenly and unexpectedly. The aetiology of the condition is not fully known but it is now recognized that there is not one simple cause. In approximately one-third of all cases, a known disease capable of causing the death is present; in another third, minimal signs of disease are found which, although unlikely to cause the death, may contribute to it. In the remaining instances, although recognized disease is absent, there is evidence of disturbed growth. *Sudden death in a completely well infant or in one which is being breast fed is very rare.*

Many cases occur in infants in social class IV and V or in families with special social problems. More occur in 'inner city' or disadvantaged areas and the reduction of such deaths may be more connected with better health visiting and more effective primary health care to such deprived areas. Prevention, in the present stage of knowledge, is inexact but studies in Sheffield suggest that it may be possible to identify families whose children may be at potential risk. Such families need more concentrated antenatal and postnatal care and health education and support from health visitors and services in such areas should be structured to enable this to occur.

Non-accidental Injury (Child Abuse)

This important subject is dealt with in detail in Chapter 23 (p. 433).

Health Visiting and the Prevention of Disease in Infants Aged One to Five Years

As the child grows older, the health visitor continues to advise and help the mother. Apart from general health education, specially important aspects include:

Immunization schedules. These are checked and everything is done to encourage completion of all immunizations and their booster doses. This is most important.

Any serious illness should be carefully followed up by the health visitor. In families, children may develop at an early age the common childhood infectious diseases such as measles, scarlet fever and whooping cough. With modern treatment the majority of such infections are of a minor nature, but occasionally such illnesses become the starting-point for various chronic inflammatory conditions—tonsilitis, bronchitis, sinusitis and otitis media. The health visitor, in her follow-up, checks on the child and if need be, arranges for the general practitioner to examine the infant. She examines the child to make certain that no squints have developed.

As the child begins to walk it is important that shoes and socks should always fit because many crippling deformities of the feet can be produced. As far as possible, shoes with wide-fitting toes should be selected. A constant watch is kept on the development of the feet of the toddler and minor deformities such as flat feet, pes cavus and rigid feet can be spotted easily. Early diagnosis is an important preventive factor, for all conditions respond much more readily to treatment at this age.

Advice to parents with disabled children. The health visitor has special responsibilities to assist and advise all parents with disabled children. The health visitor should as a *Named Person* (as defined by the Warnock Committee, see p. 138) to provide a point of contact for the parent of every child who has been found to have a disability or who is showing signs of special needs or problems.

The prevention of home accidents in young children is becoming relatively more important as other causes of child deaths (such as infectious diseases) have diminished.

In 1972, 141 000 children (under the age of 15 years) were admitted to hospital with accidental injuries and 1800 died (deaths in infants under five years of age are approximately 550 a year). More accidents occur within the home than on the roads. In infants, these accidents fall into five groups: inhalation of food or other objects leading to suffocation; mechanical suffocation; burns and scalds; falls; poisoning—by the child accidentally taking medicinal tablets or capsules. Details of these deaths are given in Table 35.

All these accidents are preventable and continual efforts are made by health visitors to reduce their incidence. Mothers are taught the dangers of letting children play with unsuitable objects. Any child from one to two years of age will automatically put things in his mouth and therefore great care is needed when

TABLE 35 Causes of deaths from home accidents, children 0–4 years, England and Wales, 1972

Suffocation (all causes)	313
Burns (and scalds)	107
Falls	58
Poisoning	23
Others	23
Hunger, thirst, exposure and neglect	14

choosing toys. Plastic bags have led to many fatalities from suffocation and must never be left about. Fireguards and flame-proof clothing (especially nightwear) are essential to avoid burning accidents. Legislation recently has insisted on flame-proof materials for children's nightwear. Unprotected stairs or balconies are most dangerous and should be guarded.

One of the most tragic accidents is poisoning. Many drugs including barbiturates and other hypnotics are marketed as brightly coloured tablets or capsules which so closely resemble sweets. Tablets of ferrous sulphate can be dangerous if taken in large doses by small children. Great care is needed to prevent these accidents and doctors and health visitors are constantly teaching mothers to lock up their drugs and medicines and to throw away those no longer needed. All containers of drugs should be fitted with the recently developed 'child-proof' caps.

Report of Court Committee on Child Health Services (Fit for the Future) Cmnd. 6684

Reference has already been made to this Committee's report in December 1976 and a number of the points raised by the Committee have been incorporated into this chapter.

Many of the Committee's recommendations have been accepted by the Government but the proposals to create new specialists such as general practitioner paediatricians, child health visitors, consultant community paediatricians and child health nurses *have not been approved* because they might make the integration of child health services more difficult.

Four main strategies are emphasized:

1. child health shows a changing pattern with more chronic illness and handicap as well as an increase in child psychiatric problems
2. much ill-health in children is preventable and social and geographical factors are very significant; there is considerable variation in local infant and perinatal mortality and morbidity
3. more importance should be paid to health and social care within families and this involves a need to promote a better partnership of care between parents and professional staff of all kinds
4. an unmistakable interrelationship exists between the health, educational and social needs of all children

To achieve these aims the Committee develops the theme that more integration of child health services is essential particularly between prevention and therapeutic care and between hospital and the community services. Health visitors are seen as key personnel in achieving this better integration and their work with children and families should become their top priority. The specialist paediatric services should be increasingly extended into the community and all general practitioners should have adequate training in child health and, in future, undertake more preventive work with children under five.

One of the more important conclusions of the Committee is their insistence on helping the children in greatest need—a crucial failing of the present child health services is that the *children who need them most use them least*. Many of these children have parents who are unemployed and many live in the deprived city areas where specially developed services are urgently needed to improve both primary health care and preventive child health services. The Government has indicated that the new Inner City Partnership programmes and Joint Financing monies should be used to improve services in such areas.

A recommendation which closely links up with the Warnock Committee recommendations (see p. 138) is that a special multidisciplinary team called a *District Handicap Team* should be established in each health district of every AHA and based on a district general hospital. The functions of such a team should include:

1. investigation and assessment of all individual children with complex disorders and coordination of their treatment
2. professional advice to parents, teachers, child care staff and others who may be directly concerned with their care and guidance to them in their management of their children
3. encouragement and help for all professional field work staff in the management and surveillance of handicapped children locally. Each team should act as part of a common service to the health, educational and social services
4. provision of primary and supporting specialist services to the local special schools

The following should always be members of any District Handicap Team: paediatrician, nursing officer for handicapped children, specialist social worker, psychologist and teacher plus supporting administrative staff.

The rejection of the recommendations by the Government to create new specialists means that *there is now a long term future for clinical medical officers* who mainly work with preschool and school children.

A new *Joint Committee for Children* has already been set up (following the Court Committee's recommendations) responsible jointly to the Personal Social Services Council and to the Central Health Services Council to keep under continuous review the needs of children and the services provided to meet them.

6 Health of the Schoolchild

The progress of any child at school depends on many factors: his parents and home, the expectation placed upon him by his environment, his intelligence, the school he attends and the teachers he works with. But an equally important factor is his health. Ill health or a serious physical or mental handicap or disability soon produces many educational problems. Thus the prevention of disease, the treatment of illness and handicap in any child is most important. Both are the concern of all branches of the health services but special arrangements are made to safeguard the health of children at school. Each AHA in conjunction with the relevant local education authority must organize a special *School Health Service*.

AIMS AND OBJECTS OF THE SCHOOL HEALTH SERVICE

The objects and functions of the school health service are:

1. To make certain that every schoolchild is as fit as possible so that each may obtain the maximum benefit from his education. The *school medical examination*, which is undertaken by doctors with special knowledge and experience of those medical conditions most likely to interfere with normal learning, aims at identifying as early as possible any departure from normal health so that effective treatment can be started before lasting ill-effects have been produced on the health of the child. In this way the school health service concentrates on providing a diagnostic service; medical

treatment for any conditions discovered is undertaken by the normal national health services although supportive treatments in the school such as speech therapy or remedial gymnastic therapy is provided by the local education authority.

2. To promote positive health in all children attending school. It is not sufficient just to check that no disease exists; there must be a definite programme designed to make every child as fit as possible. Health education in all its aspects is, therefore, most important.
3. To help with the ascertainment and treatment of various groups of *handicapped children and those with disabilities or significant difficulties and children with learning difficulties* and to assist so that every child can gain the maximum benefit from his education. The care of such children is discussed in detail in the second part of this chapter (see p. 135) but includes a wide range including those who are either partially or totally blind or deaf, suffer from the effects of some serious congenital malformation such as spastic diplegia or spina bifida, accidents, serious illness some of which are progressive and some chronic, those with serious behavioural problems who may be maladjusted, those with chest conditions such as asthma, epilepsy, neurological conditions such as autism or muscular dystrophy and endocrine diseases such as diabetes.

Organization of the School Health Service and Integration with the Pre-school and Primary Health Care Services

Special steps have been taken (in line with the Court Committee's recommendations (see p. 124) to ensure that there is greater integration of the child health services at all ages including the pre-school and schoolchild. In many instances the same health visitor acts as school nurse and the same doctor may be concerned with both. Any pre-school records must accompany the child on entry to school so that a complete, uninterrupted medical history is available. Every AHA must appoint an *Area Nurse (Child Health Services)* who is accountable to the Area Nursing Officer for all child health nursing including that within the school health service. She is also professionally responsible for all the nursing staff employed in the field of school health and must collaborate with the Area Specialist in Community Medicine (Child Health). She must also collaborate with the District Nursing Officer in the management of staff employed in child health. This post is, therefore, of great importance in assisting the fullest possible integration of the child health services.

A key doctor is the *Area Specialist in Community Medicine (Child Health) who with the Area Nurse (Child Health) has direct responsibility to the local education authority for the organization of health services to schools*. An important part of the role of this doctor is to ensure that there is a sound day-to-day link between the primary health-care team and those working in the school health services. This is being helped by increasingly employing general practitioners to work part time on a sessional basis as clinical medical officers in schools. Some full time doctors are also employed to work within the service and are specially trained to deal with handicapped children or those with disabilities or significant difficulties. The Area Specialist in Community Medicine (Child Health) should always ensure that there is a satisfactory system of interchange of essential information (some of which will be confidential) between the doctors in primary health-care teams and those in the school health services. In the same way, there should be a sound system for sharing essential information with other professionals working in the education services and especially with teachers and those who can help with information about home conditions (health visitors, education welfare officers, specialist careers officers or social workers) to ensure that there is the fullest integration between the child health, education and personal social services.

NURSERY SCHOOLS

The normal child can gain much from attending a nursery school when aged three to five years. The value of such schools, which many children only attend for half a day, is in the social contact made. The child gets used to working with others and this is especially useful for the only child, and makes the introduction into the primary school easier. Approximately 30% of children aged three years and four years attend nursery schools. The medical care of children in nursery schools is important and is undertaken by the school health service. Medical examinations are usually arranged for all such children shortly after admission. Special care must also be taken with outbreaks of communicable disease, as conditions such as dysentery can spread rapidly in nursery schools if not recognized early (see p. 210).

Pre-school Examination

Usually the initial examination takes place shortly after the child has been admitted to the infant school, but some authorities are now experimenting with the *pre-school initial medical examination*. This is carried out a year before the child is due to attend school. The mother is invited to bring the child to a convenient centre (usually a combined child health/school health clinic) and a full history collected and medical examination, including dental examination, carried out. One of the advantages of doing the initial medical examination on children aged four years is that a dental examination at this age is important if conservative dental treatment is to be successful. It also enables any medical defect discovered to be investigated and treated *before the child attends school*.

A check on the immunization received is made and, if any are needed, these can be given before entry into school. The pre-school examination is a voluntary one and can never completely replace that given on entry into the primary school. It is, however, a most valuable innovation and is likely to become more popular in the future.

School medical examinations and inspections

The present basis of the school health service is a combination of full routine examinations on all children either just before or immediately after entry into school (at five years of age) combined with selective medical examination during school life. There is a full examination at 14 years including a fitness test for employment.

Because it is essential for the doctor carrying out the medical examination to have the fullest details, it is usual for the health visitor/school nurse to complete an extensive questionnaire on each child before the five-years-old examination. This covers many points including developmental history, social development, home conditions, general muscular coordination, auditory memory.

Practice for subsequent medical examinations varies. In many instances when each child reaches the age of eight and 12 years, questionnaires are completed by parents and teachers and as a result of these answers, selective medical examinations are carried out on those children who have shown various problems.

In other schemes, in the place of subsequent periodic general medical inspections, doctors visit schools several times each term and see children brought to their attention by parents, teachers and school nurses.

The routine medical inspection takes place at school preferably in a special room by a team, consisting of school doctor, school nurse (usually also the health visitor) and a clerk to assist with clerical work. Parents are invited to attend especially at the first medical examination and are summoned on a single appointment system so that they are kept waiting as little as possible. About 12 children can usually be examined each morning or afternoon.

A careful medical history is taken from the parents and this is supplemented by child health clinic records and the health visitor's knowledge of the child and family. Where possible, general practitioner records are added and with the nurses questionnaire, a complete story of the child's progress during the first five years of life is built up, including full details of any illness, medical or surgical problems, immunizations and also a brief note of the health of the parents and family. Any unusual point in the medical history is noted and if the child is known to be at special risk (see p. 119), extra follow-up examinations are arranged. The school doctor then carries out a full medical examination in which all body systems are carefully examined including the special senses. If any illness or disability is discovered, the treatment is arranged usually at hospital after first informing the general practitioner by letter and giving him the opportunity of doing this himself. It will be seen that *the school health service is really a diagnostic service and not a treatment service*. In some instances, treatment may affect the child's ability to play a full part in some of the activities of the school such as games, but wherever possible, interference in this way is kept to a minimum.

Sight testing is carried out at the first full medical examination on five-year-olds using the Keystone machine. This tests visual acuity, colour vision and muscle balance. If any defect is found, a full ophthalmic examination is arranged. If any squint is discovered, investigation and treatment are started although many such cases will have been under treatment since infancy. In the past, most education authorities have arranged special eye clinics. This is now the responsibility of the AHA who also arrange the supply, repair and replacement of any optical appliances (spectacles) needed by schoolchildren. Special orthoptic treatment for squints is also arranged.

The hearing of each child should be tested individually at the first medical examination. This can conveniently be carried out by the school nurse using a sweep test with a pure tone audiometer, which is a light portable machine producing sounds of varying volume at frequency ranges from 128 to 8000 cycles per second. Each ear is tested independently—the child is given a small wooden mallet and asked to strike the table each time a sound is heard. Tests are carried out at each frequency starting with a loud volume of sound and gradually reducing the volume until the child can no longer hear anything. This level indicates the threshold of hearing—the lowest volume of sound at that particular frequency which the child can hear. This test is repeated for each frequency so that a pattern of hearing is quickly established for both ears at different frequencies of sound. It is important to test hearing at different frequencies as occasionally there is a loss of hearing at one particular part of the sound scale (such as a *high frequency deafness*). Testing the hearing of a five-year-old should take about three minutes. About 2% of those tested fail. Such children are referred to an Ear, Nose and Throat Department for further investigation and treatment. The AHA is responsible for the provision and repair of behind-the-ear hearing aids or, where necessary, body-worn hearing aids required by schoolchildren.

The findings of the routine medical inspection are carefully recorded and the doctor indicates when the child is to be seen again. This can be either at a convenient school clinic or at a subsequent visit to the school. Occasionally during routine medical inspection the history is so involved that there is insufficient time to carry out a full examination. In such cases, an early appointment is made for the school doctor to see the child again at a school clinic when as much time as necessary can be given. This is very important especially when examining children with difficult emotional problems or where there is a doubt about the child's intelligence. In such cases, a test of the child's intelligence should always be made either by the school doctor or psychologist.

Examples of routine medical examinations

Normal child. This child is medically examined at school when aged five years and 14 years. In addition, the school nurse visits the school each term to check on minor illnesses and cleanliness, and questionnaires are completed by parent and teacher when the child is aged eight and 12 years.

A child with a constant disability. An example would be a child with defective vision or some chronic disability such as a scoliosis or hearing defect. This child would be seen when five years old when the defect would be diagnosed. After treatment, he would be seen at least on each annual routine medical inspection. Additional frequent re-examinations are arranged for the child at the school clinic to check on progress.

Normal child on entry to school who later develops a severe illness. An example would be given by a child found to be quite normal on entry into school at five years but who developed rheumatic fever when aged seven years. Such a child would be medically examined at school on entry at five years, found normal and marked to be seen again at age 14 years. But, when he developed rheumatic fever at seven years, on his return to school he would immediately be referred to the school doctor. Subsequently he would be seen by the school doctor whenever necessary but at least annually for routine medical examinations are carried out in every school each year.

At such an inspection the following children are seen.

1. those in the various age groups selected for routine medical examination
2. any child seen previously and marked as needing to be seen that year

3. any child with recent serious illness or long absence
4. any child whom the parent, teacher or school nurse desires the school doctor to see because of unsatisfactory progress or difficulty of any kind
5. any child aged eight years or 12 years whose parental or teacher questionnaire indicates medical, behavioural or educational problems

It will be seen that the school health service carefully checks on the health of all schoolchildren and this is done in such a way as to help parents, general practitioners and teachers.

Other functions of school medical officers and school nurses

A good school medical officer and school nurse should interest themselves in many activities connected with the prevention of disease and in promoting positive good health among the children. There are four particular responsibilities of the school doctor and school nurse in this respect.

1. *Investigation of all communicable diseases in the school.* Outbreaks of communicable diseases are likely to occur from time to time especially in infant and junior schools. Prompt investigation will always reduce the chance of a large outbreak. It is not usual today to quarantine large numbers of children, for it is known that this rarely achieves much prevention of disease and invariably means a great loss of education time. If a case of tuberculosis occurs within a school complete examination of all contacts (staff and children) must be carried out to make certain that an unsuspected case has not been the cause. Contacts over the age of 15 years are X-rayed and younger contacts tuberculin tested and chest X-rays arranged on any positives (see p. 195).

The school nurse visits her schools frequently and notes which children are absent so that she can pay a home visit to gain further information, advise and help the parents.

2. *Immunization.* Immunization should always be encouraged in schoolchildren and the immunization state of every new school entrant should be carefully checked. Where needed, primary courses of immunization are arranged at school and booster doses of diphtheria and poliomyelitis vaccines should be given to five-year-olds and of poliomyelitis to 15-year-olds who have had prior courses.

BCG vaccination against tuberculosis should be offered to all schoolchildren aged 10–12 years who are tuberculin negative (see p. 198).

3. *Health education.* Health education is one of the most important functions of the school medical officer and school nurse because the aim is to promote positive health as far as possible. This means encouraging certain non-athletic and under-developed children to improve their physique in various ways and every school doctor and nurse should take an interest in the games schedules of the school. It is important not to neglect that group of children in every school who, for one reason or another (defective vision, flat feet, excessive weight) never seem able to excel at the traditional ball games, and other forms of active recreation should be encouraged both in term time and during the holidays. These include hiking, camping, cycling, rock climbing, skiing, fishing, sailing, skating and riding and these should, wherever possible, form part of the sporting activities of the school. It is possible for any school to benefit from such activities today as the Central Council of Physical Recreation runs many excellent courses in all areas of the country and these are specially designed to introduce the older child to such activities. Such an introduction during school life may later play an active part in maintaining the health of the adult after he has left school.

Special subjects in health education should be tackled in each school both by the teachers and by the school health team. Examples include sex education, family planning and general health topics including current problems such as carcinoma of the lung, carcinoma of the cervix uteri, prevention of disease by immunization, dental hygiene, etc. In this way the natural curiosity of the pupil will be aroused and, at the same time, he will be learning, as a child, sound adult health education topics. This health education should fit naturally into the ordinary pattern of education at the school. Occasionally special health education campaigns are useful (for further details see Chapter 7, p. 160).

4. *Hygiene.* The hygienic conditions of the school should be inspected periodically by the school medical officer and school nurse and this will include examination of buildings, heating plant, washing and lavatory facilities and the kitchen premises.

Regular cleanliness inspections of the children are undertaken either by the school nurse or orderly. About 2% of schoolchildren are found to have evidence of infestation with head lice, mainly in the form of nits, the eggs of the head louse. Arrangements for cleansing the child are made at a convenient school clinic and subsequent examinations are carried out to ensure that there has not been a recurrence. It is also essential for a visit to be paid to the home of the child because other members of the same family may be infested and, unless all are treated at the same time, recurrent re-infestations will occur. Particular attention on such home visits should be paid to any member of the family with long hair.

Scabies is occasionally found in schoolchildren. Treatment with benzyl benzoate is rapid and effective, but *only if all infected members of the family are treated simultaneously.*

ASCERTAINMENT AND CARE OF THE HANDICAPPED SCHOOLCHILD (THOSE WITH DISABILITIES OR SIGNIFICANT DIFFICULTIES)

The discovery, classification and care of handicapped schoolchildren is an important additional role of the school health service. In May, 1978, the report of the special committee set up by the Department of Education and Science to consider the education of Handicapped Children and Young People under the chairmanship of Mary Warnock was published. This far-seeing report puts forward many important changes in principle and these have been incorporated into this chapter.

Although the responsibility for medical services to schoolchildren is that of the AHA, the responsibility for the ascertainment of pupils needing special education remains under section 34 of the Education Act (1944) with each local education authority (LEA). At present, any LEA can legally insist on a medical examination of any child who they have reason to believe requires special education once the child has reached the age of two years, but this is likely to be altered to require any LEA to be given the power to require a multi-professional assessment of *children of any age* (after due notice to parents). A medical examination would form part of such assessment and would usually be carried out by a school doctor who has special experience and qualifications.

Definition of Handicapped Children

At present handicapped children are divided into ten categories by disability: blind, partially sighted, deaf, partially deaf, delicate, educationally subnormal (mild (M) and severe (S)), maladjusted, physically handicapped, epileptic and those with speech defects. These children in such categories who either *attend a special school or class represent 1·8% of the school population*. Considerable criticism has been levelled at these categories which are not necessarily related to the needs of the child and which tend to emphasize separate education in all instances and give no indication of multiple handicaps (i.e. a child who is both blind or deaf and has spastic diplegia). *There is a strong recommendation to abolish statutory categorization and to replace it by a recorded system of educational need.* At the same time, the planning of educational services should be based on *the assumption that about 16–17% of the school population (one in six) at any time (or 20% or one in five at some time during their school life) require some form of special educational provision.* This may take the form of special teaching techniques or equipment, a specially modified curriculum, or help with social or emotional problems. As regards terminology, it is recommended that the term 'handicapped children' be replaced by *children with disabilities or significant difficulties.* The term 'educationally subnormal' should be replaced by the term *children with learning difficulties* which should also include many children who are slow learners and who are at present assisted by the educational remedial services.

Principles applying to the care of children with disabilities or significant difficulties

There are five important principles applying to the care of children with disabilities or significant difficulties:

1. Every effort must be made to make certain that the degree of disability is diagnosed and *discovered as early as possible.* In cases such as deafness it is important that the diagnosis be made within the first year of life.
2. *Special education and care must be started early*—in deafness, as soon as diagnosed, in blindness at two years of age,

and in many other instances well before the age of five years. For many such children, it is an advantage if they can remain at school beyond the normal school leaving age.

3. The aim should always be *to make each child as independent as possible* for the final success in adult life is usually related to independence. It is important to improvise widely in dealing with individual children with a disability or significant difficulty.
4. The best solution for any schoolchild with a disability or significant difficulty is always the one that is *as near normal as possible*. For this reason integration (either fully or partly) into the ordinary school system should always be the aim (see p. 140).

The following are the ways in which a child with a disability or significant difficulty can be educated: (*a*) in an ordinary school; (*b*) in a special class in an ordinary school; (*c*) in a day special school; (*d*) in a residential special school; (*e*) at home, or in a combination of these, i.e. part time in a special class or special school with links with an ordinary school.

The aim should always be *to rehabilitate the child progressively* so that when he leaves school he is preferably in an ordinary school or, if not, in a special class or day special school.

5. The after-care of the child with a disability or significant difficulty when he leaves school is most important. If possible, special vocational training and/or work preparation should always be arranged.

Discovery of disabilities and disclosure to parents

The importance of early discovery of any disability or difficulty has already been stressed. Depending on the nature and type of problem, it may first be discovered, shortly after birth, by the parents, doctor or health visitor, during the first two or three years or during the first few months in primary school. In all instances, an explanation to the parents must be carefully and sensitively undertaken. In the case of a serious disability, most parents find it difficult to grasp the full meaning and implications and are in need of continuous support *and will require information, advice and practical help*. Parents also should know the one person whom they can contact at any time for advice and help and one individual professional should be designated the *Named Person* to act in this way. The main function of such an individual will be to introduce the parents to the right services and to ensure that any special concern about the child's development is followed up. For any child found to have a disability before attending school, the *health visitor* will normally act as the Named Person although in exceptional cases some other professional may be so designated, i.e. a peripatetic teacher in the case of a deaf child. For children found to have educational difficulties, the head teacher of the child's current school should act as the Named Person in most instances and parents should be encouraged to discuss with him any special problems or difficulties. In very large schools much of this day-to-day work may have to be carried out by another teacher, but the head teacher should still retain responsibility as the Named Person.

Occasionally, the parents may wish to discuss the suitability of the teaching provided for their child with some other professional in the education service outside the school. *The Special Education Advisory Service* of each LEA should be available to every parent of a disabled child who should always be told in writing how to contact members of this service if necessary during the school holidays.

Assessment of children with disabilities and significant difficulties

As soon as any disability or difficulty is discovered *a full assessment should be carried out* and this contains four main elements:

1. *Parents should always be involved.* No estimation of any child's needs can be complete without the fullest help from the parents. Cooperation with parents is therefore essential and the aim should be to treat parents as partners in the assessment. Therefore parents MUST be kept fully informed of expert investigations and of the results for unless the confidence of parents is maintained, the assessment will be incomplete.

2. *A multidisciplinary assessment should always be undertaken.* There will, of course, need to be the fullest medical examination and the child may need to see a hospital paediatrician or

other specialist, but the complete investigation of any disability in a child needs more than a medical examination. Doctors, health visitors, educational psychologists, teachers and social workers will all need to be involved. An attempt must be made to *discover how the child learns and responds over a period of time.* Therefore the involvement of some person who has observed the child in say a day nursery or playgroup may be very useful.

3. Assessment must include an investigation of any *aspect of a child's performance which is causing concern.* In many complicated cases, this means a wide range of professional expertise must be included in any multidisciplinary assessment.

4. *The family circumstances and home environment* should always be carefully taken into account. In very young children, the *health visitors* or a *home teacher* will usually provide most of this essential information. In older children, an *educational psychologist* will usually be involved. In most instances, a *social worker's* contribution will be required as well.

Range of special education provided

The needs of children with disabilities or significant difficulties are extremely complex and varied. It may be that quite seriously disabled children will be able to be educated in ordinary schools provided special ramps are available to accommodate wheelchairs, or special equipment (and transport) to help the child. In most severe disabilities and especially if the child has already attended a primary school and made little progress, attendance at a *special school* may be required at least for an initial period. Many different types of special school have developed run either by education authorities or voluntary bodies and some have been in existence long before there was any statutory special education for very disabled children.

In practice, special schools are needed for three groups:

1. children with very severe or complex physical disabilities. This group includes a wide range of conditions from complete blindness or deafness to children with severe congenital disabilities (spina bifida and the severe types of spastic diplegia), to children with grave progressive diseases such as certain muscular dystrophies
2. children with severe emotional or behavioural disorders

who have difficulty in forming relationships with others or whose behaviour is extreme or unpredictable (formerly such children were called 'maladjusted' but this is now a term which is rarely used)

3. children who for various reasons do badly in ordinary schools and who need the more intimate atmosphere of small teaching groups to make educational progress

Even with very severely disabled children, the aim should always be to *increase the integration of such children with normal children.* Although there are many reasons for this, one of the most important is that such mixing of disabled with normal children will do much to overcome the rather protective atmosphere of any special school. At the same time, complete mixing may be impractical or even undesirable for educational reasons—the child with severe disabilities may require a very small class and much individual attention from a teacher.

Integration

There are, however, different *forms of integration* which although falling short of complete integration (i.e. a disabled child attending an ordinary school full time) achieve some mixing of disabled and normal children for some aspects of their school activities. Three forms of such integration can be identified:

1. *Locational*, where a special school unit is sited within the same grounds as an ordinary school, but is still run, in the educational sense, as a separate school. This is a first step in integration and is helpful in reducing the isolation or even stigma felt by parents and children who attend a special school. It also allows seriously disabled children to attend the 'same school' as their brothers and sisters and, in addition, should help the children in the ordinary school better to understand the needs and problems of disabled persons.

2. *Social integration* is a further step. The children in the special school unit now play, eat and mix with the children from the ordinary school unit and may even share some of their out-of-classroom activities. There is, however, still separate classroom teaching for the children in the special and ordinary schools.

3. *Functional integration* achieves all the above but, in addition, the disabled children share some or most of their classes with ordinary children. Such an arrangement still allows some essential specialization to be practised with the severely disabled children but it also enables them to gain many of the advantages of not only mixing with normal children, but of having access to a wider range of teaching than is usually possible in a special school. It may also increase the expectation put upon the disabled child, who otherwise, particularly if he is very intelligent, may never realize anything like his full potential in a special school.

An important function of any school health service is to *assist in developing a wide range of opportunity for the disabled child.* It is possible, for instance, to develop different forms of integration between a neighbouring special and ordinary school which may not actually share the same site. Many difficulties will have to be overcome and there may well be resistance on the part of the teaching staffs of both schools. It is, however, a great help if the same school doctor, school nurse and educational psychologist look after both schools and work closely together with the head teachers and staff to achieve some degree of integration.

It is particularly important to ensure that the disabled child who has attended a special school for many years *to experience some degree of social and functional integration during the last two to three years of his formal education.* This is the only way to avoid excessive overprotection of such children which is almost inevitable in any small special school. Unless the seriously disabled school leaver mixes in this way with ordinary children, he/she will be at a great disadvantage on leaving school for their experience of mixing with ordinary people will be very limited.

Special problems of the disabled child in the transitional period from school into adult life

All children with disabilities or significant difficulties are likely to suffer special problems on leaving school. Their transition into adult life will probably be more difficult than that of a normal child for they are likely to find it less easy to get a job or to be accepted for higher education. It is therefore most important that a *careful re-assessment takes place during the child's last two to three years at school* (and certainly never later than when the child is aged 14). This reassessment should involve not only the teaching, psychological, medical and nursing staff who have been supervising the child's progress continuously, but should include *careers guidance officers, Disablement Resettlement Officers* and social workers from the social services department. At this stage, the full potential of the child should be considered and discussed with the child and parents and the help and support required estimated. It may be that the child should be advised to stay longer at school and every opportunity and encouragement should always be given to disabled children to stay at school beyond the school leaving age. The child may attend a *linked course* planned jointly by schools and colleges of further education in which the pupils spend a half day or up to two days at the college being introduced to the possibilities of further education and generally widening the child's horizons.

Another useful arrangement is '*work preparation*' whereby disabled young people still at school are placed in simulated working conditions by both visiting factories or work situations or by *work experience* in the form of a planned period of supervised employment in industry, commerce or in the public services. Such work preparation should be carefully planned as part of the school curriculum for such disabled children. For those over school leaving age, there are also *Employment Rehabilitation Centres* run by the Employment Service Division which provide work preparation courses (these are further discussed in Chapter 24, p. 443).

Assessment of a specific vocational kind should, wherever possible, be carried out locally but there are specialized residential units to which the child may go, such as the Queen Elizabeth's Foundation at Banstead Place.

Careers guidance

Special guidance is needed in career guidance for all disabled children and their parents. Specialist advice on all the problems of particular disabilities will be needed and this can best be given by a multidisciplinary team of teachers (including those with special responsibility for career guidance), the *Specialist Careers Officers* who should be available in all areas, members of the School Health Service and social services department. A link must also be maintained with the *Disablement Resettlement*

Officers employed by the Employment Service Agency who help with the employment of disabled adults (the *vocational training* of young disabled people is fully discussed in Chapter 24, p. 443).

Some young people on leaving special school (especially if their disability is of a mentally handicapped type) will be transferred to *Adult Training Centres* run by social service departments and hopefully later to sheltered workshops (see p. 482); some very severely physically disabled young persons may likewise move on to special day centres or rehabilitation units run by social services departments. In all such cases, an attempt should always be made to continue the careful health supervision of such young people and to ensure that there is *a continuing educational part of their programme* which these disabled young persons undertake (this should be directly carried out by teachers from the LEA).

It is important to realize that any disabled young person will be very vulnerable to the dangers of unemployment unless he/she is carefully trained and, if possible, can become qualified in some way. Therefore, all disabled young people leaving school should be encouraged to attend a further education college or other unit of higher education. Every effort should be made to *accommodate disabled children locally for further education* and the school health service and local social services department should assist (with transport or by providing some form of residential help if this is needed). Occasionally, however, it is necessary to seek a residential place which will provide further education and vocational training for the young person on leaving school who has a special disability. At Coventry, the LEA runs a very modern further education college (Hereward College) which provides such training and there are also many voluntary bodies who run residential colleges which LEA's can use by arrangement.

SPECIAL PROBLEMS IN CERTAIN GROUPS OF CHILDREN WITH DISABILITIES OR SIGNIFICANT DIFFICULTIES

Although disabled children are no longer formally categorized, those with certain types of disabilities will still require specialized help and brief notes are given below describing these.

Children who are Blind or Partially Sighted

Blind children have no useful sight and must be educated by non-visual methods. In practice this means that children whose sight after correction is worse than 3/60 will usually be classified as blind. Such children start their training when they are two years old in the Sunshine Homes run by the Royal National Institute for the Blind. Education in the majority of cases takes place in residential schools in the earliest years of education, except in the largest cities where other facilities are available. In older children, carefully planned integration is possible and helpful for it prepares the blind young person more completely for adult life.

Partially sighted children have very poor eyesight but, with special assistance, they can be taught using visual methods. Children whose visual acuity after correction is 3/60 to 6/24 and children with progressive myopia come into this category. Classes must be small (containing not more than 10 children) and special equipment is needed. Wherever possible, partially sighted children are taught in special day schools or special classes in ordinary schools so that the interference with the normal education programme is as little as possible.

Children who are Deaf or have only Partial Hearing

Deaf children are those who cannot be taught by auditory methods. It is most important that their education and training be started very early (as soon as diagnosed). Very specialized tuition is needed which has translated the teaching of sounds into visual tuition, and by such methods it is possible to teach totally deaf children to talk who have never heard human speech. Without such tuition, the totally deaf child would always be dumb, as speech is normally learnt by a process of copying sounds. Most deaf children are educated in special residential schools until they have acquired speech and a good mastery of lip reading. Some form of integration should then be encouraged especially in secondary schools although some extra personal teaching supervision will always be needed. Children who have partial hearing, provided they are assisted with special apparatus, can be taught by aural methods. It is usual for such children to be taught initially in small classes (not more than 10 children). These can be in special units in ordinary primary and secondary schools. Only the more severe or those with multiple disabilities are taught in special schools.

Children with Chronic Illnesses or Disabilities

This is a large mixed group containing many medical and surgical conditions which interfere with a child's education. Among the commonest medical problems are heart condition (rheumatic heart disease and congenital heart disease), chest diseases (asthma, bronchiectasis and tuberculosis), diabetes and blood diseases. Many rare diseases which make normal education difficult are also included in this category. In some instances, the unsatisfactory home conditions are an additional reason for admitting delicate children to a special residential school for a period. Often education has been badly interrupted by repeated illnesses and the child has become very backward and the parents of many such children aggravate the situation by overprotection.

Many children with chronic illness or disabilities are first admitted to a residential school to enable a full assessment to be made and correct treatment to be carried out. Once this has been done and the child's improvement stabilized, it should be possible for him to return to a day special school and/or an ordinary school. If a series of operations is needed—as in bronchiectasis or in complicated congenital conditions—the regime of a special school can help treatment by building up the child preoperatively as well as continuing his education.

Children with Learning Difficulties (formerly Educational Subnormal (Moderate), ESN (M))

This is a very large group including children who are at least two years retarded as regards educational performance in school. Learning difficulties can be caused in many ways; for instance, any child with severe hearing difficulty will be soon retarded unless a proper diagnosis is made and the correct educational help provided. But in children without physical illnesses and who are not severely emotionally disturbed, the largest simple factor in this group is a *lack of intelligence* in such children. Educational performance depends on the intelligence of the child and on his application. The level of intelligence of a child can be estimated by first calculating his mental age by carrying out an intelligence test which consists of a series of questions, puzzles and exercises designed to show knowledge gained as well as reasoning ability. These are usually carried out by educational psychologists. The Intelligence Quotient is calculated on the formula:

$$\text{Intelligence Quotient (IQ)} = \frac{\text{Mental Age}}{\text{Real Age}} \times 100$$

The following simple examples illustrate the calculation of IQ.

A child aged 10 years who has a mental age of 10 years would have an IQ of 100:

$$\text{IQ} = \frac{\text{Mental Age}}{\text{Real Age}} \times 100 = \frac{10}{10} \times 100 = 100$$

A child aged 10 years who has a mental age of 7·5 years would have an IQ of 75:

$$\text{IQ} = \frac{\text{Mental Age}}{\text{Real Age}} \times 100 = \frac{7{\cdot}5}{10} \times 100 = 75$$

A child aged 10 years who has a mental age of 13 years would have an IQ of 130:

$$\text{IQ} = \frac{\text{Mental Age}}{\text{Real Age}} \times 100 = \frac{13}{10} \times 100 = 130$$

It is thus seen that a perfectly normal child has an IQ of 100. Above average intelligence gives an IQ over 100 and below average intelligence an IQ below 100.

The distribution of IQs in the community gives a parabolic curve when plotted. In terms of usual performance, IQs will be found as follows:

Over 125	university entrant
115–124	highest stream
90–114	middle stream
80–89	lowest stream
55–79	children with learning difficulties (formerly ESN(M))

Under 50–55 children with special learning difficulties for their intelligence may be very limited (see p. 481); they were formerly classified as ESN(S)

IQs can only be used as rough guides. Performance is the decisive factor and depends on a combination of IQ and application. Mental stability, concentration and to a minor degree training, all affect application. In grading an unintelligent child, great care is needed and repeated tests will be carried out as well as a period of observation in a class or special school with a teacher highly experienced in such children. Even in cases where physical signs of mental handicap are present—a mongol child (Down's syndrome)—careful assessment is important. A very careful physical examination must also be made for any signs of an accompanying deformity especially deafness, which could be responsible for a low test result.

Children with learning difficulties usually are educated in either a special day or residential school where the curriculum contains a greater emphasis on practical teaching and where the pace of teaching is slower or they can be integrated into ordinary schools provided special help (smaller classes etc.) is available. Many such children do well and on leaving obtain and hold down sound jobs where lack of intelligence is no drawback.

A special problem with all children with learning difficulties is that they are more likely to show behaviour problems than normal children. The level of juvenile delinquency is higher in such children and the school health service and educational welfare service are always working to reduce this problem. Another difficulty is that girls with low intelligence are in greater moral danger as they are more easily led astray. Surveys of unmarried mothers always show a greater proportion with low intelligence than in the population at large and it is important that this aspect be fully discussed with parents in order to reduce this risk.

Children with Special Learning Difficulties (formerly Educationally Subnormal (Severe) ESN(S))

Following the Education (Handicapped Children) Act 1970, the care of mentally handicapped children was transferred to the education services and the junior training centre became another special school for the subnormal. Some form of transport, usually buses, is used to collect the children from convenient meeting places near their homes to carry them to and from the school. Although escorts are provided on the buses during training, emphasis is always placed on fostering independence and self-reliance in the child, and when trained and capable of doing so, each child is encouraged to make his own way from home to the collection point each day. Occasionally in rural areas five-day residential special schools for mentally handicapped children are used at which the children stay from Monday to Friday, returning home for the weekend.

The aim of each special school is to concentrate upon social training and later on preparation for workshop employment. Social habit training, including eating, care of clothes, and personal hygiene, forms an important part of the regime and in all schools midday meals are supplied. Later rudimentary lessons of arithmetic, reading and writing are held, but few ever achieve this at the end of their training. More learn to recognize simple letters and figures, handle money, and a few can do simple sums. Group activities of varying types, such as acting, games or playing in a percussion band, are stressed. The education of the older girls includes cooking and laundry work.

These children are usually educated in small mixed units (60–70 children). Each is arranged into different classes, but the children divided by aptitude rather than by age. Even so, there is a greater variation in the level of educational performance in the children of each class than at ordinary school. The level of intelligence of an entrant to such a school varies, but the majority have intelligence quotients between 40 and 50. If the behaviour of the child is uncontrollable, it may be necessary to exclude him from school, as the effect on the others attending must be considered, but fortunately exclusion rarely occurs except in the most difficult cases.

Maladjusted Children

This child is really a 'problem child' showing many behaviour difficulties, who may become retarded educationally, although his intelligence may be unimpaired. Maladjustment is caused by a multitude of factors including emotional instability in the child, psychological disorders, unstable home conditions, marital difficulties between parents including divorce or separation. A full investigation should be carried out at the *Child Guidance Clinic* where a child psychiatrist, psychologist and social worker function as a team to investigate and treat all cases. Repeated visits may be necessary before all causative facts are unravelled and therapeutic sessions are held. In many authorities the social workers at Child Guidance Clinics are now members of the social services department.

Special educational treatment may be indicated and, for maladjusted children with unsatisfactory home conditions, small residential schools containing 50 to 60 children are best with classes of ten children. The majority of maladjusted children are, however, best educated in ordinary schools as they gain from contact with normal children. In all cases, psychological disorders in the children must be treated appropriately and special attention paid to the home conditions, and, in many instances, the treatment is difficult and calls for much patience. Relapse in behaviour occurs and delinquency may be a complication. Often continued encouragement and understanding by the teaching and medical staff eventually succeed. Failure with the maladjusted child may have serious consequences later, for these children may drift into criminal behaviour and may even become habitual criminals. It is important that *social work be continued with such children after they leave school to help them settle satisfactorily in early adult life.*

Children with Epilepsy

The majority of children with epilepsy can be educated in an ordinary school provided that: (*a*) the fits do not occur too often; (*b*) the emotional stability of the child is reasonably normal and there is no marked behaviour difficulty; (*c*) there is a sympathetic teaching staff who realize that no other child in the class will be harmed by witnessing an occasional epileptic fit. Good liaison between the school doctor and teacher can help considerably.

If the child has very frequent major fits or has a marked emotional instability, admission can be arranged to a special residential school for epileptics for assessment and treatment.

Such schools are run in conjunction with an epileptic colony, as its medical and teaching staff have great experience of the problems of children with epilepsy. After assessment and correct treatment, it should be possible for a proportion of children to return to normal schools.

Other Groups of Disabled Children

There are other groups of disabled children such as those who are *spastic*. Their education will largely depend upon the degree of problem: many can be integrated into the ordinary school but the more severe and complicated cases need specialized care often in separate residential units. Children with *autism* present a small but difficult group. In the early stages of diagnosis and assessment special schools are needed, but the least affected children should be able to return eventually to ordinary school. Children with *dyslexia* can easily be misdiagnosed as 'unintelligent', which emphasizes how important a specialized multidisciplinary assessment is to unravel the real causes of the child's difficulty in reading progress. Dyslexia shows itself in a series of ways affecting spelling, reading and other language skills. There is always a marked discrepancy between the mental potential of the child (usually normal) and his educational level. The incidence is as high as 3% although many minor cases are missed. The cause of dyslexia is not fully understood, but most agree that it is caused by a lesion in the central nervous system which has been present since birth. Many children with dyslexia do well if the condition is recognized early, and attend nursery schools and later received *individual teaching* or teaching in a very small group. These children and those with *speech defects* will often develop emotional difficulties from the frustration of being unable to keep up with other children or to make themselves readily understood. This, in turn, can aggravate their reading problems or their speech defect. Special help with remedial teaching or speech therapy should be available. *Speech therapists* are employed in every school health service. Integration of children with speech defects should always be practised and it is most important that they remain in ordinary schools with normal children.

Social Education Teams

Many authorities have recently introduced an integrated service linking the child guidance, schools psychological services, remedial teaching teams and education welfare services into social education teams. The aim of these teams is to detect and help put right factors coming between children and their education. School doctors form members of the team which includes education welfare officers, psychologists, social workers, health visitor/school nurses and remedial teachers. Coordination is maintained between the teams and the social service department and social workers in social education teams are usually members of that department. Social workers in the community can also play their part in assessing the interrelationship between backwardness and social handicap.

School Dental Service

Every AHA must provide a comprehensive school dental service and the function of this is to provide both diagnostic and treatment facilities. Dental care should start in the pre-school years for it has been found that at least 20% of children first attending school have marked active dental caries (i.e. five or more decaying teeth) but 79% of such children need some dental attention.

Visits are paid by the school dental surgeon to each school every six months and every child is examined dentally and a careful record made of all defects found. Treatment is then offered and, if the parent agrees, provided from a neighbouring dental clinic, each child being called for individual treatment on an appointment system. In remote country areas, dental clinics may be mounted in a mobile caravan so that the treatment centre can be taken and parked at the school, and this enables the treatment to be undertaken without taking the children away from school for long periods. There is a shortage of dentists in the school health services and to help overcome this, dental hygienists are used. These officers have a two-year training and must work under the personal direction and supervision of a dentist. They carry out fillings, scalings and may do simple extractions under local anaesthetics, but their main function is in conservative dentistry.

Most school dental services have facilities for carrying out orthodontic treatment on children with crowded and misplaced teeth, for such treatment can prevent many dental problems later. Orthodontic treatment should always start early so that the permanent teeth may develop correctly.

An important aspect of the school dental service is the health education it undertakes and in every school it teaches sound dietary habits and dental hygiene.

7 Health Education

This book describes many ways in which disease can be prevented and the health of the community improved. But all these various preventive services can only succeed if they are widely accepted by the individual and the community. The process of persuading people to accept measures which will improve their health and to reject those which will have an adverse effect is called *health education*.

Most people are interested in factors which affect health—the reaction shown to any television or radio programme dealing with health topics demonstrates this. Indeed health education has become of more significance because individual behaviour now has a greater effect on individual health than it did 30 years ago. It is now possible for any person to improve his own life prospects and those of his children by his own behaviour. But many different factors can influence our reactions and decisions. Home and school are both powerful influences in any person's life and both can condition the ability of that person to make the right or wrong decision in regard to health matters.

Health is difficult to define; it is far more than the absence or avoidance of disease, for it is concerned with the active promotion of peak mental and physical fitness (often referred to as 'positive health').

Because the standards accepted as normal constantly vary, the science of health education itself must also be concerned with change in the behaviour and attitudes of people. Successful health education is that which succeeds in persuading an individual by a process which subtly influences not only that person, but those places which shape his attitude—his home, school or work place. Health education must, therefore, have access to as broad a section of the community as possible if it is to be successful—to parents, young children, adolescents, teachers, employees and employers and, indeed, every section of society. It is also important to realize that health education is a community responsibility—the ideal society must itself play a vital part through the power of public opinion accepting or rejecting types of behaviour. Too often in the past, health education has been considered the responsibility of the professional health educator only, whether a doctor, health visitor, nurse or health education officer and not that of the parent and child.

The role of the health educator is to convince the community and individuals of the importance of health. One of the best ways to achieve this is to ensure that many different types of individuals play a key role—parents, teachers, employers, youth leaders, social workers, church leaders, politicians, etc. so that the educating role becomes spread out and that the end effects will be equally widespread throughout the population. Because the factors which influence any community are constantly altering, a certain amount of *research* will be needed to ensure that the best results are obtained—that the impact of health education is as high as possible and proportional to the effort being made.

Organization of Health Education

Local

Health education is one of the responsibilities of the AHA under section 28 of the National Health Service Act, 1946. Health education within the school curriculum is the responsibility of the local education authority and schools. There is, however, an important continuing role for staff in the school health services in participation with teaching staff in the planning and presentation of health education programmes. This involves helping and advising pupils and their parents. It is, therefore, most important that there is the closest liaison between AHA and the local education authority. The Area Medical Officer is in overall charge of local health education, but the staff primarily responsible for the detailed work include:

1. *Health education officers*. Many of these officers have had a dual training of nursing and/or health visiting and teaching. Their function is the organization and promotion of health education within the area and this will take many forms: firstly, it must involve a considerable amount of inservice training of the staff mentioned below; secondly, the collection and distribution of suitable material and information, and, thirdly, assessment and evaluation of the impact of the health education undertaken.
2. *Health visitors*, as much of their work is educational and is carried out where teaching is most likely to be effective—within the home or with very small groups.
3. *Doctors*, which should include not only those employed by the AHA to carry out personal health services, but also every hospital doctor and general practitioner.
4. *All nursing staff* should also be involved whether working within the community or hospital.
5. *Teachers*, for their widespread influence on the lives of their pupils. School life will always play an important part in health education, as any success with children will mould the attitudes of future generations—success with children will lead to many further successes, but failure will likewise breed further failure.
6. *Social workers* are also concerned, especially those dealing with the problems of children (under the various Children's Acts), the mentally disordered, the physically handicapped and the elderly.

The wide range of different types of persons who are involved emphasizes the importance of realizing that *modern health education is a multidisciplinary task* in which the professional health educator is more of a manager enabling others to play a vital part.

National organizations

The first national organization for health education was formed in 1927 as the Central Council for Health Education. This body acted as the central advisory body until its disbandment in 1968 when its functions were taken over by the *Health Education Council*.

This body has an annual budget of approximately £450 000. Its objects and aims include the promotion and encouragement 'of education and research in the science and art of healthy living ... and to assist government departments, local authorities and other statutory and voluntary bodies in so far as their work comprises health education and propaganda directed to the promotion or safeguarding of public health or to the prevention and cure of disease....'

The organization of the Council's functions under its Director-General is shown in Fig. 11. It will be seen that there are five branches, each with its own director, dealing with:

i. Communication, research and information services.
ii. Field services.
iii. Education.
iv. Medical research.
v. Administration.

The Health Education Council is the main national source of advice and help on health education matters to local and central government, to voluntary organizations, to the press, radio and television. It also gives help to health authorities of developing countries and international organizations. It is particularly concerned with the planning and development of health education on a scientific basis. This means it evaluates the benefits of health education programmes, their impact on community health and on the community medical care and social services.

From early 1977, the Health Education Council jointly with the Family Planning Association are responsible for a *Family Planning Information Service.* This is financed by an annual grant from the DHSS and provides leaflets, posters, publications, publicity services aimed at ensuring that the public is aware of the free National Health Service Family Planning Services.

Voluntary bodies

There are many voluntary bodies which have come into being with specific aims within health education. These include the Royal Society for the Prevention of Accidents (ROSPA), a number of cancer education societies and drug societies. These bodies act as specialized centres of development for health education.

Commercial organizations

Many of the visual aids used in health education—equipment, film, filmstrips, slides, etc.—are produced by commercial firms who specialize in producing health education material. As well as these, there are also many commercial companies who make and freely lend out films which have both a health educational content and a self-advertising one for their own product. Much of this indirect commercial assistance is very discreetly carried out and is most useful.

Methods and techniques (including information and material)

Experience gained in various health education methods has made it clear that it is never sufficient just to tell people about a special subject; it is essential to ensure that not only do they understand, but that they believe the information and consider it important enough to act upon. To enable this to be carried out, considerable *skills in communication* are necessary as well as an understanding of the learning process. This means that it is necessary for the health educator to get to know as much as possible about the individual or group at whom the health education is being aimed. It is always important to understand the motivating factors in any person or group if success is to be expected. For these reasons, individual and group psychology are subjects no health educator can afford to neglect.

The technique most likely to be successful will depend both on the subject and on the group to be taught, but generally there should always be plenty of visual material. It is also important that those being taught are, in some way, brought actively into the teaching process by discussion or argument. Otherwise, the impact of any teaching material is likely to be negligible. Techniques are often conveniently divided into three main groups:

1. individual health education
2. group health education
3. mass media health education

Techniques of Health Education

Individual health education. This is always the best method of teaching as it is the most effective, particularly for continuous and permanent teaching such as ante and postnatal care, preven-

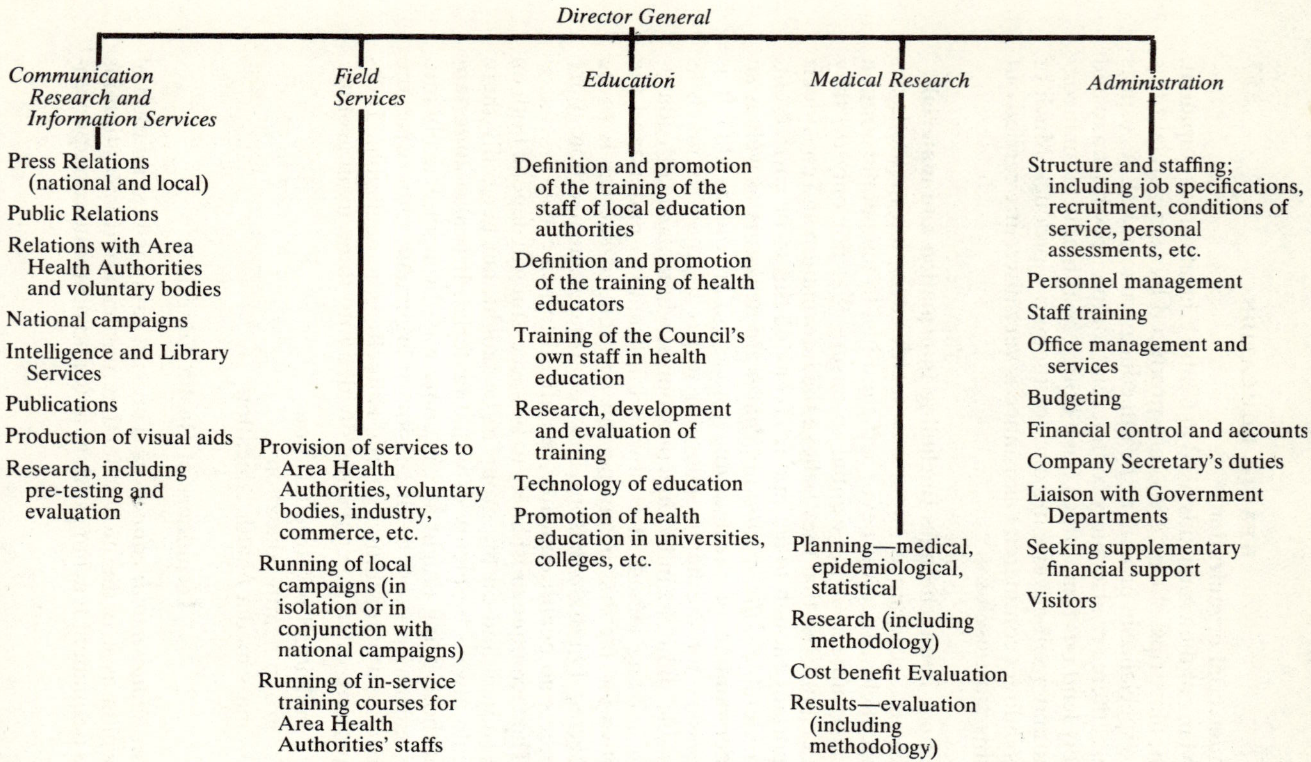

FIG. 11. Organization of the Health Education Council

tion of disease, safety, etc. Personal discussion and demonstration are commonly used in the home, surgery, hospital, school or in industry. It is always wise to follow up such teaching as many people have not understood the initial instruction or have forgotten it. Such talks should never last longer than five to ten minutes, and should concentrate on one subject at a time. Probably the *general practitioner* is in the best position to carry out individual health education as the patient has complete faith in him, which is an important factor in teaching. While treating patients for some illness, the general practitioner should notice conditions within the home and, when necessary, give advice to improve them. Examples are the avoidance of accidents, diet, food hygiene. In this way a good general practitioner will teach many patients of all ages how they can improve their health and avoid disease.

The *health visitor* is the other medical worker who carries out much individual health education. She does this in her routine work while visiting the home or while working in child health clinics (see p. 115).

Social workers and *teachers* are other professionals who have plenty of opportunity to carry out individual health education in their day-to-day work.

Group health education is used in child health clinics, schools and in some industries. Health centres also provide an ideal opportunity for such teaching. Small groups should be used, preferably about six to eight persons, and it is best to stimulate group discussions so that everyone plays an active part. Extensive use is made of various visual aids including film strips, colour slides and 16 mm sound films. Occasionally radio and television can act as a starting point for a group discussion. Provided that every effort is made to keep the groups small and that the talks are short (not longer than 10–15 minutes) and are followed by discussion, this form of health education can be valuable.

Mass media health education. Much community health education is indirect background teaching by which certain topics are constantly kept in the public eye. Posters, press publicity and features on radio and television are used extensively to instruct on a wide range of subjects such as avoidance of accidents, immunization, nutrition, dangers of smoking and venereal disease. This type of health education is limited in value but is useful if associated with other more active instruction. Recently many posters designed by the Health Education Council have tended to shock people—an element which is useful in convincing people of the importance of any subject.

Use of campaigns

Special health education campaigns may be mounted to achieve a particular aim, for example, an effort designed to boost interest in a certain topic, such as immunization or the use of safety belts in cars. In such a venture, every possible means of education should be used—posters, press articles and publicity, letters to residents, radio and television.

Occasionally shock tactics are used to emphasize a serious subject. The demonstration of dreadfully damaged cars exhibited in prominent spots beside busy roads reminds travellers of the appalling consequences of road accidents.

Concentration on special problems

From time to time it is necessary to concentrate health education on new problems which are developing within a community to prevent them becoming inbuilt and permanent. An example is drug misuse which is currently an increasing menace and which it is important to prevent before it becomes widespread and possibly permanent. In the tackling of such a problem, there will always be two main facets:

1. *primary prevention* to reduce the likelihood of more victims becoming involved
2. *secondary prevention* to help those already misusing drugs and to prevent deterioration of their condition

In the case cited—controlling drug misuse—communication with those already taking drugs may be one of the greatest problems and demonstrates how important it is to recognize that health education must use a wide range of helpers. A special social worker and volunteer who is actually visiting those taking drugs is obviously likely to be one of the most effective workers in this instance.

Examples of Health Education

All the preventive medical/social topics discussed in this book can be greatly influenced by health education. To avoid duplication, the reader is referred to the appropriate chapter, but the list is long and includes:

1. Maternity care especially antenatal care (Chapter 4)
2. Child health/care services in all their aspects (Chapters 5 and 23)
3. Prevention of disease by immunization—in children and in adults especially when travelling (Chapter 10)
4. Accident prevention, especially in children (Chapter 5), at work (Chapter 15) and in old age (Chapter 26)
5. Nutrition (Chapter 16)
6. Prevention of infectious diseases (Chapter 7)
7. Smoking (Chapter 14)
8. Sexually transmitted diseases (Chapter 13)
9. Sex education, including avoidance of marital problems and illegitimacy (Chapter 15)
10. Cancer education, especially in relation to cervical cytology, cancer of lung, cancer of skin and breast cancer (Chapter 14)
11. Dental care (Chapter 4)
12. Alcoholism (Chapter 25)
13. Health check-ups and screening—if these are to be used more in future, then the public should be prepared by health education to make effective use of them (Chapter 15)
14. Food hygiene and the prevention of food poisoning (Chapter 12)
15. First aid, including mouth to mouth breathing (Chapter 8)
16. Atmospheric pollution prevention (Chapter 17)
17. Preparation for retirement (Chapter 26)
18. Drug addiction (Chapter 25)

8 Other Community Health Services

HEALTH CENTRES

Health Centres are units where family doctor services, child health (including school health) and health education services are carried out and are the premises now most favoured by the DHSS in the development of modern primary health care. Each AHA has the responsibility of providing and servicing health centres (including the provision of caretaking staff and cleaners). In most, the general practitioners provide their own receptionists and secretarial staff. At present, approximately 21% of general practitioners practice from health centres and the building programme is such that about 2% of general practitioners each year are rehoused in new health centres.

Originally health centres were designed with a separate general practitioner wing and a separate child health and school health wing. However, the modern trend is for the development of an integrated centre in which the general practitioners and nursing staff work in the same part. This has been a natural development following the closer working relationship which has developed with the secondment of health visitors and home nurses to general practice to form the primary health care team. 80% of all community nursing staff (health visitors, district nurses and midwives) now work in association with general practitioners in such teams and the growth of health centres has helped this development.

Considerable flexibility has also been encouraged by the DHSS in the size of health centres and in the number of general practitioners working there as well as in the scope of community health services provided. Factors which influence health centre development include the number of doctors in the area keen and willing to participate and the provision of existing facilities such as child health clinics in the neighbouring districts. The most usual number of doctors working in a health centre is between four and six though this may vary from three to twelve, with a full integration of health visitors/school nurses and home nurses.

Such a unit would undertake most of the community health services of the area and the general practitioners would carry out all child health and school health clinics in the centre. With the secondment of health visitors and home nurses, doctors in such a health centre should be in an ideal position to encourage preventive medicine in their practices. The centre acts as a natural meeting place for other community services including the social services and there should be a close link between the general practitioners working there and the area social service team. Partial attachment of a social worker to a primary health care team based on a health centre is becoming commoner.

Smaller health centres often contain minimal community health services especially if there is already a large child health clinic close by. The smallest health centre must at least provide rooms for health visitors and home nurses.

Although there are many excellent examples of health centres in every part of the country, there are still many general practitioners who are not yet prepared to work in them, although the opposition to health centres is far less than formerly especially in younger general practitioners. It is important that the staff who will eventually work in a health centre should meet well in advance to discuss and define their future roles.

The DHSS published an excellent Health Centre Design Guide in 1970, and this document, which considers the problems and plans of health centres in great detail, should be studied carefully by all who are planning such developments.

Home Nursing

A comprehensive home nursing service must be provided by each AHA to assist in the treatment of disease at home. In practice, it is the district organization (the District Nursing Officer) who has the day to day responsibility for this service.

Home nursing (or 'community nursing' as it is now being called) has changed a great deal during the last fifteen years, mainly because of the consequences for home nursing which followed the attachment of home nurses to the primary health care team in general practice.

In England, in 1976, 11 665 nurses (whole time equivalents) were employed as home nurses. Many were full time but there were also a proportion of part time nurses. Their work, which shows a marked increase over the last five years, was spread out between different age groups of the population with the majority of work (in proportion) being undertaken for the elderly as shown by Table 36.

TABLE 36 Home nursing, England, 1976

Age	*Total of persons nursed*
0–4 years	171 200
5–64 years	1 479 300
65 + years	1 301 100
	2 951 600

(from *Health and Personal Social Service Statistics England*, 1977, DHSS)

Traditionally, home nursing provides nursing care for the patient being treated at home by the general practitioner. Comprehensive nursing care is provided for both acute and chronic patients. Special late night visits are arranged to assist very ill patients who may need a late injection of morphia. In some areas a special service has been provided to enable continuous care to be given at night to patients very ill at home—often to persons suffering from a terminal illness.

With elderly chronic patients who may be incontinent and bedridden, a special soiled laundry service has been developed in conjunction with the home nursing services for daily changes of clean linen to be provided. This is a great asset to relatives looking after any bedridden incontinent patient and enables the elderly person to remain at home for a longer time.

The Health Services and Public Health Act, 1968 extended the law regarding the provision of home nurses, for it made 'the attendance of nurses on persons who require nursing elsewhere than in their own homes' an explicit responsibility.

Many primary health care teams then introduced a 'treatment room' and the home nurse attached to the practice was put in charge of many of the procedures carried out there. Many variations of practice have developed but tasks which the home nurse now undertakes include:

1. diagnostic and progress tests in the treatment room in addition to the more conventional nursing duties. These include venepuncture, inoculations and the taking of electrocardiograms
2. organization of the nursing needs of the practice
3. the undertaking of 'first' visits, carried out in close cooperation with the doctor. Such visits may be for a variety of reasons:
   a. to assess the situation and to report back to the doctor who then decides if he should visit personally
   b. to children with common infectious diseases in place of a doctor
   c. routine follow-up of the long-term patients who do not require regular nursing care

In all cases strict criteria are laid down for the type of case the home nurse sees. In many instances patients benefit from such arrangements. Not only is the doctor's time saved for more urgent duties, but the home nurse will probably undertake a dressing better than a doctor and be able to spend a little more time with the patient explaining medical instructions or advising him on his health care. It is interesting to note that experimental systems tried in general practice where patients can choose whether they first see the doctor or home nurse have worked well and, in many instances, the patient prefers to see the home nurse first.

One of the features of these developments is that less home visiting is undertaken and more patients attend the treatment room of the practice. There is also a better degree of coordination between the doctor and home nurse.

Role of home nurse in hospital practice

Marked changes have also occurred in the role of home nurses in hospital practice with the development of day hospitals, the community hospital and day surgery.

Day hospitals have become an important feature of a comprehensive geriatric hospital service. The home nurse is in an excellent position to follow up the patient at home. In this respect, she may tend to overlap with the health visitor who, in some cases, may later take the case over. But as both the home nurse and health visitor are members of the primary health-care team, this is not a disadvantage.

Community hospitals (as demonstrated at Peppard Hospital, Oxfordshire) are a relatively new concept. Occupying similar buildings to the older cottage hospitals, their function is quite different because they are not replicas of a large hospital, but part of the total bed allocation of the area *being staffed by the practice health team.* Not only does the general practitioner provide the medical expertise but the home nurse the nursing expertise.

The community hospital is linked to the health centre and has a small number of in-patient beds and a day ward. It receives various groups of patients:

1. physically and mentally handicapped patients and those in need of social support .
2. acute medical cases not requiring intensive care
3. predischarge postoperative patients
4. certain geriatric patients
5. 'holiday' admissions of certain chronically handicapped patients
6. terminal care patients

This community hospital has dealt with many elderly and handicapped patients who could become long stay patients in a chronic geriatric ward. In the rehabilitative functions of such a unit the role of the home nurse has proved to be most important.

Day surgery and conventional surgery. Day surgery is developing in many areas. A crucial member of any day surgery team is the home nurse, who visits before the operation to assess the patient's suitability for day surgery. She gives him preoperative advice and visits him on the evening of the operation soon after his return home. She observes, gives advice and sedation if prescribed. She also acts as a most important link with the hospital.

In the same way, a number of conventional surgical units have a home nurse attached to them. She visits patients at home before surgical treatment; she can give the patient any explanation if he requires it, allays fears and acquaints him with hospital routine. In addition, *she can assess the quality of aftercare* he is likely to get from the home and this is crucial in determining the discharge date of the patient.

CHIROPODY

Chiropody services are provided by AHAs for elderly and handicapped persons. Most old people suffer from a variety of minor foot defects such as ingrowing toe nails, corns, hallux valgus and hammer toes which lead to much pain on walking, and to some degree limit movement. This may even result in the old person being made housebound with all the subsequent problems, i.e. difficulty with shopping leading eventually to malnutrition. Most of these foot defects can be considerably helped by regular chiropody. Arrangements vary in different districts, but there are two main ways of providing chiropody: (1) special chiropody sessions are arranged in clinics and old people's clubs where free treatment is given. A domiciliary treatment service is also provided in serious cases, but it is better to encourage the elderly to come to a nearby centre for chiropody because the outing is beneficial. This is now a free service. Occasionally, where there is great frailty, home treatment is the only practical solution. (2) Chiropody treatment may be carried out at the private surgeries of chiropodists. In this case, the AHA meets the cost.

To obtain maximum value, chiropody treatment must be carried out regularly—once every six to eight weeks—otherwise the condition of the old person's feet will rapidly deteriorate.

In England, during 1976, 1261 000 people were treated by chiropodists in this service. Of these, 1161 000 were elderly, 57 000 children and 25 000 physically disabled. Many of the chiropodists provided this service on a part-time basis.

FAMILY PLANNING

Since July 1975 free family planning advice, treatment and supplies (the arrangements relate to female methods of contraception) have been provided by AHAs through their family planning clinics and by general practitioners and pharmacists under the national health service. About 90% of general practitioner principals are providing such services and about 25% had inserted intrauterine devices within the first two years.

At the same time, free family planning services (including vasectomy and female sterilization) was made available to all in hospitals. *A distinction is no longer made between family planning work on medical or other grounds.*

By 1976, the transfer of all clinics and domiciliary family planning services previously run on an agency basis by the Family Planning Association was completed and AHAs became responsible for direct provision. By the beginning of 1977, there were nearly 1700 family planning clinics in England giving a family planning service to over 1·4 million people. Another 19 000 were seen in the domiciliary service and 1·9 million women were receiving family planning services from their general practitioners (see p. 271). It is believed that the extended free family planning services have contributed to the reduction in the numbers of women of all ages having a pregnancy terminated by abortion.

Cervical Cytology

The number of women having a cervical cytology test has continued to increase and in 1976 nearly 2·5 million women were tested in England. The results are shown in Table 37 and show that *about six positive cases are detected per 1000 examined over the age of 30 years.*

Full details of this test are given on p. 268. Because the incidence of cancer of the cervix is so much higher in women of social class V, it is most important to ensure that such women are tested. Many AHAs have planned special industrial services in which a health visitor arranges for a doctor to attend a factory to carry out these tests there.

TABLE 37 Cervical Cytology, England, 1976

Age	*No. of cases examined*	*Positive cases (per 1000 examined)*
Under 25	546 000	2·4
25–29	455 000	5·1
30–34	406 000	6·1
35 and over	1 041 000	6·3
All ages	2 448 000	5·2

(from *Health and Personal Social Services Statistics England*, 1977)

AMBULANCE SERVICES

Since the reorganization of the health services, the ambulance services are now an integral part of the nationalized health service. In England the ambulance services are arranged mainly in two ways.

In the largest conurbations, there is one ambulance service—the Metropolitan Ambulance Service—usually bearing the name of the Metropolitan county, i.e. Merseyside, West Midlands, etc. This service is under the control of a Metropolitan Ambulance Officer. In the non-metropolitan counties (i.e. the AHAs outside the conurbations) there is an Area Ambulance Service under an Area Ambulance Officer.

Both services are controlled for planning and for financial purposes by a Regional Ambulance Service (under a Regional Ambulance Officer) who covers the area of each of the RHAs.

Ambulance services transport ill persons from home to hospital (or hospital to home) or from the scene of an accident to hospital. Their medical condition must be sufficiently serious to prevent them from travelling by public transport. National Health Service ambulances do not transport persons from home to another house or from home to a doctor's or dentist's surgery.

Two types of ambulance are normally used—stretcher ambulances and sitting case vehicles. The former carry ill patients to and from hospital when requiring admission, and the latter are used to transport sitting patients to hospital out-patient departments or physiotherapy or occupational therapy departments of hospitals. In large cities and towns, separate stretcher ambulances are manned to deal with accidents and emergencies.

All ambulance personnel are trained in first aid and each ambulance should carry modern automatic oxygen resuscitation apparatus. Skilful first aid, such as properly conducted mouth to mouth breathing, followed by oxygen therapy can be a life-saving procedure in emergencies such as drowning, gas poisoning or electrical shock. To increase efficiency it is usual for all stretcher ambulances to be radio controlled.

The deployment of ambulances is often difficult because of the unequal demand throughout the day. The peak periods are between 8 and 10 a.m., 12 a.m. and 1 p.m., 1.30 and 2.30 p.m., and 4.30 and 5.30 p.m. due to the demand of out-patient departments. Considerable help can be obtained by stationing at each large hospital a full-time ambulance control officer to coordinate the reception and removal of patients by ambulance.

Special arrangements are usually made to meet a large emergency due to a major civilian disaster such as a train accident and large supplies of medical and nursing equipment are always available at ambulance headquarters to rush to the scene of such incidents. This ensures that any doctors who are at the scene of the disaster or are called out as mobile medical teams from hospitals can function successfully.

9 Epidemiology of Communicable Diseases

Communicable or infectious diseases are those which can be spread either from person to person or from animal or insect to a human. Such diseases are caused by infection of the body with bacteria or viruses or their products. *Epidemiology* is the study of all the factors connected with the incidence and spread of such diseases—it includes the causation of the illness (*aetiology*).

When many cases of the same infectious disease occur simultaneously, an *epidemic* is said to exist. A series of similar epidemics throughout the world is a *pandemic*. Scattered cases of infectious disease with no connection between them are said to be *sporadic*. When a communicable disease is constantly present in any area, it is said to be *endemic*.

CLASSIFICATION OF COMMUNICABLE DISEASES

One of the best methods of classifying communicable diseases is by their mode of spread. There are five main groups.

Air-borne or Droplet Infections

Bacterial diseases

Streptococcal infections—scarlet fever, erysipelas, puerperal fever, tonsillitis, rheumatic fever
Staphylococcal infections—pemphigus neonatorum
Diphtheria
Bacterial meningitis
Whooping cough

Tuberculosis
Pneumonia

Virus diseases

Smallpox
Influenza
Encephalitis
Common childhood infections: measles, rubella, mumps and chickenpox
Glandular fever
Virus meningitis
Virus respiratory infections
Common cold

Faecal-borne or Gastrointestinal Infections

Bacterial diseases

Typhoid and paratyphoid fever
Dysentery
Food poisoning
Infantile gastroenteritis
Cholera

Virus diseases

Poliomyelitis
Infective hepatitis

From Animals

Anthrax
Leptospirosis
Rabies
Q fever
Toxoplasmosis
Via milk—bovine tuberculosis, brucellosis
Viral haemorrhagic diseases (Lassa fever, Marburg disease and Ebola virus disease)

Contact

(Man)—Venereal diseases (syphilis and gonorrhoea)
(Injury)—Tetanus

Insects

Plague
Malaria
Yellow fever
Typhus

Note. In addition, in serum hepatitis infection is caused by transfer of virus to blood stream by injection or blood transfusion.

Epidemiological Investigation of Communicable Diseases

A full investigation of all serious communicable diseases should always be undertaken to find the cause of the infection and to study the factors which contributed to its spread. A successful investigation will often prevent further cases by defining a continuing source of infection. Epidemiological investigations should include a careful history of the patient and his close contacts and any link between the patient and other cases should be investigated. If the disease is not normally present in the country (e.g. smallpox) it is important to establish if contact has been made with someone who has recently travelled abroad. In gastrointestinal infections (typhoid fever or food poisoning) which are usually the result of a food contamination, a complete record is collected of the food eaten.

Incubation period

In all communicable disease, there is a latent period, between infection and the first symptoms or signs of the disease, called the *incubation period*. A person infected with typhoid fever will show no symptoms for 14 days. An accurate knowledge of this incubation period is most important for it allows investigations to be concentrated on the food eaten 14 days before the first symptoms, for this was the time of infection.

Incubation periods are never easy to remember and may vary in the same disease. They can most conveniently be divided into three groups.

Very short incubation periods, 2 to 18 hours

Staphylococcal food poisoning (2 to 4 hours)
Clostridium perfringens food poisoning (10 to 20 hours)
Salmonella food poisoning (12 to 18 hours)

Short incubation periods, 2 to 9 days

- Streptococcal infections—scarlet fever, erysipelas, puerperal infection, tonsillitis
- Staphylococcal air-borne infections—pemphigus neonatorum
- Pneumonia
- Diphtheria
- Influenza
- Meningitis
- Dysentery
- Infantile gastroenteritis
- Paratyphoid
- Anthrax
- Gonorrhoea

Long incubation periods, 10 to 21 days

- Lassa fever—usually 10 days
- Smallpox—usually 12 days
- Chickenpox—usually 17 to 21 days
- Rubella—usually 17 to 20 days
- Measles—usually 12 days
- Whooping cough—usually 14 days
- Mumps—usually 17 to 20 days
- Typhoid—usually 14 days
- Poliomyelitis—usually 11 to 14 days
- Q fever—usually 19 days
- Syphilis—usually 21 to 25 days
- Rabies—14–42 days
- Infective hepatitis—usually 18 to 45 days

Bacteriological or Virological Investigations

These are most important in all investigations of communicable disease. They aim at:

1. confirming the diagnosis
2. discovering which close contacts are carriers
3. demonstrating a source of infection, e.g. a contaminated foodstuff in food poisoning

If possible, the pathogenic organism should be isolated. This may be by blood culture (typhoid, meningococcal septicaemia), nose and throat swabs (streptococcal infections, diphtheria), sputum (tuberculosis, pneumonia), faeces (typhoid, dysentery, poliomyelitis) or throat washing (influenza).

In air-borne bacterial disease, nose and throat swabs are taken. In tuberculosis, sputum tests, both by direct examination and culture, should be carried out on all patients. In faecal-borne disease specimens of faeces or rectal swabs of patients and contacts should always be examined. In most outbreaks, it is usual to find a symptomless carrier. If such a person works with foodstuffs, he may easily cause further infections. In some virus diseases, electron microscopy is used to study the morphology of the virus particles (this is used in the identification of smallpox virus).

Blood tests on antigen-antibody reactions often provide valuable diagnostic aids. These include precipitation tests as in grouping and typing of streptococci, or agglutination tests, e.g. Widal tests for salmonella infections. Usually, such tests only give a retrospective diagnosis. This is because a positive result depends on demonstrating a rising titre of antibody in the patient's blood in specimens collected (*a*) very early in the disease and (*b*) about six weeks later.

In some instances, the source of infection may be a human carrier. A carrier is a person who is harbouring and excreting the pathogenic bacteria or virus without suffering from any symptoms. Human carriers are of two kinds:

1. *Convalescent carriers* have had the disease recently and, during their convalescence, still excrete the causative organism. In many infectious diseases, such as diphtheria, streptococcal infections, typhoid fever, dysentery and poliomyelitis, convalescent carriers are common. But such carriers are usually temporary and excrete organisms for a few weeks only. Occasionally, convalescent carriers may become permanent carriers. An example is a chronic typhoid carrier who will intermittently excrete typhoid bacilli in the faeces all his life.

2. *Symptomless carriers.* These are people who have never suffered from the disease or had any symptoms but who are excreting the pathogenic organism. Such carriers probably have had a sub-clinical attack of the disease. Examples include typhoid, dysentery, salmonella food poisoning, and poliomyelitis. Symptomless carriers may be temporary or permanent. Carriers may be further classified as:

1. nasal carriers: streptococcal and staphylococcal infections, diphtheria
2. throat carriers: streptococcal infections, diphtheria, meningococcal infections
3. faecal carriers: typhoid, poliomyelitis, dysentery
4. urinary carriers: typhoid

Before any investigation can be started, it is essential to know the location of every case. For this reason, the majority of infectious diseases are compulsorily notifiable—they must be reported immediately to the 'proper officer', a doctor on the staff of the AHA nominated for this purpose. In metropolitan districts, single London districts and in single district AHAs, this will normally be the *Area Specialist in Community Medicine (Environmental Health)*. In other areas, the doctor will be the appropriate District Community Physician. A small fee is paid to the doctor for each notification. The complete list of notifiable diseases is:

Acute meningitis
Anthrax
Cholera
Diphtheria
Dysentery (amoebic or bacillary)
Encephalitis (acute)
Food poisoning
Infective jaundice
Lassa fever
Leptospirosis
Leprosy
Malaria
Marburg disease
Measles
Ophthalmia neonatorum
Plague
Poliomyelitis (acute)
Rabies
Relapsing fever
Scarlet fever
Smallpox
Tetanus
Tuberculosis
Typhoid and paratyphoid
Typhus
Whooping cough
Viral haemorrhagic diseases
Yellow fever

It is helpful to remember the few communicable diseases which are *not* notifiable:

Common cold
Chickenpox
Rubella (German measles)
Sexually transmitted diseases
Mumps
Influenza
Pneumonia

Sexually transmitted (venereal) diseases have never been made notifiable in the United Kingdom because it is feared that to do so would result in much concealment of infections and encourage inadequate treatment. Certainly those countries which have insisted upon notification have a higher rate of infection.

Factors Connected with the Development of Communicable Diseases

There are three main factors which determine the development of communicable disease:

Environment

The ease of spread of communicable disease depends on the environment. Air-borne infections are commoner in winter time when cold conditions encourage overcrowding in houses with a subsequent greater risk of aerial infection. Gastrointestinal diseases, on the other hand, are commoner during the summer months when warm weather assists bacterial multiplication in infected foodstuffs or when insects, such as flies, are found. This seasonal incidence is an example of the effect of environment.

Bad housing conditions including overcrowding and lack of adequate ventilation will further aid the spread of communicable diseases. Many tropical diseases are spread by insects and the presence or absence of such vectors determines the level of disease.

Properties of the infecting bacteria or viruses

The two main factors are the *virulence of the bacteria or virus* and the *size of the infecting dose*. With a bacteria of high virulence, the size of the infecting dose will be small and *vice versa.*

Characteristics of the patient being attacked

This is mainly connected with the resistance of the patient to the disease and depends on both local and general immunity, which may be natural or artificial.

In an individual subject with risk of infection, the end result may be: development of serious attack; development of mild attack; development of subclinical attack; development of a symptomless carrier state; escape of infection.

Which of these five possibilities occurs mainly depends upon the relative importance of the environmental factors, the properties of the infecting organism and the immunity of the patient. In very adverse conditions where there are bad environmental or living conditions, or where very virulent bacteria or viruses attack a person with no immunity, a serious case of the disease will probably develop rapidly. On the other hand, an infection with a mildly virulent bacterium in a person with a good resistance will probably result in no development of disease. Between these two extremes all types of result may follow—a normal attack of the disease, a very mild attack which may not be recognized (subclinical attack) or the development of a carrier state.

Complete avoidance of the risk of infection is not usually possible with many common infectious diseases. But in some instances (e.g. Lassa fever) avoidance of importation of the disease or control of any imported source (travellers who have been in contact with the disease) is one of the best ways to prevent the disease.

The virulence of the bacterium or virus is always important. The sudden emergence of a new strain of a bacterium or virus with an increased invasiveness can be a major factor in producing an epidemic. The unexpected development of a serious streptococcal septicaemia is usually explained by accidental infection with a very virulent organism.

The size of the infecting dose is also important and varies in different infectious diseases. In smallpox, measles, typhoid and cholera, the minimum dose of organism which will lead to infection is small. In such diseases, the *threshold of infection* is said to be low—the diseases are extremely infectious. In other illnesses, such as whooping cough or salmonella food poisoning, the threshold of infection is higher—it is necessary for the minimum infecting dose to be much bigger and, consequently, such diseases are not as infectious.

Local resistance can be lowered by factors such as injury or cold. The development of a common cold after chilling in winter is probably due to a temporary lowering of local resistance. However, the most important factor is the presence or absence of general immunity.

Natural immunity may be genetic, for there are differences in the resistance shown by different races in the world. Such immunity is connected with genetic factors and these are responsible for much variation in the natural resistance of different members of the same race. Thus, some families and individuals seem naturally to escape attacks while others readily fall victims to many communicable diseases. Artificial immunity is discussed in the next chapter.

10 Prevention of Disease by Immunization

In many communicable diseases an attack is followed by a varying period of immunity from further attacks. Not all communicable diseases are followed by such an immunity (e.g. the common cold), but in many the length of immunity is substantial and may last many years or even a lifetime. Whenever a person develops an immunity in this way, he does so by manufacturing special disease resistant bodies in his blood called *antibodies*. It is possible to copy this mechanism artificially by introducing into the human body modified bacteria, viruses or their products so that the individual does not suffer from the disease but develops antibodies and, therefore, an immunity to a natural attack. Artificial immunization and vaccination rely on this principle.

ARTIFICIAL IMMUNIZATION

Artificial immunization can be either active or passive. In *active immunity* a special product of the bacterium or virus (antigen) is introduced into the body, often by injection, but occasionally by mouth, which stimulates the human body to manufacture its own protective antibodies. In this way the patient makes his own protection. Artificial active immunity produced in this way is more satisfactory as it lasts a long time. Its only drawback is that it often takes one to two months for the human body to build up immunity actively.

In *passive immunity*, antibodies which have been made by first immunizing an animal or man are used to protect the patient. The great value of this method is that it gives immediate immunity, but this is very transient and rarely lasts longer than four to six weeks. It is, however, very useful either to treat a patient suffering from a disease, such as the giving of diphtheria antitoxin, or to give a temporary immunity to a person who has been in close contact with the disease and who may be incubating it. A disadvantage of passive immunity, which uses antibodies from animals, is that the patient may easily be sensitized to the protein of the animal and suffer from serum sickness. A more satisfactory passive immunity is obtained by using immunoglobulin, the active constituent of human blood which contains antibodies.

In preventive medicine, great use is made of active immunization but little of passive immunization.

Active Immunization and Vaccination

Communicable diseases attack in two main ways:

1. By a direct invasion process usually of a certain part of the body. Examples include the inflammation of the lung in whooping cough, of the small intestine in typhoid, or of part of the central nervous system in poliomyelitis.

2. By the bacteria producing a very powerful poison (toxin) as they multiply in the body. Examples include diphtheria and tetanus.

The first group of diseases can be prevented by immunizing with an antigen consisting of either the dead bacteria or viruses concerned (examples, typhoid prevented by typhoid-paratyphoid A and B vaccine (TAB)) or else by a modified or changed bacterium or virus such as Bacillus-Calmette-Guerin (BCG) in tuberculosis, Sabin vaccine in poliomyelitis, measles or rubella vaccines. In the latter four cases, the live bacterium or virus has undergone a mutation which results in the modified bacterium or virus being unable to produce the real disease in humans, but it can produce a modified reaction which will then be followed by an immunity.

In the second group of diseases a modified toxin (toxoid) is injected. Toxoid is harmless but has retained the antigenic properties of toxin so that its injection results in the patient actively developing his own antibodies which can counteract toxins.

After immunization or vaccination, the levels of antibodies

present (and therefore the level of immunity) will vary in different persons. Over a number of years, protection will gradually wear off as the level of antibodies declines. In people who originally had a low level of antibody production after immunization, this will occur earlier than in a patient who had an excellent antibody response. It is for this reason that even after immunization it is never possible to guarantee complete protection. Most diseases are usually prevented at least in 90% of people immunized. Even in those who do develop an attack after immunization, this is usually very mild.

Active immunization schedule for a child

Table 38 gives the usual programme of active immunization arranged for a child. At present in the UK, computer-linked immunization recording and computer-assisted appointment systems are available for approximately 58% of the child population.

TABLE 38 Active immunization for a child

Age	*Immunization*
3 months	Combined diphtheria, whooping cough and tetanus plus oral poliomyelitis (1)
5 months	Combined diphtheria, whooping cough and tetanus plus oral poliomyelitis (2)
11 months	Combined diphtheria, whooping cough and tetanus plus oral poliomyelitis (3)
12–18 months	Measles
5 years	Booster: Diphtheria, tetanus, poliomyelitis (oral or inactivated)
11–13 years	(Girls only) Rubella
10–13 years	BCG (to protect against tuberculosis; for tuberculin-negative children)
15 years	Booster: Tetanus, poliomyelitis (oral or inactivated).

Triple immunization against diphtheria, whooping cough and tetanus

These immunizations are combined for convenience. They are given first to the young baby at three to six months because it is important to prevent whooping cough early in life, when it can be a dangerous disease. The diphtheria and tetanus portions of this immunization are toxoids (the antigen produced by action of formalin on toxin). The whooping cough portion is a true vaccine—a mixture of killed pertussis bacteria. Injection of triple vaccine gives a sound immunity for four or five years.

Booster doses for diphtheria, tetanus and poliomyelitis vaccination are given when the child is aged five years, and again when the child is aged 15 years. It is also wise to give a booster dose of tetanus toxoid following any injury.

It is most important to realize that all three doses of the primary immunization must be given to ensure complete protection. The first injection is followed by hardly any immunity, the second produces a fair protection, while the third dose gives the most lasting protection. The ideal interval between injections is two months but it must never be less than one month or longer than four months.

Poliomyelitis immunization

It is usual today to use oral Sabin vaccine, which has the following advantages over the inactivated vaccine.

1. it is easier to administer—by mouth rather than by injection
2. it produces an immunity not only to a clinical attack of poliomyelitis, but also to a carrier state in the intestine
3. it can be given to close contacts to reduce the danger of an epidemic
4. it is free from the danger of allergic reactions which may accompany other administrative routes

All three types of poliomyelitis virus—types I, II and III—must be included in the immunization which should be offered to all the population up to the age of 40 years. It is usual to give three doses of a trivalent vaccine (containing all three types of virus). Each dose seeds the small intestine with one of the types of poliomyelitis virus which then grows rapidly and colonizes in the villi of the intestine. This produces a marked immunity against that type of virus. Once the intestine has been seeded by poliomyelitis virus of a particular type, it cannot be colonized again with the same type. So the second dose leads to colonization of one of the other types and the third dose with colonization and protection against all three types. *It is thus essential that three doses are given to ensure complete protection*. The vaccine can be conveniently given on a lump of sugar.

Measles immunization

Live vaccines only are now used as the killed vaccines failed to produce long-lasting immunity. The Scharz strain of live vaccine is used.

Immunization is by a single injection preferably at the age of one year and this is usually followed by a satisfactory immunity. Measles vaccines should not be given to any child with active tuberculosis or with an allergic history.

BCG vaccination against tuberculosis

Immunization against tuberculosis is undertaken using a live vaccine of the Bacillus-Calmette-Guerin (BCG) type. It is a modified (attenuated) bovine strain of *Mycobacterium tuberculosis* which has lost its power to cause disease in man but can still produce a small trivial skin lesion. The vaccine is inoculated intradermally and, after a short period, an immunity against tuberculosis develops. BCG immunization is only used on persons who are *tuberculin negative*—persons who have no skin sensitivity to tuberculin as shown by Mantoux or Heaf test. Four main groups of persons are immunized.

1. *Close contacts* (i.e. other members of the family) of a case of tuberculosis. This group includes the newborn baby if either parent has had tuberculosis.
2. *School children who are tuberculin negative* at the age of 10 to 13 years.
3. *Nurses and medical students who, in their occupations, are liable to run a greater risk of infection from tuberculosis*.
4. Children of certain immigrants (see p. 195).
   All groups should be tuberculin tested and those who are negative immediately vaccinated with BCG.

After vaccination with BCG, it is usual for a small discharging ulcer to develop which clears up in two to three months. This is quite normal and all that is required is for the lesion to be covered with a dry dressing. Occasionally BCG is accompanied by an axillary adenitis which normally resolves without further complications.

Anthrax

Immunization against anthrax has now been introduced for all workers at risk. A killed vaccine is used and primary immunization should be carried out by three doses of vaccine injected intramuscularly: the second injection is given six weeks after the first and the third 20 weeks later. One booster injection should be given annually.

Rubella immunization

After successful trials in the USA, active rubella immunization was started in the UK in 1970 for girls aged 11 to 13 years. A freeze-dried live attenuated virus vaccine is used of the Cendehill strain. A single dose is used and the vaccine has a storage life of one year at 2 to 8°C.

Vaccination of women of childbearing age is not recommended routinely as it is not known whether vaccine virus can reach or harm the fetus. If vaccination of such women is requested, a serological test, which can be carried out by the Public Health Laboratory Service, should always be undertaken. Vaccination should only be offered to those who are seronegative (approximately 75% women aged 16 to 40 years have immunity already). It is most important that a woman is not pregnant at the time of vaccination or becomes pregnant for at least two months after protection. Probably the immediate post-partum period is safest, but even at such a time, a further pregnancy must be excluded.

Immunization following injury

Tetanus

A booster dose of tetanus toxoid should be given following any injury and particularly a street accident or any injury where the wound could have been contaminated with soil.

Rabies

Active immunization is arranged immediately after a patient has been bitten by a rabid animal. Human diploid cell rabies vaccine is used and the course consists of 14 daily subcutaneous injections into the abdominal wall with booster dose 10 days later and a final booster dose 20 days after that. For persons at special risk (i.e. handling animals that may be rabid) two immunizations are used and are given four to six weeks apart. Booster doses follow six months later and subsequently every three years.

Immunization for Persons Travelling Outside the UK

Immunization against typhoid and paratyphoid fevers. Typhoid and paratyphoid fevers can be prevented by giving a course of typhoid paratyphoid ABC vaccine (TAB) which is a suspension of killed typhoid and paratyphoid bacteria. Two doses are given at intervals of not less than 10 days or more than two months. Booster doses should be given every two years.

TAB immunization should be given to all who are going to travel in countries in which primitive water supplies are common. These include all tropical countries, Italy, Spain and North Africa. It is also a wise precaution if camping in Europe.

It is usual to suffer from a mild reaction after TAB inoculations—the patient complains of a headache and has a slight pyrexia for a few hours.

Immunization against yellow fever. Yellow fever is a serious tropical disease which is limited to a narrow band of country in mid-Africa and central South America. A most effective immunization is given by injection of a live attenuated strain of virus which produces immunity. Very stringent storage conditions are essential for this vaccine which is freeze-dried. For this reason, special centres have been set up in this country to give yellow fever vaccination and it can only be given at such centres. Immunization is only necessary for persons visiting those parts of Africa or South America where the disease occurs but for all such travellers, immunization against yellow fever is compulsory.

Immunization against cholera. Cholera vaccine is of less value in controlling the spread of cholera than in conferring some temporary protection against clinical illness in individuals who travel to countries where the disease occurs. Immunization against cholera is only necessary for travellers visiting certain parts of India or other countries where cholera occurs. The immunization is by means of a vaccine (a suspension of killed cholera bacteria in equal parts of Ogawa and Inaba serotypes prepared from smooth cultures of the classical biotype of *Vibrio cholerae*), and consists of two inoculations with at least two weeks in between each dose. Moderately severe reactions may follow this inoculation. Recently the effectiveness of such vaccines has been reported by WHO to be low and of short duration.

Smallpox vaccination. With the virtual disappearance of smallpox, this is now very rarely used. The vaccination depends on the substantial protection given within 10–14 days to any person by artificially infecting (or vaccinating) a small area of the skin with the relatively mild disease cowpox. Re-vaccination has to be carried out every three years.

General Contraindications to Immunization

Wherever possible, immunization should not be carried out in patients who have recently been ill or are in poor health.

Live vaccines (oral poliomyelitis, measles, smallpox, rubella, BCG) should *not* be given to children suffering from: leukaemia, Hodgkin's disease, other malignant conditions, hypogammaglobulinaemia; or undergoing corticosteroid or immunosuppressive treatment; or women in the early months of pregnancy.

Passive Immunization

Human immunoglobulin can be used for passive immunization to prevent infections in the close contacts of three diseases, rubella, measles and infective hepatitis.

In rubella (German measles) passive immunization can be used to prevent infection in a woman contact in the first 12 weeks of pregnancy. It is, of course, not used if the woman has either had the disease or has been immunized actively when aged 11 to 13 years (see p. 185). An attack of rubella at this stage of pregnancy often leads to a miscarriage or to the birth of a congenitally malformed child (see p. 112). Because of this, any woman at this time who has been in contact with a case of rubella and who has never suffered from the disease should be given 2·0 g of immunoglobulin.

In measles, immunoglobulin is only used to protect a child already ill who has been in contact with the disease and in whom the additional strain of an attack of measles might be very serious. In practice, this immunization is usually only given to contacts in a paediatric ward when measles occurs. The normal protecting dose of immunoglobulin is 0·4 g for children under two years and 0·75 g for older children.

In infective hepatitis, a small vulnerable population (such as those attending a day centre for physically or mentally handicapped persons) can be protected against an epidemic of infective hepatitis by using immunoglobulin. The dosage used is 500 mg for everyone except those under the age of 10 years when it is 250 mg.

11 Epidemiology of Air-borne or Droplet Infections

BACTERIAL DISEASES

Streptococcal Infections

Causative organism: Streptococcus haemolyticus Group A.
Incubation period: (Short) 2 to 7 days.

These include such varied diseases as scarlet fever, erysipelas, puerperal fever, tonsillitis, cellulitis, septicaemia and rheumatic fever. Infection usually spreads from another case or from a nasal or throat carrier either directly by droplets or indirectly by infected dust. It is most important to realize that the same type of streptococcus may cause scarlet fever in one patient, tonsillitis in another and even puerperal pyrexia in a woman recently confined.

Scarlet Fever

Incidence

Scarlet fever is still commonly seen in the United Kingdom but is usually mild. In the three years 1974–6 an average of 10 400 cases were notified in Great Britain. It is commoner in winter than summer and is caused by infection with a strain of *haemolytic streptococcus which produces an erythrogenic toxin in a patient who has no immunity to this toxin*. If the patient has an immunity to the erythrogenic toxin, no skin rash develops although other symptoms (e.g. tonsillitis) will occur. Such a case can readily infect another person who, if he has no immunity, will develop a rash and be diagnosed as scarlet fever. For this reason, the source of infection may be a carrier, a patient with tonsillitis or another case of scarlet fever.

Method of spread

Scarlet fever is spread by air-borne infection via droplets and dusts.

Control

Home isolation is sufficient except in severe cases or unless there are special dangers of further infection, e.g. a home attached to a food shop or dairy.

Children can return to school when complete clinical recovery occurs.

Secondary Streptococcal Infections

Secondary streptococcal infections used to be a major problem in puerperal pelvic infection and in cross infection within hospitals. Because of the sensitivity of streptococci to antibiotics and chemotherapy, secondary streptococcal infections are now far less serious than staphylococcal and other infections (see below). The danger is still present and is greatest in surgical wards where great care must be taken in dressing wounds. No wound should be dressed shortly after the ward has been cleaned or beds made because of the danger of circulating infected dusts.

Since many normal persons carry pathogenic streptococci in their noses and throats, it is still most important to maintain aseptic conditions in surgical theatres and in midwifery practice. Sterile masks, caps, gowns and gloves must always be worn by doctors and midwives attending deliveries in home or hospital. Special sterilized packs are supplied free for all home confinements. No midwife with a nasal or throat infection should attend a mother in her confinement. In such circumstances, the midwife must remain off duty until bacteriological examination of her nasal and throat swabs are normal. If an unexpected puerperal infection occurs, the nasal and throat swabs of all who attended the birth must be examined to exclude carriers.

Staphylococcal Infections

Causative organism: Staphylococcus aureus.
Incubation period: 4 to 7 days.

Staphylococcal infections are responsible for pemphigus neonatorum, for a number of cross infections in hospitals, some cases of bacterial infections and for a small proportion of toxin food poisonings (see pp. 211–212).

Pemphigus Neonatorum

This highly infectious and dangerous disease is, fortunately, rare, but mortality from complications may be considerable in some outbreaks. It is spread by:

a. contact with a person with a purulent staphylococcal lesion *or*
b. air-borne infection

It is important to isolate the infant immediately and, if possible, away from the maternity unit; it is best to admit the mother and child to an infectious disease hospital.

Prevention

The following are important preventive measures:

1. early diagnosis to enable prompt isolation—all skin blisters in infants should be swabbed
2. early discharge home of remaining mothers and babies to reduce the chance of cross infection
3. in outbreaks which are not immediately controlled, new admissions to the maternity unit should be stopped

Hospital Infections

Many different types of bacteria can produce hospital infections. Strains of *Staphylococcus aureus* that are resistant to antibiotics are an important cause of hospital infection. Recently many Gram-negative bacilli, including *Pseudomonas pyocyanea*, *Escherichia coli*, *B. proteus*, have become more troublesome in this respect.

Whenever cases of hospital cross infection suddenly occur, a full bacteriological survey must be undertaken. It is also important to isolate the patient, as removal of the source of bacterial infection is essential to control further infections especially in cases of *Pseudomonas pyocyanea*.

It is helpful to appoint a *Hospital Infection Control Officer* who may be a bacteriologist or hospital sister who coordinates the work of controlling the spread of infection. The function of such an officer includes:

1. collection of records of hospital infections
2. encouraging prompt recognition and isolation of infected patients
3. checking ward techniques (barrier nursing)
4. supervising routine checks of staphylococcal carrier rates in staffs in operating theatres
5. following up and coordinating with the investigation of discharged patients. In this respect close links must be built with the *Area Specialist in Community Medicine (Environmental Health)*—or *District Community Physician* responsible for investigating outbreaks of communicable disease in the community

Diphtheria

Causative organism: Corynebacterium diphtheriae.

Incubation period: 2 to 7 days.

This disease is now very rare. In the last five years the yearly average number of cases in Great Britain was 6. This compares with an annual average of 55 000 in the 10 years before the introduction of immunization in 1942 which produced this dramatic decline.

Prevention

Widespread active immunization in infancy is essential to maintain a low level of incidence.

Immediately a case is reported, an investigation should be started to discover the source of the infection (this is usually another case or carrier). Nasal and throat swabs should be taken from all close contacts (members of same household or class).

Other children in the same family should be excluded from school until bacteriological tests are completed and any close contacts who are food handlers should also be excluded from work. Child contacts previously immunized should be given an immediate booster immunization. Adult contacts should be Schick tested to find susceptible contacts (all Schick positives are susceptible), but children who have never been immunized can be assumed to be susceptible. All susceptible contacts should be given a small dose of antitoxin (500 units).

Daily visits should be paid to the family by a health visitor to check whether any contact has developed symptoms. This is important as early diagnosis is essential if treatment with antitoxin is to be effective.

If any of the contacts are found to be carriers, a virulence test must be carried out on the *Corynebacterium diphtheriae* isolated as a minority of them are avirulent. No carrier should be implicated as a source of infection until it has been confirmed that he is a carrier of virulent organisms. Positive carriers should be treated with antibiotics and no carrier should be assumed to be clear until a succession of negative nasal and throat swabs have been reported.

Meningitis

Causative organisms: various bacteria

In 1976, 1876 cases were notified in England and Wales. Many different bacteria have been responsible for bacterial meningitis—the largest group (718 cases) were caused by meningococci (*Neisseria meningitidis*) with pneumococci and haemophilus being the next commonest causes. Other bacteria responsible include staphylococci, *Escherichia coli*, *Klebsiella aerogenes*, *Pseudomonas pyocyanea*, *Proteus* spp. and *Mycobacterium tuberculosis*.

Tuberculosis

Causative organism: Mycobacterium tuberculosis.

Incubation period: Unknown but probably weeks.

In England and Wales in 1976, 7712 cases of pulmonary tuberculosis were traced; 4944 occurred in men and 2768 in women and, in the same year, 576 persons died from the disease.

The present ratio in incidence between the sexes of almost 2:1 males:females has been a characteristic for the last 10 years in the UK. It is also interesting to note that approximately 51% of male cases occurred in those aged 45 years and over and this trend is increasing, for tuberculosis is becoming more and more a disease of middle-aged and elderly men. There has been a marked reduction in new cases during the last 25 years—in 1950, 42 435 infections were traced (23 752 in men and 18 683 in women) with 15 969 deaths.

Regional and international differences

It is not always realized that the incidence of tuberculosis varies considerably within the UK. A clear indication of this variation is given by comparing the standardized mortality ratio (SMR) for the UK for 1971 (see Table 39).

TABLE 39 Standardized mortality ratio tuberculosis, 1971 (UK = 100)

	Males	*Females*
England and Wales	95	94
Scotland	153	157
Northern Ireland	98	98

It will be seen that the rate in Scotland is significantly higher than that in England and Wales and in Ireland.

The lowest notification rates are in East Anglia (6 per 100 000 and the *highest in North West Thames Region (27 per 100 000)*. The main factor in these differences is thought to be the proportion of Asian immigrants in these communities.

There is a higher incidence in Finland, Geımany, France, Italy and in all the Eastern European countries. The rate in England is similar or rather higher than that of Holland, Denmark, Norway or Sweden.

Tuberculosis in immigrants

There have been many investigations recently which have demonstrated that the level of infection of tuberculosis is much higher in Afro-Asian immigrants into the UK. The problem is, however, only a serious medical one in certain urban communities in the north and midlands and in London. Pakistani immigrants have been shown to have an incidence at least 26 times greater than the native born population and Indian immigrants 12 times greater. Other immigrants show a much lower incidence—six times greater. These surveys have shown ample evidence of spread of infection among the immigrant populations themselves although *there is no evidence of spread from the immigrants to the native born population*. Because of these facts, an extra-careful check is made on entry of all immigrants who should be X-rayed on arrival. Non-pulmonary forms of tuberculosis are relatively much commoner in young adult immigrants and may give rise to atypical manifestations of the disease.

Method of spread

Occurs by droplets via infected sputum from a known or an unsuspected case. Bovine tuberculosis has virtually disappeared in the UK and milk is no longer a vehicle of infection. In countries with a bovine tuberculosis problem, milk can be an important source if drunk raw. Consumption of infected meat can also spread tuberculosis, but proper meat inspection should prevent this problem.

Prevention of tuberculosis

The responsibility for prevention of tuberculosis rests with chest physicians, community physicians, specially trained health visitors called tuberculosis visitors, who are usually attached to chest clinic teams for preventive work, and general medical practitioners. Early diagnosis and the discovery of unsuspected infections are of great value. Detailed preventive work includes:

Tracing of infection

When any new case is diagnosed, it is essential to search for the cause of infection, which is likely to be someone living or working with the patient. This 'contact tracing' is the basis of prevention and consists of X-raying, usually by mass miniature radiography, all adult contacts. For children under the age of 15 years, a tuberculin skin test should be carried out and a large chest X-ray film taken of those with a positive reaction.

Prevention of tuberculosis will only succeed if *all* contacts are

X-rayed, as there is a tendency for those with minor symptoms to be reticent about having an X-ray and it is one of the tasks of tuberculosis visitors to ensure that this is done. As there is a preponderance of tuberculosis infection in men over the age of 50 years, special attention is paid to this group. It is *most important to realize that a person may have a heavily infected sputum and yet be able to carry on a normal life*. Therefore, the absence of any symptoms should never be used as an excuse to dispense with an X-ray in a contact.

Steps to reduce the chance of infection

Sputum disposal. The tuberculosis visitor should teach every patient about the safe disposal of sputum. Expectoration should always be into a plastic sputum bottle containing a small amount of sterilizing fluid and later the contents should be washed down a water closet and never brought into the kitchen.

Housing. Overcrowded housing and sleeping accommodation produce conditions favouring the spread of tuberculosis. Unless the patient is married, he should *always* have his own bedroom. Where the patient is married, the couple can share the same room but should use twin beds. It is most important that no parent who has had tuberculosis should ever sleep in the same room as a child. Equally no child with tuberculosis should share a room with other children. If the home of the patient is not large enough to allow the patient to have a separate bedroom, immediate rehousing is essential to avoid infection spreading through the family. Most local authorities have special priority housing schemes which enable such patients to be rapidly rehoused.

Occupation. Special precautions are taken to ensure that no one with tuberculosis is employed in an occupation where he is likely to spread the disease. All entrants to Teachers' Training Colleges must have a clear chest X-ray and periodic check-ups for teachers are encouraged. Routine chest X-rays are carried out on nursery nurses, and other persons working with young children.

It is illegal for a person with open tuberculosis to be employed in the food trade.

Follow up. All patients are carefully followed up for at least five years after infection and this should include: (*a*) visits to a chest clinic (for clinical check-up with X-rays) and (*b*) home visits by tuberculosis visitor to ensure that social factors there have not deteriorated, for if this happens a relapse is more likely. A watch is kept on the nutrition of the patient, who is also advised not to become overtired. Home visits should be made once in six months even when the patient's condition is quiescent. In women patients, this will ensure that any pregnancy will be known to the tuberculosis visitor before full term.

Pregnancy in a patient whose tuberculosis is controlled is likely to do no harm, but everything must be done to help the mother to meet this extra challenge. Delivery should take place in hospital and she should have five to six weeks' convalescence afterwards. Her baby should be vaccinated with BCG. If the problem of pregnancy is known early, it is usually possible to make satisfactory arrangements for the care of the baby and family. But if the history of past tuberculosis is only discovered in the puerperium, the mother may discharge herself to look after her baby and family, and in this way runs a risk of relapse and of spreading infection to her family.

Chemoprophylaxis

The use of drugs to prevent infection is now widespread. *Primary chemoprophylaxis* is the use of drugs to prevent infection in those particularly at risk, e.g. newborn babies of mothers with positive sputum. *Secondary chemoprophylaxis* is the use of drugs in tuberculin-positive persons who have no clinical evidence of tuberculosis, to prevent the development of clinical disease.

In treatment of clinical cases, the use of drugs is effective both in curing the individual and in reducing infectivity at an early stage. *Constancy of drug treatment is essential.*

Recent studies have shown that many such patients fail to take their drugs regularly and this not only reduces the efficacy of the treatment but increases the chance of drug resistance developing.

Immunization with BCG

The ingestion of live *Mycobacterium tuberculosis* may or may not result in a recognizable clinical infection of tuberculosis. In many instances the patient develops sufficient resistance and immunity to prevent a clinical infection, but in every case a skin sensitivity develops. If later a minute quantity of old tuberculin or purified protein derivative (PPD) is introduced into the skin of such a person by intradermal injection (Mantoux test) or by multiple puncture (Heaf test), a sharp reaction or flare occurs. This is called a positive tuberculin skin test. It means that, at some time in the past, the patient has ingested live *Mycobacterium tuberculosis* and all such persons should be X-rayed, as occasionally a latent infection will be found. If no disease is discovered, it can be assumed that there is enough immunity to resist infection. In this way, the tuberculin skin tests, although tests of hypersensitivity, can be used as indicators of immunity to tuberculosis.

Immunization should be offered to all negative reactors in the following groups:

1. all family contacts of cases
2. all medical students and nurses
3. all schoolchildren aged 10 to 13 years
4. children of immigrants (and especially newborn babies) in whose communities there is a high incidence of tuberculosis irrespective of their age

Weak positive reactions to the tuberculin test are no longer regarded as a contraindication to BCG vaccination. Heaf Grade 1 reactors should be offered BCG.

In 1972 the Medical Research Council published its report on its 20-year controlled trial of BCG vaccination. 55 000 children aged 14 to 15½ who were negative reactors were either vaccinated with BCG or vole bacillus vaccine or left unvaccinated. In practice it has proved to be an effective vaccine, with only minor side effects, giving protection which certainly lasts 13 years and probably longer.

Mass miniature radiography

The main danger of spreading tuberculosis comes from undetected cases who are sputum-positive but as yet undiagnosed. In some cases, the disease can become so chronic that such a patient may be infectious for years without anyone discovering the fact. Once diagnosed, the danger of infection can quickly be minimized by both treatment and preventive measures. Mass radiography plays an important part in discovering these unknown infections, and about 15% of all tuberculosis infections discovered were diagnosed as a result of mass miniature radiography. Over 95% of those X-rayed can be cleared on the small film and the remaining 5% are recalled for a large film on which a final diagnosis is made. Mass radiography can be used: (*a*) in the investigation of cases to screen contacts; (*b*) to allow general practitioners to order routine chest X-rays; (*c*) in special industrial surveys; (*d*) in surveys to examine special age groups.

Widespread community surveys are no longer used. The most effective results are in screening contacts and in the general practitioner referral group—the incidence of cases found needing treatment is four times that of the industrial survey.

VIRUS DISEASES

Influenza

Causative organism: Influenza viruses are now typed into three strains, A, B and C. Most epidemics are caused by strain A, strain B being a secondary cause. Strain C does not cause epidemics.

Incubation period: 1 to 3 days.

Incidence

The disease is endemic during the winter. Epidemics occur irregularly every two to six years and often are worldwide in distribution (pandemic). Influenza is spread by droplet infection.

Prevention

The rather limited success of active immunization has in the past been due to vaccine being prepared from strains which are different from the virus causing the current epidemic. Recently viruses have been developed by genetic recombination of naturally occurring strains of influenza A virus with a low yield in laboratory culture with high-yielding laboratory-adapted strains. These recombinant strains are indistinguishable from the naturally occurring parent and are used to prepare vaccine. The advantage of this process is that vaccines can now be prepared reasonably quickly after the appearance of a new variant of influenza A virus.

The WHO plays an important role in influenza prevention.

Recently many new variants have first appeared in the southern hemisphere or Far East and this has enabled vaccines to be prepared against these new strains to protect individuals in the UK.

Even with new techniques effective vaccines may be in short supply, so essential workers should be protected first together with other 'at risk' groups of the community such as the elderly, persons with asthma and those suffering from certain chronic diseases.

Measles

Causative organism: A virus.
Incubation period: 10 to 14 days (usually 12).

Incidence

Large-scale epidemics occur among children usually with a peak outbreak on average every two years, especially in large towns.

Since the introduction of immunization in 1966, a reducing trend of incidence of measles has been noted in Great Britain—cases notified varying in the last six years from 55 498 to 168 228.

A droplet infection, measles is usually relatively mild, the most serious feature being the complication of pneumonia or encephalitis. Provided the mother has had measles, the disease is rarely seen in children under six months of age.

Prevention

Immunization with measles virus vaccine (live attenuated) given at the age of one year (see p. 184). In ward infections in paediatric hospitals, passive immunization with immunoglobulin can be used (0·4 g for children under two years of age and 0·75 g for older children).

Rubella (German Measles)

Causative organism: A virus.
Incubation period: 17 to 20 days.

This is a mild disease the only significance of which is in differential diagnosis and the danger of congenital malformations developing in the baby if a woman develops rubella in the first three months of pregnancy. This risk only occurs during this stage of pregnancy.

Prevention

1. Avoidance of contact by any woman in early pregnancy with cases of rubella.
2. Active immunization of all girls aged 11 to 13 years. If older women are immunized, *it is essential to ensure that pregnancy does not occur for at least three months* following vaccination.
3. Passive immunization with immunoglobulin can be attempted for a woman who has never had the disease and has been in contact with a case during the first three months of pregnancy *but dosage must be high* (2·0 g).

Smallpox

Smallpox was on the brink of extinction from the world when a single case occurred following a laboratory infection in Birmingham, UK in August 1978. The following brief description is therefore still given.

Causative organism: Variola virus.

Incubation period: 10 to 14 days (usually 12).

Method of spread

Air-borne infection or contact with the disease. Smallpox is extremely infectious and air-borne infection has been traced over long distances. Indirect spread has often occurred through articles of clothing contaminated by patients and infection has been traced through laundries.

Diagnosis

This may be easy or very difficult depending on the degree of modification due to previous vaccination. The history of the patient's recent movements is most important and, as smallpox is invariably imported into the UK, there must be a connection with travel. It is also essential to know accurately the vaccination state of the contact, for anyone vaccinated a few years ago may show signs of 'modified smallpox'. The differential diagnosis from chickenpox may be difficult. In the classical attack with a well-developed rash, the distribution and type of rash are important points. Smallpox has a centrifugal rash, chickenpox a centripetal rash. Smallpox rash has deeper seated lesions than chickenpox and the rash in smallpox tends to develop steadily through its four stages—macule, papule, vesicle, pustule—in the same area of the body. The opposite occurs in chickenpox where the rash often shows 'cropping' with lesions of all stages present at the same time in the same area of the body.

Laboratory diagnosis in smallpox is a most helpful aid and must always be undertaken if there is any doubt. An unnecessary laboratory diagnosis is a small inconvenience compared with the serious mistake of a missed case of smallpox. Material for laboratory diagnosis should be collected as follows:

1. Maculopapular stage—clean skin with ether, scrape at least six lesions and make six thick smears on four glass slides. Allow to dry (*no heat*). Take 10 ml clotted blood in dry sterile bottle.
2. At vesicular and pustular stage—remove six to ten lesions and place in small bottle. Collect fluid from lesions in capillary tubes. Scrape base of six lesions and make six smears on four slides. Take 10 ml blood.
3. At crusting stage—remove as many scabs as possible (up to twelve) and place in a small bottle. These should be sent to the Public Health Laboratory.

Laboratory tests include egg-culture of blood, complement fixation tests using material collected and culture on the chorioallantoic membrane of 10 to 12-day-old fertile hen's eggs. This latter test is most sensitive but the result takes up to 72 hours. Growth is obtained with smallpox, cowpox and herpes simplex viruses but not with chickenpox. Examination by electron microscope gives the most rapid result.

Period of infectivity

The patient remains infectious until the separation of the last scab. This usually means the separation of the lesions on the feet.

Segregation of patient

All patients with smallpox *must* be nursed in a smallpox hospital. Under section 169 of Public Health Act 1936, there is power to remove patients to hospital who are suffering from a notifiable disease and this power should be used in the unlikely event of a smallpox patient refusing hospital admission.

Prevention

The prevention of smallpox at present depends on avoiding any laboratory infections. As smallpox only attacks human beings (no animal can be infected) the control of stocks of virus is crucial. Soon stocks will have to be concentrated in very few laboratories and then destroyed, under the control of WHO.

Prevention in any outbreak depends on early and correct diagnosis of any case and control of the spread of the disease by contact tracing and surveillance.

1. The steps to ensure *early and correct diagnosis* have been discussed above. Laboratory diagnosis is of great importance.

A panel of 'smallpox consultants' is maintained by the Department of Health and Social Security and they are available to advise any Area Medical Officer or 'proper officer' who is doubtful about the diagnosis.

2. Once a case of smallpox has occurred, further spread of the disease is prevented by: immediate revaccination or vaccination of all contacts; prophylactic treatment of close contacts with thiosemicarbazone (Marboran) or passive immunization with hyperimmune immunoglobulin; close daily surveillance of all contacts for 16 to 21 days.

a. If a person is successfully revaccinated within four days of contact his immunity will be boosted sufficiently to prevent him developing smallpox. Successful primary vaccination will usually protect him in the same way provided it is performed within three days of contact.

b. Very encouraging results have been reported by treating close contacts of a case of smallpox with thiosemicarbazone (Marboran). Each contact should be given two doses of 3 g by mouth after meals within a period of 12 hours. The tablets are very large and need to be chewed by the contact. To be of value, this drug *must* be given in the incubation period, usually on the eighth day. It is of no value if given after symptoms have developed.

c. Every contact must be traced, medically examined and vaccinated. Arrangements are then made to visit each contact daily, when an examination is made to ascertain that he is well and has not developed any symptoms or rash. This visit (surveillance) is repeated daily for 16 to 21 days after the last contact. If the patient develops any symptoms or signs, he must be immediately isolated.

Daily surveillance succeeds in preventing spread of infection because no patient developing smallpox becomes infectious until at least two to three days after his first symptom. Therefore, provided the patient is immediately isolated on developing the first symptoms, he is being removed and admitted to a smallpox hospital at least 24 hours before he becomes infectious. During this period of surveillance, there is no need for the movements of the contact to be restricted. If he is travelling he must tell the Area Medical Officer his itinerary so that arrangements can be made to continue his surveillance which must continue for at least 16 days. Because attenuated smallpox occasionally shows an extended incubation period it is safer to continue it for 21 days.

Widespread immediate vaccination of the general public will never control infection as it is never possible to immunize everyone. Availability of staff and materials rarely make mass vaccination practicable, but even if this could be undertaken there would be an increased risk of the rare but dangerous complication of encephalitis.

During an outbreak of smallpox, it is most important for the Area Medical Officer to: (*a*) notify all general practitioners of occurrence; (*b*) arrange for a domiciliary consultation service for any general practitioner who has doubtful cases; (*c*) notify immediately the DHSS on *suspicion* of a case; (*d*) keep in touch with Area Medical Officers of neighbouring areas.

During widespread outbreaks, chickenpox can be made locally notifiable.

12 Epidemiology of Faecal-borne and Food-borne Infections

BACTERIAL DISEASES

Typhoid or Paratyphoid Fevers

Causative organisms: Salmonella typhi casing typhoid fever and *Salmonella paratyphi* A, B or C, giving rise to paratyphoid.

Incubation period: Typhoid fever, 12 to 21 days (usually 14 days), paratyphoid fever, 2 to 7 days.

Incidence

Recently 100 to 182 cases of typhoid fever have usually occurred annually in England and Wales (182 in 1976). Many of these cases are in small isolated outbreaks. About 85% of the cases of typhoid occur in travellers who have contracted their infection abroad, especially in Italy, Yugoslavia, Portugal, Spain and North Africa. Only one-fifth of the cases of paratyphoid are infected abroad. Most cases traced in the UK have been caused by a food-borne infection. The mortality of typhoid fever has been reduced to about 1% by antibiotic therapy. In a large-scale epidemic, mortality is often lower due to rapid diagnosis and treatment.

Paratyphoid fever is now less common and is always associated with food-borne outbreaks and carriers play an important part in the spread of infection.

Method of spread

The eventual source of every infection is the faeces of a human case or carrier. Typhoid fever has a *low threshold of infection*.

This means that it can be spread by a very small dose of bacteria. Paratyphoid, however, has a much higher threshold of infection. The methods of spread include: (1) *Direct transmission*. This is rarely seen, but there is always a danger of infection to those nursing typhoid cases. For this reason, all cases of typhoid *must* be treated in an infectious disease hospital by staff previously immunized. It is hazardous to treat typhoid fever in a side ward of a general hospital; (2) *Indirect transmission*. This is, for example, by water, food, shellfish, milk and flies.

Water

In the last century, this was the most usual method of infection, but with the control of water supplies, it is very rare in well-developed countries to find such an outbreak, although it is still the usual method of spread in more primitive communities. The last serious water-borne outbreak of typhoid fever in this country was in Croydon in 1937 when 290 cases of typhoid fever occurred. It was caused by a urinary carrier contaminating the water supply while he worked on a deep well. In 1963 a water-borne outbreak in Zermatt, Switzerland, resulted in 434 cases.

Food

This is the main vehicle of infection today. Any foodstuff may be involved but prepared/cooked meat products are among the commonest. Although much publicity was given to the 1964 Aberdeen outbreak, which was caused by a 6 lb tin of corned beef which became infected with *Salmonella typhi* through the use of unchlorinated water during the cooling process following sterilization, canned foods generally are a rare cause of typhoid fever. Foodstuffs are most commonly infected by a carrier working in the kitchen and contaminating food. Ice cream can cause typhoid if contaminated with typhoid during manufacture (Aberystwyth outbreak in 1945). Compulsory pasteurization of ice cream in the UK prevents a recurrence of this method of spread.

Shellfish growing in polluted water may contain typhoid bacilli as it is usual for them to filter large quantities of water through their shells. Any bacteria in the water will remain in the shellfish. Subsequent consumption may lead to typhoid or paratyphoid fever.

Milk. Since widespread pasteurization of supplies, milk-borne typhoid fever has never been reported in this country. With primitive production methods, typhoid fever could be spread by milk contaminated directly or indirectly by a carrier.

Flies may, in primitive conditions, contaminate food by carrying *Salmonella typhi* from human faeces to foodstuffs. This is only likely where there are very primitive methods of faecal disposal such as trench latrines.

Period of infectivity

As long as *Salmonella typhi* or *S. paratyphi* are excreted in either the faeces or urine, the patient is infectious. It is usual for the uncomplicated case to excrete bacteria in the faeces for a few weeks, but about 7% continue to do so for three months and from 2 to 5% become chronic carriers. Faecal carriers far outnumber urinary carriers, who are rare. Faecal carriers are invariably intermittent, carrying for a short time, then ceasing to carry for a few weeks, so that routine random sampling will uncover few carriers.

Prevention

It is essential that all typhoid patients should be admitted to an infectious disease hospital. Early diagnosis is an important factor in prevention. Laboratory aids to diagnosis include:

Blood culture

The best time is first week of disease when over 80% of cases are positive. Subsequently the number of failures increases. Collect 5 to 10 ml blood.

Stool cultures

Positive results are found in the second week.

Urinary cultures

In a minority of patients, a positive culture in the urine is obtained usually during the third week.

Agglutination tests (*Widal reaction*)

Contrary to widespread belief, agglutination tests are less valuable diagnostic tests than culture of the organism in the blood, faeces or urine. To be conclusive, a rising titre of H and O agglutinins must be demonstrated. Blood must be collected as early as possible (first week) and compared with the results of samples collected four to six weeks later. This means that conclusive diagnosis is only possible retrospectively by this method. In an uninoculated person, an H titre of 1 in 50 and an O titre of 1 in 100 are highly suspicious of infection. It is most important to realize that previous inoculation (TAB) can cause ambiguous results especially with H agglutinins. The 'Vi' agglutination is useful to help trace carriers as often a carrier will have a high Vi titre (1 in 10).

In tracing the source of infection, a knowledge of the *phage type* of typhoid or paratyphoid organism responsible is essential. There are now 90 recognized and different phage types of *Salmonella typhi*, 50 of *Salmonella paratyphi* B and six of *Salmonella paratyphi* A. Isolation of the organism in blood, stool or urine enables this typing to be carried out.

The prevention of typhoid and paratyphoid fevers depends on: (*a*) full immediate investigation of cases to discover the cause; (*b*) control of chronic carriers; (*c*) food control—sampling at docks, pasteurization of milk and ice cream, prohibition of infected shellfish; (*d*) environmental hygiene; (*e*) immunization of holiday visitors to Italy, Yugoslavia, Portugal, Spain and Africa.

a. Carriers are responsible for most infections and any carrier who handles food of any description or who is employed by a water supply department may be most dangerous. For this reason, whenever a case of typhoid or paratyphoid fever occurs, a complete investigation must immediately be carried out to find the cause of the infection. A careful history is taken to discover what food was eaten by the victim and close contacts at the start of the incubation period, which is 14 days before the first symptoms in typhoid fever, and seven days in paratyphoid fever.

Immediate stool examinations must be carried out on all close contacts and especially on kitchen personnel. If a carrier is discovered, the typhoid bacteria are identified and typed by phage typing. This is then compared with that causing the outbreak. If the type is different, the carrier could *not* be the cause of the infection, but if it is the same, the carrier *may* have been responsible. The discovery of a carrier of the same type does not prove the cause and further epidemiological investigations are necessary.

The treatment of typhoid carriers is difficult. Prolonged antibiotic treatment occasionally cures the condition but usually is ineffective. Many faecal carriers are cured by cholecystectomy, but not all, as the bile duct may also be infected and cholecystectomy should not be advocated in carriers unless indicated clinically.

b. The only certain method of finding carriers is to follow up every case for many months after infection by regular fortnightly sampling of faeces and urine. By this means the chronic intermittent carrier will be identified.

Once a carrier is diagnosed, a careful check is kept on his occupation and family. *By law, no chronic carrier of typhoid or paratyphoid may be employed in the food trade.* Nor should a carrier be allowed to work in any kitchen, water department or school or similar institution.

c. Constant sampling of foodstuffs, pasteurization of milk and ice cream supplies and cleansing of shellfish are all important preventive measures. These are discussed in Chapter 16.

d. Careful methods of sewage disposal and purification and sterilization of water supplies have reduced the likelihood of any further water-borne outbreaks in the UK (see p. 305). The failure, however, to maintain such standards can be disastrous, as was illustrated by the Zermatt water-borne outbreak of typhoid.

e. Reference has already been made to the value of TAB immunization for travellers (see p. 186). It is also important to immunize: (i) family contacts of a chronic carrier; (ii) nurses in fever hospitals who must nurse any typhoid cases.

Dysentery (Bacillary)

Causative organism: There are four main groups of dysentery bacteria. *Shigella dysenteriae* and *Shigella bodyii* are largely confined to the Far East. In the UK *Shigella flexneri* is occasionally reported, but most of the cases are caused by *Shigella sonnei*.

Incubation period: 1 to 7 days (usually 3 to 4 days).

Incidence

Usually about 6000 to 9000 cases are notified annually in England and Wales (6217 in 1976). Deaths from dysentery now number under 10 per year (1 in 1976), and occur mainly in the very young or old. The disease is usually mild, and only serious in young babies or debilitated elderly people.

Method of spread

Sonne dysentery is spread by direct contamination from person to person. In a closed community, such as a ward or nursery, it spreads slowly at first but, as soon as a substantial proportion is infected, the outbreak develops much more quickly.

Prevention

Outbreaks of dysentery can be prevented by: (*a*) early diagnosis of first cases; (*b*) home isolation of cases and symptomless (contact) carriers.

a. This is especially important in day nurseries and hospital wards. All cases of diarrhoea, however mild or transient, should be bacteriologically examined (stool specimens or rectal swabs) to make certain that early cases are identified. It is usual to find a proportion of symptomless carriers among close contacts, but this carrier state only lasts from two to three weeks. Chronic carriers are unknown.

b. Provided action is taken early, careful investigation and isolation of all sources of infection (cases and carriers) will prevent a serious widespread outbreak. If a widespread outbreak has already developed, isolation will achieve little.

Food Poisoning

Apart from the rare chemical (tin, antimony) or fungal food poisonings (poisoning with *Aminata phalloides* or *Aminata muscaria*) bacterial food poisonings may be divided into:

1. toxic food poisoning caused by staphylococci; *Clostridium perfringens (cl. welchii)*; and botulism.
2. infective food poisoning, e.g. salmonellosis.

Toxin food poisonings

Toxin food poisonings are those in which the poisonous substance ingested is a bacterial enterotoxin produced by prior bacterial multiplication in the food. Once this toxin is present, the further role of the bacteria is unimportant and subsequent destruction of the bacteria (by heat—pasteurization) will not usually destroy the toxin, which is heat stabile, or render the food safe.

Staphylococcal toxin food poisoning

The ingestion of food containing an enterotoxin which has been produced by the multiplication of certain strains of staphylococci causes this type of food poisoning.

Incubation period: Very short--2 to 4 hours.

Incidence. Although varying from year to year, usually 1–2% of food poisoning episodes are traced to this cause. Fatalities have resulted from staphylococcal toxin food poisoning but are very rare.

Method of spread. In most instances, human staphylococcal lesions such as abscesses, paronychia, nasal infections or infected nails are the source of the contamination. Very occasionally, an outbreak has been traced to a staphylococcal lesion of the udder of cows leading to heavy contamination of milk.

The foods which are most often implicated in staphylococcal food poisoning are prepared meats. All types of cooked meats have been traced as vehicles of infection, the commonest being ham. Other foods which may be involved include canned foodstuffs—meats, fish and vegetables and, much less commonly, unpasteurized milk and its products.

Staphylococcal toxin food poisoning can occur only after a combination of the following events:

1. Contamination of the foodstuff with a strain of *Staphylococcus aureus* which is capable of producing an enterotoxin. Fortunately only a few strains can do this.
2. Food must provide a suitable culture medium—cold meats are a good medium for staphylococci and growth is not inhibited by the presence of salt in the meat.
3. Food must be stored at a sufficiently high temperature, 10 to 49°C, to encourage growth of the staphylococci—*enterotoxin is produced during multiplication of staphylococci in the food, and 8 to 12 hours' multiplication is necessary for production of a substantial amount of toxin.* Once staphylococcal enterotoxin has been produced in any food, it is difficult to destroy as it is heat stabile. This means

that even boiling a foodstuff already contaminated with enterotoxin would only destroy a small and insignificant amount of that toxin, although all staphylococci would be destroyed.

Although the simultaneous combination of factors (1), (2) and (3) occur only infrequently, the fact that over 10% of persons carry staphylococci in their noses means that potentially dangerous pathogenic bacteria will contaminate foods occasionally.

Prevention. Staphylococcal food poisoning can best be avoided by: (*a*) consuming foodstuffs wherever possible within two hours of preparation; (*b*) where this is not possible, food must *always* be stored in cool, refrigerated conditions which are too cold for bacterial multiplication (if no multiplication occurs, toxin will not be produced). (*c*) by ensuring scrupulously clean conditions while handling or preparing foods. A high degree of personal hygiene is important. Hands must be frequently washed and habits avoided which would encourage transfer of staphylococci from the nose and mouth of the food handler to foodstuffs. (Many of the rules laid down by the Food Hygiene Regulations cover these points.)

Clostridium perfringens (Cl. welchii) toxin food poisoning

This is an anaerobic spore-bearing bacterium which on multiplication can produce a heat stabile toxin which causes a mild food poisoning. There is increasing evidence that heating the spores tends to activate their germination. This 'heat shock' may well explain why so many outbreaks of this food poisoning follow heating up of precooked foods.

Incubation period: 10 to 20 hours.

Incidence and method of spread. The incidence of *Clostridium perfringens* food poisoning is increasing and the number of cases traced annually in England and Wales represent approximately 15% of all outbreaks. The spores of *Clostridium perfringens* are very widely disseminated in earth and faeces. *Anaerobic conditions are needed* for multiplication and toxin production. Meat dishes (stews, soups, boiled meats) are usually found to be the cause, especially if prepared some hours before consumption.

Prevention. It must be realized that it is almost inevitable that spores of *Clostridium perfringens* will gain access to kitchens on raw meat. This means that infection can only be avoided if the following strict rules are followed:

1. avoidance of precooking of meats
2. avoidance of storage of any food between 49°C and 10°C for more than three hours
3. if meats have to be precooked, it is essential that they are rapidly cooled and maintained below 10°C in a domestic refrigerator
4. care should always be taken when gutting animals such as rabbits to avoid contamination of the flesh with faeces in the intestines

Botulism

This is a very rare disease caused by toxins produced by the anaerobic *Clostridium botulinum*. It is a very serious disease with a high mortality. Cases are very rare in the UK (until the 1978 outbreak there had been no case for over 40 years). In 1978, four cases of botulism occurred (with one fatality and three other very serious paralysed cases) following consumption of a tin of red salmon. Cases are still reported in America and Europe. Most botulism in America has been traced to home-bottled vegetables in which there is inadequate sterilization with anaerobic conditions being produced. Prevention includes avoidance of bottling of any vegetables and proper control of commercial canning.

Infective food poisoning—salmonellosis

Infective food poisoning is a true bacterial infection in which the small intestine is attacked by various salmonella bacteria producing a gastroenteritis.

Causative organisms: Many types of salmonella organisms produce this food poisoning. There are over 1000 different serotypes but the commonest is *Salmonella typhimurium* which is responsible for about 40% of all cases. The next commonest serotypes are *S. heidelberg, S. agona, S. enteritidis* or *S. hadar.* Rare types of salmonellae are classified at the Salmonella Reference Laboratory at the Public Health Laboratory Service Headquarters at Colindale.

Incubation period: Usually 12 to 14 hours (limits, 8 to 48 hours).

Incidence

In the past 10 years salmonellosis has been the commonest food poisoning traced in the UK and is responsible for about 70% of all food poisoning outbreaks.

There is a wide variation in the severity of cases but the average patient has an illness of two to three days. Occasionally a severe case occurs in young children or the elderly. The mortality rate is usually in the order of 0·3%.

Method of spread

There are five main sources of infection: (1) human cases and carriers; (2) domestic animals and rodents; (3) eggs of ducks and hens; (4) pigs; (5) chickens.

Any one of these sources may lead to contamination of food. Evidence of typing of salmonella is tending to incriminate more and more the latter two sources and pork pies have been responsible for some of the latest large outbreaks. Heavy infections occur in ducks in which the oviduct is often involved leading to very heavily contaminated eggs. Hens' eggs are, fortunately, rarely infected and then usually with a light contamination.

Abattoirs can be important sources of salmonella contamination, as well as poultry farms. Recently it has been shown that there may be a high incidence of salmonellae in animal feeding stuffs, sundried fish meal and imported bone products. *Salmonella agona* first appeared in the UK in 1970 being imported in fish meal. As this product is widely used in feeding chickens and pigs reared by intensive farming methods, it spread rapidly.

Prevention

A complete epidemiological investigation must be undertaken whenever an outbreak of salmonellosis occurs. Specimens for bacteriological examination should be collected from all close contacts and kitchen personnel and any salmonellae isolated must be typed. If a carrier is found, it must *not* be assumed that he or she is necessarily the cause, for such a carrier may also have been infected in the outbreak. Any carriers who are food handlers must be kept away from work until they are clear. It is rare for salmonella carriers to become chronic as the carrier state usually lasts for only a few weeks.

Duck eggs are particularly liable to become heavily contaminated and should only be eaten as hard-boiled eggs (10 minutes boiling). Cases have been traced where duck eggs have been used for making cakes—the cooking may not completely destroy any salmonellae due to poor conduction of heat in cake mixtures. Egg products such as imported egg albumen should be pasteurized as laid down by the Liquid Egg (Pasteurization) Regulations, 1963. Similarly coconut products are best heat treated.

The risk of salmonella food poisoning can be reduced by the following:

1. Careful storage methods must be observed. Refrigeration of foods liable to contamination is most important to reduce the multiplication of any contaminating bacteria. This is especially important with *prepared meat products—meat or pork pies and cooked meats*. In shops such foods should constantly be kept in refrigerated conditions—special refrigerated display cabinets make this possible.
2. Extreme care must be taken in the handling and preparation of food, for this reduces the chance of a faecal carrier accidentally contaminating food.
3. Immediate bacteriological investigation of any diarrhoea or gastroenteritis, however mild, among food handlers. While awaiting results, such personnel should stop working.
4. Avoidance of unnecessary storage of prepared foods. If only all prepared foods were eaten promptly, or if any left over portions were thrown away (*not* stored), there would be a considerable reduction in such food poisoning. In this respect, it is most unwise to prepare the sweet today for lunch tomorrow unless it can be stored in a refrigerator.
5. Gamma radiation from a cobalt-60 source has been shown to be very useful in destroying salmonellae in frozen whole egg, coconut, imported meats and animal feeding stuffs.
6. Pasteurization of liquid milk as raw milk has been traced as the infecting agent in about 2–3% of cases.

Cholera

Causative organism: Vibrio cholerae including Eltor biotype, serotype Ogawa and serotype Inaba.

Incubation period: 2 to 3 days.

Incidence

Cholera last occurred in epidemic form in the UK in 1866 and was virtually absent from most Westernized communities until the recent Eltor outbreaks. It is endemic in India, Burma and the Philippines, but in 1970 a considerable epidemic of the Eltor strain spread outside this region to parts of Africa, Middle East and Turkey and parts of Europe. In 1971, three cases of imported cholera (Eltor serotype Ogawa) were treated in England. Modern rapid air travel facilitates the spread of such cases, and three more cases with the serotype Inaba occurred in 1974. No secondary cases occurred in either outbreak.

Method of spread

Contaminated water in the early stages of an epidemic and direct contact from cases later both contribute to the spread of the disease. Flies may also be responsible. The disease becomes epidemic in areas in India and the Far East during the hot, moist seasons before the rains and then rapidly subsides.

Period of infectivity

This depends on the presence of cholera vibrios in the stools—usually for 14 days but occasionally up to three months. Recent work in Eltor epidemics has shown that many infections with this serotype have no symptoms and that some may excrete the organism for up to four years.

Prevention

This depends on purification of water supplies and safe disposal of sewage and it is this factor which has been responsible for the disappearance of the disease in highly developed countries. In epidemics water or milk should be boiled (unless pasteurized) and careful segregation of all patients arranged with terminal and concurrent disinfection.

Active immunization should be arranged for those at special

risk (doctors, nurses) and for travellers. Immunization provides approximately 50% protection for a short period (few months). Re-immunization is, therefore, advisable for those at risk after six months. Under International Sanitary Regulations, the validity of a cholera vaccination certificate lasts for six months beginning six days after the first injection of vaccine.

Mass vaccination has proved of limited value because of the short period of protection and of the cost.

Infantile Gastroenteritis

This is a general description of a mixed group of severe gastrointestinal infections in young infants. Most have a short incubation period, two to five days. The exact causes include certain pathogenic strains of *Escherichia coli* including O 26, O 55, O 111, O 125, O 126, O 127, O 128 and O 229. Many enteroviruses (ECHO and Coxsackie B viruses) have also been identified as causes.

The disease is fortunately much less common now than it was 40–50 years ago. The incidence is greater in bottle-fed babies than in breast-fed children. Poverty and the associated conditions are important factors, for most cases of the disease occur in the overcrowded homes of social classes IV and V. Infantile gastroenteritis can be a very serious problem in paediatric hospitals and maternity units.

Prevention

Encouragement of breast feeding can do much to reduce the incidence of infantile gastroenteritis and *every effort should be made to keep breast feeding going if the infant develops an illness.* If the baby must enter hospital his mother should also be admitted so that breast feeding may be maintained.

The risk of hospital outbreaks can be minimized by arranging for all young babies to spend as little time as possible in hospital as there is no doubt that many attacks result from cross infection from infant to infant in the ward. It is therefore important that any infant with diarrhoea is immediately isolated and that no child with a history of diarrhoea be admitted to a clean infants' ward but sent to an isolation unit.

There is a particularly dangerous type of unidentified gastroenteritis which occasionally breaks out in the nursery unit of a maternity ward. As soon as such an attack is confirmed, *all new admissions to the maternity ward should be stopped and the ward emptied as soon as possible*—mothers and babies being discharged home early. By this action, the danger of widespread infection will be reduced.

Attempts to control the spread of infantile gastroenteritis by strict barrier nursing usually fail, probably due to the intensity of infection, the physiological incontinence of infants and the role that infected dusts play in spreading the disease.

VIRUS DISEASES

Poliomyelitis

Causative organism: A virus with three distinct types.
Incubation period: 10 to 16 days.

Since mass immunization started in the early 1960s, poliomyelitis has been a rare disease and less than 14 cases have occurred annually in Great Britain during the last 10 years. This virtual disappearance of the disease is dependent upon a continued high rate of immunization in young children followed by booster doses when aged 5 and 15 years. Poliomyelitis has a very marked seasonal incidence, the majority of cases occurring in late summer and early autumn. July to September, in the northern hemisphere and February and March in the southern hemisphere.

Those now attacked include people of all ages (originally the disease was only seen in very young children). There is a tendency for the disease to be more severe when older persons develop it.

Method of spread

Poliomyelitis is a faecal-borne disease spread mainly by close human contact. The following factors may precipitate attacks:

1. Tonsillectomy or tooth extraction if undertaken while the patient is carrying the virus in his throat or faeces. For this reason, in serious epidemics, or in close contacts, it is usual to suspend such operations.

2. Certain prophylactic injections if carried out *while the*

patient is incubating the disease. This type of attack, often called 'provocation' poliomyelitis, is not often seen and is usually mild, only affecting the group of muscles into which the injection was given. Lumbar puncture is contraindicated.

3. Violent exercise can lead to a more serious attack *if undertaken in the early meningitic phase of the disease.* Because of the danger of close contacts developing poliomyelitis, it is wise to limit violent exercise in the close contacts during the incubation period.

Prevention

Active immunization is the most effective method of preventing poliomyelitis and *efforts should be made to immunize all the population including booster doses at 5 and 15 years of age.* If a case develops, all the following should immediately be given an oral dose of poliomyelitis vaccine whether previously immunized or not:

1. all contacts at home, work and school
2. all persons living within an approximate radius of a quarter of a mile of the patient

This not only serves to boost their immunity, but also blocks the entrance of 'wild' or epidemic virus into their intestines and thus reduces the chance of further infection.

As far as possible, the family contacts of a case should be segregated from the general population during the incubation period and any children among them should be kept away from school for three weeks. Household contacts should also be placed under daily surveillance for three weeks and a health visitor should visit daily to check temperatures and to see whether they have any symptoms. If any abnormality is noted, the contact should be put to bed immediately and kept as quiet as possible.

Restrictions among the general population regarding swimming baths are probably useless in preventing poliomyelitis. However, swimming is a fairly violent form of exercise and should be avoided for three weeks by contacts. Reference has already been made to the postponement of elective tonsillectomy and dental extractions at epidemic times.

Segregation of patient

Paralytic cases should be admitted to a special unit in an infectious disease hospital. Mild cases treated at home should be segregated for at least three weeks.

Infective Hepatitis

Causative organism: Virus of at least two types and probably a third.

Incubation period: Exceptionally long, 15 to 45 days. (Much longer in serum hepatitis.)

Incidence

Sporadic cases and small outbreaks of infective hepatitis occur annually in the United Kingdom mainly in autumn and winter. *Infective jaundice* is now generally notifiable in England and Wales but this term includes infective hepatitis and serum hepatitis. This is caused by a different type of virus, a different epidemiology and is discussed on p. 231. 5954 cases of infective jaundice were notified in 1976. In all outbreaks a number of cases of infection without clinical jaundice can be traced.

Prevention

There is no method of active immunization. In contacts who are already ill with another disease, immunoglobulin has been used as a passive immunization and there is evidence that it has modified the severity of the resultant disease. Serum hepatitis which has an entirely different epidemiology and is caused by a different type of virus is discussed on p. 231.

Toxoplasmosis

Causative organism: Unicellular parasite: *Toxoplasma gondii.*

This disease is caused by infection of certain tissues of the body by the unicellular parasite, *Toxoplasma gondii*, approximately 700 cases occur each year in the UK. In adults, the infection follows the eating of raw or partly cooked meats containing the parasite and is often asymptomless but may produce a chronic chlororetinitis. It can also be spread to the human fetus *in utero* from an infected mother and symptoms in infants include jaundice with enlargement of liver and spleen, an encephalomyelitis, followed by hydrocephalus, microcephaly and retinochoroiditis. Most cases are diagnosed in infants, but skin tests have shown evidence of pest infection in adults. There is widespread infection in pork and mutton, but rarely in beef. Most infections in adults are caused by eating raw or inadequately cooked meats.

Prevention is mainly by destruction of *T. gondii* by:

1. heat—the parasite is killed on normal cooking
2. refrigeration—fortunately the parasite is particularly sensitive to low temperatures
3. radiation—low doses of gamma radiation will kill the parasites

Trichiniasis

This disease, which is worldwide but rarely seen in the UK, is caused by infestation with the worm *Trichinella spiralis*.

The adult worm is usually found attached to the intestinal wall of the pig or rat. Embryo worms are then deposited in the intestinal wall and later migrate, via the bloodstream, to the muscles where they develop small cysts (1 mm long)—the dormant stage. Occasionally man becomes infected by eating partially cooked pork which contains such cysts, and the same cycle then occurs in man with the adult worm developing in the intestine and embryo worms migrating to various muscles. Symptoms are produced during this migration—fever, muscular pains, tenderness and oedema of eyelids. If cardiac muscle is invaded, sudden heart failure may occur at this stage.

Control is maintained by careful meat inspection, including regular sampling of pig muscles by microscopic examination. Snippets of muscle from the diaphragm, flanks and cheeks are cut from the pig carcases after final inspection has been completed. Particular attention should be paid to sow carcases which are often used in sausage manufacture. Recently it has been shown that low doses of gamma radiation to carcases will kill any parasites. Probably the most certain method of avoiding this disease is to ensure that all pork products are properly cooked. Many recent outbreaks have been traced to the ingestion of infested partly cooked sausage meat. The disease is more common among the Germans, probably due to the habit of eating under-cooked pork.

13 Epidemiology of Other Communicable Diseases

DISEASES SPREAD FROM ANIMALS

Anthrax

Causative organism: Spore-bearing *Bacillus anthracis*.
Incubation period: 2 to 5 days.

Incidence

Anthrax is primarily a disease of animals (sheep and cattle). It is not commonly found in animals in the UK, but is widespread in many Middle East and Eastern countries. Most cases of anthrax in the UK are associated with imported animal products such as wool and hair, bristles, hides and bone meal. It is primarily an industrial disease, affecting those who run special risks attached to their occupation. Men working in wool sorting, dockers handling hides, abattoir workers and those working with bone meal products are most likely to develop the disease.

About ten cases of cutaneous anthrax occur annually in England and Wales, but cases of the more dangerous pneumonic form are extremely rare. *Bacillus anthracis* rapidly produces spores on contact with oxygen and these spores then become widely disseminated in air and soil. In countries where the disease is endemic, infection spreads via such spores.

Segregation of patient

All patients should be treated in an infectious disease hospital. Because of the difficulty in diagnosis, cases may accidentally be admitted to general hospitals. Fortunately effective antibiotic treatment is usually prescribed early and the danger of cross infection is virtually non-existent.

Prevention

As anthrax is a special hazard in the occupations mentioned, it is important to ensure that such workers understand the dangers they face. Diagrams illustrating symptoms are prominently displayed so that, if anyone develops the skin lesion of anthrax, it is more likely to be recognized and diagnosed early. In addition, all such workers carry a small 'identification type' of card on his person to show to any doctor attending them, so that the doctor is warned of this industrial hazard. Early diagnosis is most important as modern antibiotic treatment can quickly cut short an attack. Further preventive measures include:

1. Cleansing treatment of wool imports is now carried out at a number of centres close to the mills.
2. Protective clothing should be worn by persons handling hides and bones. There is evidence to suggest that the handling of wet hides is safer than dried hides.
3. There are special regulations regarding the disposal of carcases of animals who have died from anthrax (Anthrax Order 1938). If any animal has died from a disease suspected to be anthrax, a veterinary surgeon should confirm the diagnosis by collecting a specimen of blood from the ear. Once anthrax is confirmed, it is most important that no autopsy is performed as this would encourage widespread formation and dissemination of spores. Carcases of animals should be burned or buried deep in quick lime.
4. Immunization against anthrax (see p. 185).

Brucellosis

The name covers a group of diseases spread from animals to man and is caused by small, short, non-mobile Gram-negative coccobacilli. Brucellae are primarily animal pathogens and man becomes infected by contact with animals or their products—especially milk.

Causative organisms. These belong to three distinct

types—*Brucella abortus* which produces a disease of cattle and also causes brucellosis (undulant fever), the only type found in the UK; *Brucella melitensis* infects goats, and is common in Malta and various Mediterranean countries; *Brucella suis* infects pigs and occasionally man—it is found in the USA, Denmark and Switzerland.

Incubation period: Very variable. It is thought to be usually 7 to 21 days but may be considerably longer.

Incidence

As the disease is only notifiable in 10 areas in the UK, it is impossible to be certain of its incidence. A further difficulty is that in some cases the symptoms are vague and probably many infections are missed. It was estimated that 500 to 1300 cases occurred annually. Brucellosis is commoner in certain parts of the country—the highest level of infection in England and Wales is probably in the Lake District.

Method of spread

In the UK there are two methods of spread: (*a*) contact by farm workers and others with infected material (about 65% of cases); (*b*) by drinking raw milk containing *Brucella abortus* because cows infected with this disease excrete the bacteria in their milk (about 35%).

Prevention

The prevention of brucellosis depends on: (1) eradication of the disease from animals; (2) heat treatment of milk supplies.

1. As infection in cattle leads to abortion, there is a great incentive for farmers to do all they can to reduce infection. Widespread vaccination of newborn calves is encouraged using a non-virulent live vaccine (S.19). Vaccination of adult cows should not be undertaken because of the difficulty of later using skin tests for diagnosis of possible infection. Complete segregation of a herd of cattle has repeatedly been shown to fail in preventing infection—probably other animals, such as rodents, play a part in spreading the disease.

There is a Brucellosis Incentive Scheme run by the Ministry of Agriculture, Fisheries and Food whereby money incentives are paid to farmers whose herds show three clear blood tests at four monthly intervals.

2. Once a case has been reported a complete bacteriological investigation of the herd must be undertaken and this is usually a lengthy procedure. While the milk is being tested, local deliveries should be stopped and pasteurized supplies substituted. The infected milk should be sent to a large central dairy for pasteurization. The divisional inspector of the Ministry of Agriculture, Fisheries and Food will arrange for the testing of the herd.

In an outbreak, the local authority can apply for a 'pasteurization order' under Reg. 20 of the Milk and Dairies (General) Regulations, 1959 if the milk sampled shows the presence of *Br. abortus*. Milk from the infected cows must then be sent for pasteurization.

Leptospirosis (Weil's disease)

Causative organism: Leptospira icterohaemorrhagiae.
Incubation period: 9 to 19 days (usually 10 to 11).

Incidence

This is primarily a disease of rats and, to a lesser degree, dogs. In the rat, it often leads to a chronic urinary carrier state. About 30 to 45 cases are treated annually in the UK and are mainly seen in men whose occupations bring them into contact with rats—sewage and abattoir workers.

Method of spread

The source of infection is the urine of rats which may contain large numbers of leptospira. Infection usually occurs by the leptospira entering the skin and gaining access to the bloodstream. Bathing in ditches, walking barefoot in pig sties or even swimming in water known to be rat-infested is hazardous and may produce an infection.

Prevention

Personnel at risk should always be warned of the dangers of infection and the method of contamination. It is useful to provide each worker with an 'identification type' of card giving warning symptoms and ask him to show this to any doctor he consults. Such an arrangement helps early diagnosis.

It is important that workers liable to contamination use protective clothing, rubber gloves and rubber thigh boots for sewer workers especially when they are working in an area known to be heavily rat infested.

The public and especially children should never be allowed to wade or bathe in a ditch or pond known to be rat infested. Occasionally infections have been traced to bathing in slow-moving rivers. Everything should be done to destroy the rats (see p. 309).

Canicola Fever

Causative organism: Leptospira canicola.

This disease, with similar but milder symptoms to leptospirosis, is spread from infected dogs. Many patients also show signs of meningitis. It is thought that infection is caused by skin contamination with dog's urine from an infected animal. Many confirmed cases show a close contact with a dog, usually a household pet. In all such instances, the serum of such a dog should be examined. Symptomless carriers among dogs are not uncommon. Careful handwashing after handling dogs and cats is thought to be an important preventive measure.

Rabies

Causative organism: Virus

Incubation period: 2 to 6 weeks but occasionally longer.

At present, considerable concern is being shown about the dangers and problems of rabies because of the increase of this disease on the continent of Europe. Many different wild animals can be infected (including foxes, otters and many rodents) but the vast majority of cases in wild animals have occurred in foxes (about 90% in European countries). An epizootic in foxes has spread during the last 12 years to France from Germany, Switzerland, Austria, Denmark and Belgium. About three-quarters of all animal outbreaks traced on the continent have occurred among wild animals and the remaining among domestic animals. Dogs are most commonly affected in the group but cats and bovines are also infected.

Two imported cases of rabies occurred in the UK in 1975. Both patients had been bitten by rabid dogs before arrival in this country and, although both received intensive treatment both died. Another case from abroad died early in 1977.

Prevention

The virus of rabies is present in the saliva of a rabid animal. After a bite from such an animal, the virus spreads in humans to the central nervous system producing the characteristic symptoms. The disease has a high mortality and anyone bitten by a rabid animal must be immunized (see p. 185). Although rabies is not usually transmitted from man to man, the longer survival times now reported from intensive care units and the nature of the treatment given there raises the possibility that *hospital staff are now more exposed to the risk of infection than previously.* In the event of a number of cases being treated at a specialist hospital, key nursing and medical staff may require immunization.

Rabies Act 1974

Under this Act, there is a compulsory six months quarantine for all animals entering the country. Effective precautions must also be taken against the transmission of the disease within quarantine kennels. All dogs and cats entering quarantine must be vaccinated on entry with a proved potency tested inactivated vaccine; they must also be revaccinated after one month in quarantine to extend immunity.

Dogs and cats will be allowed to enter Britain only at a limited number of ports. Animals landed illegally may be destroyed on landing and the Act provides severe penalties, including up to one year's imprisonment for offences against the orders under the Act.

Further orders provide for a wide range of measures to control any outbreak of rabies in Britain. These include destruction of foxes, controls on the movement of domestic pets and their vaccination, the seizure of strays and the banning of hunting and cat and dog shows.

Prophylactic vaccination against rabies (see p. 185) should be offered to all persons who in their work are at risk including:

1. those employed at quarantine kennels
2. those working in quarantine premises in zoos
3. agents who are authorized to carry such animals
4. those working in research and acclimatization centres where primates and other imported mammals are housed
5. those working in ports regularly importing animals

Booster immunization should be given every two or three years.

Q Fever

Causative organism: Coxiella burneti.
Incubation period: 19 to 20 days.

Q fever is a disease usually presenting as a pneumonia. Pyrexia, shivering, pains in the legs and anorexia are other symptoms commonly reported.

Method of spread

The disease is widespread in animals and birds and is often spread by milk. The organism is also present in very large numbers in the placenta. Consequently it is usually seen in farm or abattoir workers. About 50 to 60 cases are traced each year in the UK.

Prevention

Pasteurization of milk will prevent any milk-borne infections, but most cases now result from contact with infected cows and sheep. The wearing of rubber gloves provides a protection for those having to handle the placenta during calving or lambing.

Prompt diagnosis is by means of a rising titre in the complement fixation test. Prompt treatment with chloramphenicol or tetracyclines is usually effective and will reduce the risk of further direct infections.

SPREAD BY HUMAN CONTACT—SEXUALLY TRANSMITTED DISEASES

There are three infectious sexually transmitted or venereal diseases endemic in the United Kingdom—*syphilis*, *gonorrhoea* and *non-specific urethritis*. None of these diseases is notifiable, but accurate records are kept by all large hospital treatment centres.

Syphilis

Incubation period: approximately 25 days.

In 1976, there were 1468 new cases of primary and secondary syphilis in England. The gradual increase especially in males is shown in Table 40. About 14% of these cases have been contracted abroad.

TABLE 40 New cases of primary and secondary syphilis by sex and age group, England, 1968–76

	1968	*1970*	*1972*	*1974*	*1976*
Males	1937	938	1005	1395	1468
Females	224	185	182	253	214
Total	1261	1123	1187	1648	1628

There are very few early congenital cases (less than 20 each year) due to the efficacy of serological tests in pregnancy.

Gonorrhoea

Incubation period: 3 to 10 days (usually 5).

The overall trend for gonorrhoea has been similarly upward. There were 58 676 new cases traced in 1976 in England (Table 41).

TABLE 41 New cases of gonorrhoea (post pubertal infections) by sex and age groups, England, 1968–76

	1968	*1970*	*1972*	*1974*	*1976*
Males	31 829	36 969	35 033	37 337	37 179
Females	12 006	16 556	18 341	20 734	21 497
Total	43 835	53 525	53 374	58 071	58 676

Non-specific Genital Infections (Non-specific Urethritis)

Incubation period: 10 to 28 days.

The incidence of non-specific genital infections also is rising and there were 92 976 cases in England in 1976 (73 425 men and 19 551 women). This compares with 72 870 in 1971.

There appears to be a world-wide increase in sexually transmitted diseases, although the *rate of increase* in the UK is less than that in the 1960s.

Method of spread

All these diseases are spread by direct contact during sexual intercourse—one partner infecting the other.

Prevention

The prevention of sexually transmitted disease depends on: (1) complete and efficient diagnosis and treatment of all cases; (2) the examination, if possible, of the cohabiting partner to discover unsuspected infections; in males, homosexual relations are responsible for some cases; (3) complete serological tests for all pregnant women; (4) avoidance of casual, promiscuous sexual contact.

1. In women, diagnosis of gonorrhoea is not easy in many cases and a woman may remain infectious for a lengthy period without realizing she has the disease. In doubtful cases of vaginal discharge the doctor should refer the patient to a hospital out-patient department for bacteriological and serological tests.

Recent advice from the DHSS has stressed that any woman who has had casual sexual intercourse, even if only once, should attend a VD clinic for examination even though she has no symptoms. From a recent survey, records show that out of 198 symptomless women who attended a large London clinic, no less than 124 were found to have gonorrhoea and 80 of these were under 25 years of age.

An intensive pilot campaign was started in two London Boroughs in 1972 with the aid of the Health Education Council to encourage people to cooperate in the control of gonorrhoea by attending clinics for medical examination and supplying information to aid in the tracing of potentially infected contacts. Much of this work has concentrated upon the younger age groups. As approximately half the infections of gonorrhoea occur within the London area, a special campaign is being mounted by AHAs and Area Medical Officers to improve contact tracing.

Treatment by inexperienced doctors is dangerous, for it may lead to incomplete cure or the suppression of symptoms. The possibility of a double infection—gonorrhoea and syphilis in the same patient—must be excluded.

2. Whenever a case of venereal disease is diagnosed, a careful history should be taken and arrangements made for the cohabiting partner to be medically examined as soon as possible. To carry out this contact tracing, specially trained nurses and welfare officers are employed by AHAs and attached to all venereal disease departments. Their task is to trace the cohabiting partner wherever possible and persuade him or her to come to the clinic for a full examination. This contact tracing is done on a voluntary basis—the contact cannot be compelled to attend. These nurses and welfare officers also follow up cases who default while under treatment.

3. A serological test (Wassermann or Khan) should be carried out on every woman when three months pregnant. It is important to test at this stage of pregnancy, for if the woman has latent syphilis and if treatment is started promptly, congenital syphilis in the child will be prevented.

4. Better education is required to reduce the incidence of promiscuous sexual intercourse as this is undoubtedly a major factor in encouraging infection. Health education of young persons in schools and youth clubs is desirable.

DISEASE SPREAD BY INJECTION

Serum Hepatitis

This disease is caused by accidentally injecting virus during an injection or transfusion of human blood, plasma or serum. It is not unusual for the virus of hepatitis to be present in the bloodstream and it can therefore quite easily contaminate needles or syringes and be passed on to other patients. It is most important to use a separate sterile needle and syringe for every injection as washing the syringe or needle through with hot water is quite inadequate. Also, it is dangerous to change only the needle for different patients, as there may have been regurgitation of blood (and virus) into the body of the syringe. Sterile plastic disposable syringes are now widely used to prevent any chance of infection.

Blood donors should never be used if there is a history of contact with hepatitis during the past six months or if the donor has himself had a transfusion in this period. Tattooing should be discouraged as it may also lead to infection.

Considerable interest has been focused recently on:

1. The increase in serum hepatitis in drug addicts probably due to infection being spread by shared syringes and needles.
2. The problems found in renal dialysis units in which the staff have been found to have an exceptionally high rate of infection. Outbreaks have been identified in a number of such units and have resulted in the death of staff working there. *This emphasizes the dangers involved in the handling of blood from possibly infected patients.*

   In urological units dealing with renal dialysis, it is now usual to test all patients for antibodies. Those found to have been infected in the past are dialysed separately from the main unit if possible, by staff who have an immunity from serum hepatitis.

SPREAD FROM ANIMALS AND BY ACCIDENTAL INOCULATION—VIRAL HAEMORRHAGIC DISEASES

There are three viral haemorrhagic diseases known to have caused cases in Europe and America: Lassa fever, Marburg disease and Ebola virus disease.

Lassa fever

Causative organism: Virus similar morphologically and serologically to the viruses of lymphocytic choriomeningitis and of Argentinian and Bolivian haemorrhagic fevers.

Incubation period: 3 to 21 days (usually 7 to 10 days).

The virus causing Lassa fever, which was first identified in a missionary nurse in Lassa in Nigeria, is naturally endemic in a species of rat in Nigeria. Lassa fever is a serious disease characterized by malaise, muscular pains, exudative pharyngitis and haemorrhagic maculo-papular rash, with a mortality rate of 27% (from 1969 to 1977, 386 cases traced with 104 deaths). The common rats and mice of the UK are not susceptible but white mice can be infected in laboratories.

Infection in man occurs in two main ways:

1. by food or dusts contaminated by virus from the Nigerian rat (the usual method of primary infection in Nigeria);
2. by person-to-person infection in hospitals and this is the most likely method of infection by which the disease could be spread in the UK.

In view of the danger of (2), special precautions are now laid down for dealing with suspected cases:

1. Early diagnosis of any imported cases—any unsuspected fever in a traveller from Nigeria should be investigated to exclude Lassa fever, by blood culture and isolation of the virus and by evidence of antibody development.
2. Immediate removal of any suspected cases to special isolation hospitals by special ambulances. One such unit has been set up in London and probably four more will be developed in the UK.
3. Strict precautions for all staff nursing such patients (spread has been traced to accidental inoculation by needles or instruments).
4. Daily surveillance of all close contacts for 21 days. Temperatures should be taken daily and special note made of any signs of pharyngitis.

Special laboratories and hospitals have been designated for investigation of Lassa fever, and the Specialist in Community Medicine (Environmental Health) or the District Community Physician has full details.

Experience in Sierra Leone and outside West Africa has generally indicated that isolation and barrier nursing are *effective in preventing the spread of infection* in hospitals although occasionally patients with *severe pulmonary involvement may be infectious* by the airborne route by droplets and droplet nuclei. Such cases therefore require the use of special isolation units or Trexler isolation.

Marburg Disease and Ebola Virus Disease

Causative organism: Viruses similar in type to Lassa fever but antigenically different.

Incubation period: 3 to 21 days (usually 3 to 9 days).

Marburg disease was first recognized in 25 laboratory staff in Marburg, Germany in 1967 after they had handled a consignment of African green monkeys. All developed a febrile illness, with extreme malaise, headache and pains in the limbs with a characteristic macular papular haemorrhagic rash between the fifth and eighth day of illness. Seven died. The disease again appeared in South Africa in 1975 when three cases (one fatal) occurred in a hitch-hiking party.

In 1976, two very extensive outbreaks of a clinically similar disease occurred in south Sudan and northern Zaire and was shown to be due to a similar but antigenically different virus and was named *Ebola virus disease*. The disease spread quickly *but only by close prolonged household contact or by contact with patients' blood*. In 1977, a single case of laboratory infection was reported in England, following an accidental prick of the thumb of a laboratory worker handling infected tissues.

Prevention of Viral Haemorrhagic Diseases

All three diseases are zoonoses with a high mortality rate in man. The main preventive health problems in the UK and other Western countries are the methods to be used to recognize and then to nurse any suspected cases. A problem of differential diagnosis exists—a study of the history of imported viral haemorrhagic diseases has shown *that 45% had been given a diagnosis of malaria.* The occurrence of any febrile illness in a person who has travelled within the last 21 days from Nigeria calls for a careful and wide investigation. At this stage unless there are many indications that the disease is one of the virus haemorrhagic diseases, hospital isolation is indicated rather than widespread community surveillance of contacts. Within Nigeria, the greatest risk of natural infection occurs in persons arriving from areas or hospitals where viral haemorrhagic diseases are known to be present and when the person is known to have been in contact. The lowest risk is in persons arriving from cities in Nigeria with no known contact with the disease.

By far the *greatest risks of infection in the UK is to laboratory and health staff either handling patients, or infected blood, secretions and tissues.* Such staff who are likely to look after patients and material from Central and West Africa should be carefully trained in the hazards and in the use of special equipment (i.e. how to use special isolation units or Trexler isolation).

Patients from Central and West Africa with febrile diseases should *never* be admitted to district general hospitals without any isolation unit being available.

Surveillance of close contacts

Close family and other contacts should be visited daily at home for 21 days, in a rather similar way to the past surveillance of smallpox contacts. Any developing a febrile illness should be isolated for further investigation.

It is, however, most important to realize that the risks of community spread (as with smallpox in the past) have been exaggerated for airborne infection is very rare and only likely to take place with a very ill patient with pulmonary involvement. The real dangers are to hospital and laboratory staff becoming accidentally infected.

INSECT-BORNE DISEASES

There are no insect-borne diseases endemic in the UK. Insect-borne diseases include a number of tropical diseases including malaria, yellow fever, dengue spread by mosquitoes, plague spread by the rat flea and typhus spread by lice. It is beyond the scope of this book to deal with tropical diseases, but brief descriptions of the epidemiology of malaria, plague and typhus are given as these diseases occasionally occur in temperate countries.

Malaria

Malaria is spread through the bite of an infected female *Anopheles* mosquito. The malarial parasite has two cycles, an asexual one occurring in man and a sexual one in the mosquito. Thus, the mosquito is not only the vehicle of infection but is necessary for the completion of the life cycle of the malarial parasite.

Incubation periods vary with the type of malarial parasite. The average incubation period for *Plasmodium falciparum* is 12 days, for *Pl. vivax* and *Pl. orale* 14 days and up to 30 days for *Pl. malariae*.

The period of communicability in an infected human is as long as the infective gametocytes are present in the bloodstream. This period is, of course, dependent on treatment given.

Prevention

About 1100 imported cases of malaria occur annually in the UK and about 300 of these are persons who contract the disease on short holidays or business trips to malarious areas abroad. These figures emphasize the need for such visitors to take precautions including the regular use of suppressive drugs and protection from mosquito bites especially at night.

The international eradication measures are discussed on p. 323.

Plague

Plague last occurred in the UK in 1910, when there was a small outbreak in Suffolk. The disease is endemic in Asia, India, South America and in Central Africa. It is primarily a disease of rats, and man becomes infected when bitten by the rat flea, *Xenopsylla cheopis*.

In the UK, plague was commonly epidemic in the 13th to 17th centuries as outbreaks of the Black Death. At this period, the only species of rat in the United Kingdom was the ship rat—the black rat (*Rattus rattus*). This rat likes climbing and lives in close proximity to man and so facilitates the spread of plague. At the beginning of the 18th century, the larger brown rat migrated across Europe and reached the UK. It quickly established itself and reduced the number of black rats which soon became rare. This change led to a marked reduction in plague as the different habits of the brown rat, which prefers to burrow rather than climb, meant that it rarely came into close contact with man. There was thus little chance of rat fleas contaminating man and of spreading the disease.

Prevention

Preventive measures against plague in the UK include widespread measures to destroy rats in ports. A careful watch is also maintained to see if any infected rats are present. All ships have to be 'de-ratted', completely fumigated to destroy all rats, every six months. Rat-proofing is also insisted upon for every ship berthing to reduce the possibility of rats migrating from the ship to shore.

Typhus Fever

Classic typhus fever is caused by *Rickettsia prowazeki*. This organism infects the alimentary canal of the louse and the faeces of an infected louse contain *Rickettsia*. Skin is contaminated with louse faeces and then scratching causes typhus.

This disease has caused considerable mortality in the past. During the period 1917–21 typhus ravaged Russia and it has been estimated that, in this period, over 24 million cases occurred with 3 million deaths.

Until the discovery of modern insecticides, it was difficult for combat troops in cold climates to remain free from lice, and this was the reason why most serious epidemics of typhus accompanied winter military campaigns.

Prevention

The main method of avoiding typhus in endemic areas and at epidemic times is to ensure that the population remains free from lice. Widespread prophylactic treatment of clothing and persons using DDT became routine practice in the 1939–45 war and was responsible more than any other single factor in preventing any serious outbreaks of typhus. In 1944, an outbreak of typhus did start in Naples but was completely controlled and further cases prevented by a widespread de-lousing operation using DDT.

The use of DDT has now been stopped and it has been replaced by 5% gamma benzene hexachloride (see p. 312).

14 Epidemiology and the Prevention of Non-communicable Diseases

EPIDEMIOLOGY

Diseases can only be effectively prevented if all the various factors which cause them are fully understood. In the last chapters, it has been shown how communicable diseases can be prevented by understanding the qualities of the various infecting organisms—bacteria or viruses—and the reaction of the human body when invaded by them.

With non-infectious illnesses the greatest barrier to prevention is that, in many instances, so little is known about the cause of disease. Yet, even when the exact cause of the disease process is imperfectly understood (as with a neoplastic disease), much can be learnt about it by a study of the many factors that influence it. The complete study of these various complex factors is called *epidemiology*. As well as covering the causation of disease (aetiology), epidemiology includes the following:

1. Variations of the disease *in time*, which covers a brief study of the way the disease has altered in incidence and severity over the past few generations.
2. Present-day *morbidity* (or incidence) of the disease including comparisons between different countries, different areas of the same country and in different strata of the same community. The following factors are connected with morbidity:

   a. seasonal incidence
   b. the effect of heredity or race
   c. geographical factors

d. predisposing causes—these may be either in the occupation of the patient or connected with his social and recreational life or habits
e. sex differences
f. the personality of the patient—psychosomatic factors

3. Social factors in the disease.
4. Mortality of the disease.
5. Estimation of the chances of an individual developing the disease.
6. Methods of preventing the disease.

In this short book, no attempt will be made to discuss even briefly the epidemiology of all groups of non-communicable diseases. Instead, a few diseases will be discussed which illustrate many of the fascinating aspects of epidemiological study and how methods of prevention may be developed.

Epidemiology often concentrates attention on a disease because of some significant change in its incidence which leads to more research and brings to light further features and finally an important causative factor may be defined. Cancer of the lung is an example. Because of its marked increase more and more research has been undertaken and a connection with cigarette smoking has been demonstrated. Such a causative factor could never have been discovered by the investigation of a series of single clinical cases—*it needed a study of the whole community to bring it to light.*

Epidemiology can also be said to help define the problems of disease. In most cases, there is a *multiplicity of factors* affecting its incidence. The clinician studies the various pathological factors concerned, but his treatment must fit into the life of the patient. The *social factors in the patient's environment are all important* and may well be responsible for a relapse (a good example is given by duodenal ulcer). The field of epidemiology enlarges the scope of investigation into disease. It also covers many more cases than could ever be seen by any individual clinician.

The Cancers

The true causation of neoplastic disease is unknown. There are, however, many associated factors now recognized which predispose to the development of cancers and most of these are connected with some chronic recurring form of irritation. It has long been known that various skin cancers can be caused by irritation of oils, and cancer of the tongue by the irritation of a clay pipe. Inhalation of chronic asbestos dust leads to a pneumoconiosis called asbestosis and this may be followed by cancer of the lung. The severely torn cervix uteri may be the seat of chronic infection and later develop cancer. There is an association between cancer of the bladder and contact with antioxidants containing benzidine or naphthylamine.

Prevention in such instances can best be achieved by removing or avoiding the predisposing factor. If this is not possible, prevention depends on recognizing a very early *precancerous condition* which, if then radically treated, can prevent the subsequent cancer. This is the basis of screening tests, e.g. exfoliate cytology for cancer of the cervix uteri.

Incidence of cancers

In England and Wales, there are various regional cancer registration schemes usually run by specialized hospital units dealing with the treatment of such cases. It is estimated that the annual incidence of new cancers in England and Wales is in the region of 150 000. Nearly one-quarter of all deaths are caused by some form of cancer.

The deaths from cancer are known accurately and in 1975 numbered 123 738 (66 376 men and 57 352 women). Table 42, which lists deaths from cancer in England and Wales in 1975, shows many interesting points.

It will be seen that there are many differences between the sexes. Among the most obvious is the great preponderance of male deaths from cancer of the lung. Men also die more frequently from cancers of the bladder. Female preponderance occurs in breast and genital organs. In other organs minor differences occur.

It is not often realized that there are quite considerable variations in the mortality from various neoplastic diseases in different parts of the country. In Table 43 the mortality from certain cancers is compared in five different areas. It will be seen that most cancer mortality is low in East Anglia and in the South West and high in the North West. London shows high levels of cancer of the lung while Wales has a high figure of cancer of the stomach.

TABLE 42 Principal causes of cancer deaths, England and Wales, 1975

Site	*Male*	*Female*
Lung	26 075	6756
Stomach	6983	5000
Breast	82	11 637
Large intestine (except rectum)	4245	6269
Rectum	3247	2856
Pancreas	2963	2607
Prostate	4421	—
Bladder	2837	1227
Ovary	—	3621
Leukaemia	1753	1441
Cervix uteri	—	2143
Brain	1077	771

(from *Mortality Statistics*, 1975, OPCS)

TABLE 43 Standardized mortality rates (SMR) for cancers for different parts of England and Wales, 1975

Disease	*North West*	*East Anglia*	*South West*	*Greater London*	*Wales*
Males					
Cancer of buccal cavity and pharynx	131	47	82	105	105
Cancer of stomach	119	86	84	103	113
Cancer of intestine and rectum	111	88	99	91	108
Cancer of lung	111	88	83	116	94
Females					
Cancer of cervix uteri	125	92	89	78	93
Cancer of breast	99	101	100	103	96

(from *Mortality Statistics (area)*, 1975, OPCS)

Social class

Cancers also showed marked variations with the social classes (see Fig. 12).

There are marked differences between the social classes as regards mortality. In men there is a greater variation with mortality greatest in social class V and least in social class I.

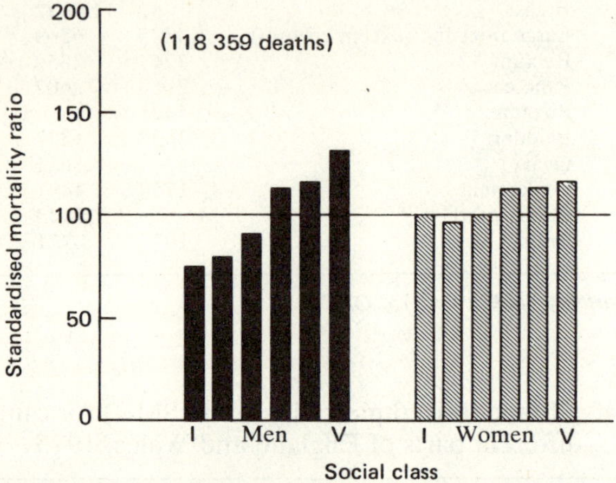

FIG. 12. Mortality from malignant neoplasms by social class for men and married women aged 15–64, England and Wales, 1970–2. (From *Occupation Mortality*, 1970–2, OPCS)

International cancer mortality

It is also revealing to compare the cancer mortality of different countries (Table 45).

Some of the most striking differences are between Japan and England and Wales. It is interesting to note that although the differences are too large to be explained by varying degrees of diagnosis or treatment concerned, the rates of cancer of the stomach, lung and leukaemia are significantly greater in men than in women.

There is an exceptionally low rate for cancer of the lung and breast in Japan, but, on the other hand, cancer of the stomach is commoner there. Although not shown in Table 45, it is also interesting to note that the death rate of Japanese who emigrate to the USA quickly approximates to the American levels.

Age incidence of cancers

It is well known that all types of cancers are rare before the age of 20 years; after this the incidence increases rapidly until 75–80 years when it again falls markedly.

A rather similar relationship has been shown in radiation-induced leukaemia which reaches a maximum five to eight years after radiation and then the incidence begins to fall rapidly.

The relationship between exposure to β-naphthylamine and allied aromatic amines and the consequent development of bladder cancers is well known (see p. 249). What is not so commonly recognized is that there is a higher incidence in those men who were exposed at the older ages.

Cancer of the lung

There has been a dramatic increase in cancer of the lung in England and Wales during the last 30 years as shown by Table 44. The disease is four times commoner in men.

TABLE 44 Deaths from cancer of the lung, England and Wales, 1947–76

1947	9204	1961	22 810
1949	10 979	1963	24 434
1951	13 347	1965	26 399
1953	15 132	1967	28 188
1955	17 272	1969	29 768
1957	19 028	1971	30 754
1959	12 063	1976	33 524

There is also a marked social class gradient with the disease three times commoner in social classes II and V (Fig. 13).

The upward trend in cancer of the lung has been reported from many countries and has resulted in much research designed to investigate the factors which may be responsible. Although these include atmospheric pollution, all the surveys and research in different parts of the world have shown that more lung cancer

TABLE 45 Cancer death rates per 100 000 population, 1973

	USA	*Austria*	*France*	*Netherlands*	*England and Wales*	*Australia*	*Japan*	*Ireland (1972)*
Stomach								
Males	9·0	48·7	23·1	27·9	29·7	13·7	57·4	6·3
Females	5·6	38·1	17·0	17·8	20·1	9·0	36·3	6·3
Trachea/Bronchus								
Males	57·9	27·5	45·1	83·3	108·8	46·7	17·4	50·8
Females	14·6	12·9	6·5	5·5	24·3	8·6	6·5	16·9
Breast	29·6	34·2	28·8	37·0	45·2	24·6	5·4	31·2
Cervix uteri	5·6	7·8	3·7	5·4	8·9	6·0	2·5	5·1
Leukaemia								
Males	8·1	7·8	8·5	7·8	7·1	6·9	4·1	7·1
Females	5·8	6·7	6·8	5·8	5·3	5·0	3·1	4·1

(from *Annual Epidemiological and Vital Statistics Report*, World Health Organization, 1976)

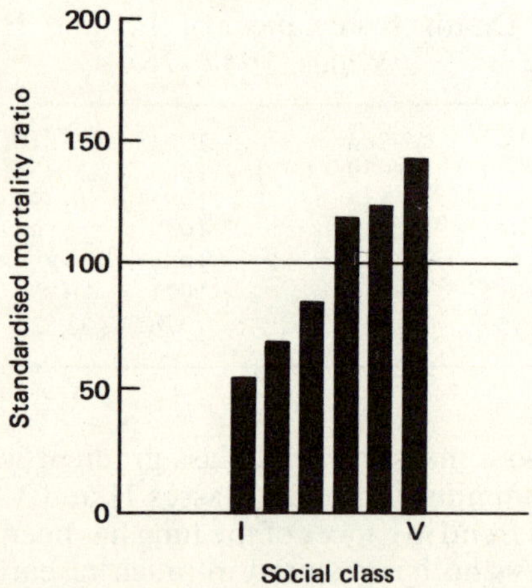

FIG 13. Mortality from cancer of the lung by social class for men aged 15–64, England and Wales, 1970–2. (From *Occupational Mortality*, 1970–2, OPCS)

patients are smokers of cigarettes than are the controls in the experiments. It has also been shown that the death rates from lung cancer increase steeply as consumption of cigarettes increases. Heavy cigarette smokers have thirty times the death rate from cancer of the lung compared with non-smokers. From 1962 to 1970 the Royal College of Physicians studied this problem and their reports stated that 'cigarette smoking is an important cause of lung cancer. If the habit ceased, the number of deaths caused by the disease should fall steeply in the course of time.' *The prevention of lung cancer must be closely connected with the smoking habits of any community.* Cigarette smoking is much more dangerous than cigar, cheroot or pipe smoking and cigarettes with a low tar content are safer than those with a high tar content. Lung cancer deaths represent 40% of all deaths from cancer in men but only 11% in women. In spite of the weight of evidence incriminating cigarette smoking as a main causative factor, people are still prepared to run the risk. Ignorance may play a part for, in a professional group who have expert knowledge of the risks, such as male doctors, the incidence of smoking has been dramatically reduced and so has the death rate from cancer of the lung.

It is interesting to note that studies have now shown that the *incidence of lung cancer falls off as early as five years after smoking has stopped* and that after 10 to 15 years the incidence has fallen to a figure very close to that of the non-smoker.

Atmospheric pollution also is a small contributory factor and is responsible for the higher incidence of cancer of the lung in the UK compared with its occurrence in other parts of the world (see p. 244).

Cancer of the breast

In women, cancer of the breast is an important cause of death—in 1976, 11 763 women died from this disease in England and Wales. In Table 45 it has already been pointed out that the mortality varies between different countries. The United Kingdom has the highest death rate, 42·4 deaths per 1 000 000 population compared with 34·7 in Holland, 27·9 in the USA, 27·4 in France and 4·7 in Japan. The causation of cancer of the breast is imperfectly understood, but there is considerable evidence that the incidence is much lower in women who have breast fed their children and it is thought that this fact may be responsible for the very low rate in Japan where breast feeding is common. However, all the mortality rates for cancer of the breast are rising in these countries—by about 12% in England and Wales in six years, but by approximately 25% in Japan over the same period.

The reduction in the mortality from cancer of the breast is closely linked with early diagnosis which is essential if operative treatment is to be successful. *The type of carcinoma also is an important factor*—the most rapidly spreading types being those which occur during pregnancy and lactation.

Cancer of the stomach

The second commonest cancer in England and Wales is of the stomach. In 1976 11 869 persons died from this disease (6925 men and 4944 women). It is interesting to note that in cancer of the stomach there is:

1. A well-marked variation in the social classes rising steadily from a Standardized Mortality Ratio of 50 for class I to 153 for class V (Fig. 14).

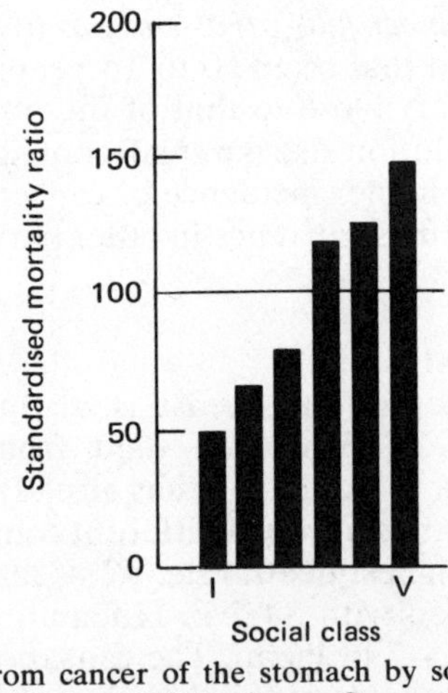

FIG. 14. Mortality from cancer of the stomach by social class for men aged 15–64, England and Wales, 1970–2. (From *Occupational Mortality*, 1970–2, OPCS)

2. A well-marked geographical association and the highest rates are in the rural areas of North Wales.

3. An association between chronic gastric irritation—chronic gastritis or even a previous gastric ulcer—and the subsequent development of a cancer.

The geographical variation which is so striking has stimulated much research to find out whether the residents of the rural areas of North Wales show special preferences for certain foods, but so far little has been found. A clue to the causation of this disease probably lies in its geographic and social class differences.

Cancer of the cervix

Cancer of the cervix was responsible for 2143 deaths in women in 1975 but the death rate from this condition has been falling. There is a very well-marked variation in the social classes.

It is known that repetitive damage to the cervix uteri in childbirth is a predisposing cause of this cancer and this probably explains much of the variation noted in the social classes, as it is more usual for women in class V to have larger families with the correspondingly greater risk of cervical damage. Cervical cytology tests should therefore be concentrated upon examining women of social classes IV and V. The test is described on p. 268.

Leukaemia

The incidence of leukaemia increased considerably from 1950 to 1968, but has been steady since. This is shown by the following rise in the Standardized Mortality Ratio for the disease for England and Wales (Table 46).

TABLE 46 Standardized mortality ratio for leukaemia, males, England and Wales (1968 = 100)

1950–1	71
1961	90
1966	95
1968	100
1970	96
1975	100

Leukaemia is one of the unusual diseases in that *there is a reverse social class gradient: it is slightly higher in social classes I and II than in V* (Fig. 15).

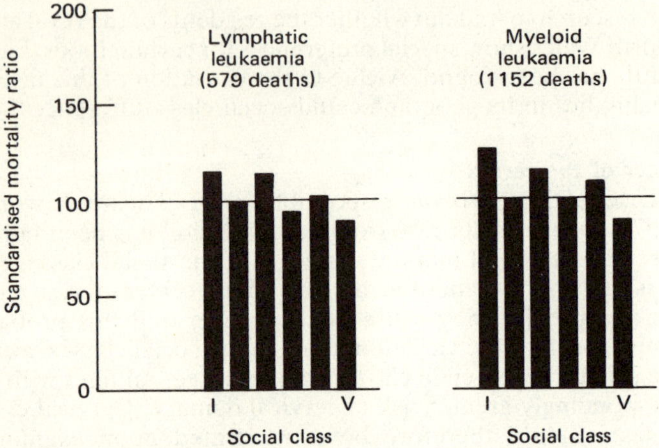

FIG. 15. Mortality from leukaemia by social class for men aged 15–64, England and Wales, 1970–2. (From *Occupational Mortality*, 1978, OPCS)

There is epidemiological evidence that increased incidence of leukaemia is associated with an excess of radiation—leukaemia is more often found among radiologists compared with other doctors and the general public, and among patients who have had a long period of X-ray treatment, e.g. for ankylosing spondylitis. There has been a high incidence of the disease in survivors of the atomic bomb attacks on Hiroshima and Nagasaki. A higher level of leukaemia has also been noted among children whose mothers had been X-rayed during pregnancy. Investigations are still progressing and the association between leukaemia in childhood and antenatal X-rays has not yet been proved.

An interesting finding is that mongolism is more likely to be associated with leukaemia, and it has been estimated that the age-specific leukaemia death rate for mongols is in the region of thirty times that of normal children.

Cancer of the bladder

Cases of cancer of the bladder are more marked in males than in females (in 1975, 2837 male and 1227 female deaths were reported in England and Wales).

Part of the difference is occupational for there is a connection with cancer of the bladder and long exposure to hardeners or anti-oxidants containing benzidine or β-naphthylamine based derivatives which used to be used in the rubber and cable manufacturing industries. After initial exposure to such chemicals, there may be a latent period of 12 to 20 years before a cancer of the bladder appears. At present, men who have been exposed to such chemicals at work are being followed up by twice-yearly urinary examinations for evidence of exfoliated tumour cells in the urine. In this way it is hoped to recognize very early tumours which may develop.

There is a marked difference between the incidence of cancer of the bladder in men and women and in different parts of the United Kingdom (Table 47).

TABLE 47 Incidence of cancer of bladder, UK, 1971 (SMR 1968 = 100)

	Males	*Females*
England and Wales	100	97
Scotland	105	136
Northern Ireland	67	78

There is a social class gradient but this is less marked than for other cancers (Fig. 16).

Ischaemic heart disease

The incidence of ischaemic heart disease has increased markedly during the last 20 years. The Standardized Mortality Ratio for this disease in England and Wales rose by 41% for males between 1950 and 1960. The increase since 1960 has been more gradual and is shown in Table 48.

The social class gradient is shown in Table 30, p. 88. Note that it is much steeper in women: SMR 58 in social class I and 146 in social class V.

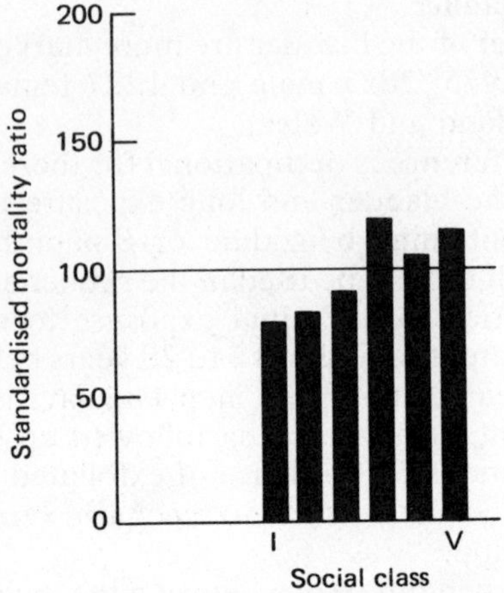

FIG. 16. Mortality from cancer of the bladder by social class for men aged 15–64, England and Wales, 1970–2. (From *Occupational Mortality,* 1970–2, OPCS)

TABLE 48 SMR for ischaemic heart disease, England and Wales (1968 = 100)

	1961	*1965*	*1966*	*1968*	*1971*	*1975*
Males	89	98	97	100	101	104
Females	95	93	96	100	97	101

The disease in persons under the age of 45 is much commoner (eight times) in men than women and in the older age groups this male predominance continues but is much less marked. It is interesting to note that deaths from ischaemic heart disease are increasing at the same rate in men and women. Throughout the world, there are large differences noted in the level of ischaemic heart disease as shown in Table 49.

In all countries male deaths exceed those in females. The rates in England and Wales, USA and Scotland are high while those in Japan and France are low.

There are many different factors associated with the development of ischaemic heart disease including the following:

1. high blood lipid levels
2. hypertension
3. cigarette smoking
4. genetic factors
5. physical inactivity
6. increase in body weight
7. diabetes
8. nervous stress

TABLE 49 Deaths from ischaemic heart disease per 100 000 population, both sexes, 1973

Japan	39·0	Israel	216·1
Yugoslavia	65·6	Netherlands	217·7
Spain	67·2	Canada	228·8
Poland	67·8	Austria	235·2
Greece	79·3	Hungary	236·0
France	88·0	Australia	251·2
Portugal	91·9	England and Wales	308·9
Switzerland	107·8	Denmark	325·2
Italy	150·3	USA	326·0
Belgium	187·0	Scotland	363·1
Germany (Federal Republic)	196·5	Sweden	378·1

(from *Annual Epidemiological and Vital Statistics Report*, World Health Organization, 1976)

In most instances there are important relationships between these two factors so that the likelihood of an attack is increased where many adverse factors operate.

It has been suggested that there is a link between the amount of animal fats consumed and the level of atheroma and consequent ischaemic heart disease. Some have suggested that the low level of the disease in Japan is connected with the low animal fat consumption and conversely the high levels in the USA, Sweden and Scotland are associated with high levels of consumption. It is, however, more likely that a combination of the above eight factors is the explanation. Certainly the incidence is greater in sedentary, overweight, cigarette-smoking men. On the genetic side, the short heavier type of man (mesomorph) is more likely to suffer an *early* attack than the tall thin person. Regular exercise seems to have a protective effect and farmers and others leading physically active lives have a lower incidence than sedentary workers (even though their animal fat consumption may be greater). The present day popularity of the motor car which discourages exercise is an environmental factor which tends to increase the incidence of this disease.

There is certainly an endocrine factor which is probably responsible for the higher rate in younger men than in younger women (before age 50). After the menopause the rate in women gradually increases until by the age of 70 years it is similar to that of men. Women who have their ovaries removed surgically have a higher incidence. There is also definite experimental evidence in birds that oestrogen therapy can clear an induced atheroma.

Prevention. There is no agreement about prophylactic measures to prevent ischaemic heart disease. It has been suggested that routine blood cholesterol tests should be carried out on all men aged 35 years and over. This would define the small group with high blood cholesterol levels who have a special risk of developing early coronary thrombosis. Such cases could then undertake remedial measures such as: (i) acceptance of a diet in which animal fats are replaced by vegetable fats; (ii) dieting to avoid overweight; (iii) steady constant exercise such as walking; (iv) giving up cigarette smoking (there is evidence of a great risk among heavy smokers). Some physicians, however, fear that such a regime might only worry many patients unduly and, in the end, do more harm than good.

Although there is an increased risk of ischaemic heart disease in the heavy smoker, *if that person stops smoking, these risks will fall to the level of the non-smoker within 48 hours* (this is quite different from the risks of cancer of the lung (see p. 245)).

Bronchitis

Bronchitis was responsible for 25 730 deaths (18 699 men, 7031 women) in 1976 in England. This is a marked decrease from the 31 763 deaths in 1969. The trend of deaths in England and Wales is shown in Table 50.

Table 51 shows the mortality rates of bronchitis, emphysema and asthma in different countries. The reason why chronic bronchitis is called the 'English disease' is obvious, as the death rate is

TABLE 50 Standardized mortality ratios, bronchitis, England and Wales, 1960 to 70 (1968 = 100)

	Males	*Females*
1961	104	115
1965	97	91
1967	90	84
1968	100	100
1969	105	98
1970	90	87
1971	85	79
1976	72	66

TABLE 51 Deaths from bronchitis, emphysema and asthma, 1973 (per 100 000 population)

	Males	*Females*	*Total*
France	17·1	7·4	12·7
USA	22·2	6·5	14·2
Netherlands	36·2	10·7	23·4
Australia	49·9	12·7	31·4
England and Wales	85·1	28·3	55·9

(from *Annual Epidemiological and Vital Statistics Report*, World Health Organization, 1976)

so much higher. The climate of the UK has often been blamed, but it is curious to see that Australia (a sunny climate) is another country with relatively high figures. The two lowest, the USA and Japan, have recently had serious atmospheric pollution problems, yet their incidence of chronic bronchitis is low.

The great preponderance of bronchitis deaths in men rather than women (2·5 to 1) is probably connected with the effect of cigarette smoking, for men smoke more than women and this aggravates bronchitis.

Atmospheric pollution in acute episodes has produced a marked increase in the deaths from bronchitis; in December 1952 it was estimated that in the London area just under 4000 deaths from bronchitis resulted from a very serious four-day smog. Improvements in atmospheric pollution have followed action under the Clean Air Act 1956 (see p. 298). In the control of atmospheric pollution, it is important to control both smoke and the emission of noxious gases such as sulphur dioxide and trioxide, as these are irritant to the bronchial mucosa.

There is no doubt that smoking is another contributory factor and all smokers, especially heavy cigarette smokers, are much more affected by bronchitis. The connection is so marked that as a prophylactic measure it is essential that anyone with a tendency to early bronchitis or asthma should never smoke.

Peptic Ulceration

It is difficult to estimate accurately the incidence of peptic ulceration in England and Wales. Recently in 4000 consecutive post-mortem examinations 9·5% showed evidence of a chronic peptic ulcer either healed or unhealed. But this gives little indication of incidence in younger adults today. There is a marked gradient in mortality (see Fig. 17) for both gastric and duodenal ulceration.

The mortality in women and men is changing (Table 52). In men the SMR has fallen for both but, in women, it is rising.

It is known that there are wide international differences in the incidence although no satisfactory explanation has yet been put forward.

Diabetes

One of the most interesting epidemiological features of diabetes is how the disease is *now commonest in social classes IV and V, whereas 50 years ago the gradient was the reverse* (Table 53).

The reason for this change of pattern is unknown: it may be linked with more effective treatment in social classes I and II since the introduction of insulin in the 1920s or it may be partly dietetic or it may be due to changes in the standard of diagnosis. There is a greater incidence in females than in males.

The causation of diabetes is still unknown, but two very important factors have been defined (1) *hereditary*; (2) *overnutrition.*

1. Diabetes has often been traced among members of the

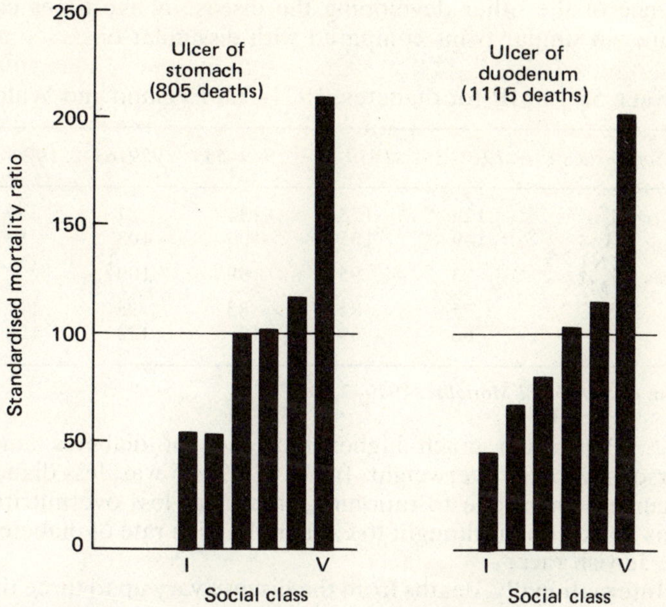

FIG. 17. Mortality from ulcer of the stomach of duodenum by social class for men aged 15–64, England and Wales, 1970–2. (From *Occupational Mortality*, 1970–2, OPCS)

TABLE 52 SMR for gastric and duodenal ulceration England, 1968–76 (1968 = 100)

	1968	*1970*	*1972*	*1974*	*1975*
Ulcer of stomach					
Males	100	85	77	80	78
Females	100	94	97	102	108
Ulcer of duodenum					
Males	100	82	86	87	83
Females	100	87	107	109	118

(from *Health and Personal Social Services Statistics*, 1977, DHSS)

same family. It has been shown that if one twin has diabetes, the chance of the other developing the disease is five times commoner in similar twins compared with dissimilar ones.

TABLE 53 SMR for diabetes, 1921–72, England and Wales

Social class	*1921–3*	*1930–2*	*1949–53*	*1959–63*	*1970–2*
I	129	122	134	81	83
II	149	155	100	103	93
III N	93	95	99	100	111
III M					98
IV	75	82	85	98	111
V	66	69	105	122	128

(from *Occupational Mortality*, 1970–2, OPCS)

2. There is a much higher incidence of diabetes among persons who are overweight. In the 1939–45 war, less diabetes occurred when, due to rationing, there was less overnutrition. This association is thought to explain the high rate of diabetes in the Jewish race.

Internationally, deaths from the disease vary up to three times in the major countries (Table 54). Japan has the lowest rates and the USA the highest. It is interesting to note that diabetes is one of the few diseases in which there is a consistently higher death rate in women than in men.

The prevention of the serious type of diabetes in young people may be impossible if there is a strong hereditary factor. The 'adult' milder type of diabetes can, however, be considerably reduced by the avoidance of overnutrition and overweight. Serious disease can also be prevented by ensuring that the treatment prescribed is properly carried out. This can best be done by arranging for a health visitor to call regularly on all diabetic patients. An excellent administrative arrangement is for such a health visitor to be attached to the diabetic out-patient clinic where she will be able to get to know the treatment prescribed for each patient. On her visits later, she can check whether the treatment is being followed and can also ensure that adverse social conditions do not prevent effective treatment. She can advise the physician treating the patient of any difficulties at home and keep a watch for the development of complications. In this way, deterioration in the patient's condition can be prevented.

TABLE 54 Deaths from diabetes mellitus (per 100 000 population) 1973

	Males	*Females*	*Total*
Japan	7·6	7·7	7·7
England and Wales	8·3	12·5	10·4
Ireland	11·4	16·1	13·7
Australia	12·6	14·7	13·6
France	10·9	17·9	14·5
USA	15·3	20·9	18·2

(from the *Annual Epidemiological and Vital Statistics Report*, World Health Organization, 1976)

Cirrhosis of the Liver

The wide variations in the mortality from cirrhosis of the liver are shown in Table 55.

It will be seen that England and Wales have the lowest figures and Italy, Germany and France the highest. The population of these three countries drink large quantities of wine and this is likely to be the main reason for the high incidence. An extremely

TABLE 55 Deaths from cirrhosis of the liver (per 100 000 population), 1973

	Males	*Females*	*Total*
England and Wales	3·9	3·4	3·7
Finland	6·0	3·2	4·6
Scotland	5·7	4·5	5·1
USA	21·3	10·7	15·9
Germany (Federal Republic)	35·9	16·3	25·7
Italy	47·2	18·1	32·3
France	49·2	20·3	34·5

(from the *Annual Epidemiological and Vital Statistics Report*, World Health Organization, 1976)

interesting figure is that from Finland. That country had a high incidence of alcoholism but this has been markedly reduced by the state controlling the sale of alcoholic drinks.

Cirrhosis of the liver is a disease where the SMR compared by social class can give a misleading impression. As seen from Fig. 18 the SMR is highest in social class II. However, this is due to the exceptionally high mortality from cirrhosis of the liver in publicans and inn keepers (SMR 1576) who are now included in social class II.

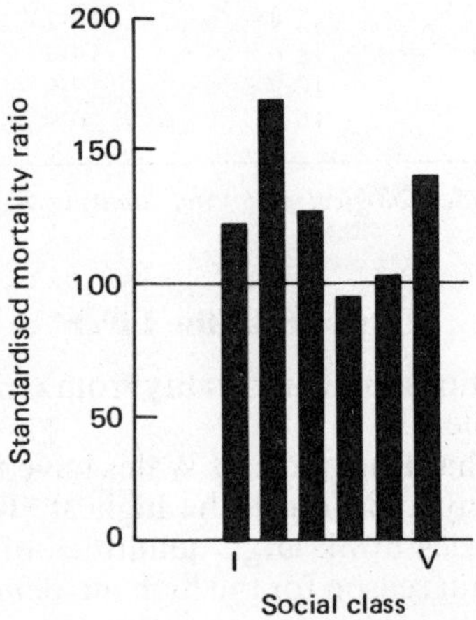

FIG. 18. Mortality from cirrhosis of the liver by social class for men aged 15–64, England and Wales, 1970–2. (From *Occupational Mortality*, 1970–2, OPCS)

Mental Illness

In 1975, in the UK, out of a total population of 56 million, 87 000 persons (37 000 men and 50 000 women) were receiving in-patient care in hospitals. Approximately 70% of these have been in hospital one year or more and 49% five years or more. Approximately 300 000 persons receive care from local authorities because of mental illness.

Reference has already been made to the large number of days lost per year from mental illness in women than in men (see Table 25, p. 82).

The social class pattern shows a curious difference between the sexes (Fig. 19). In men, there is a substantial increase in social class V which is entirely absent from the histogram for women.

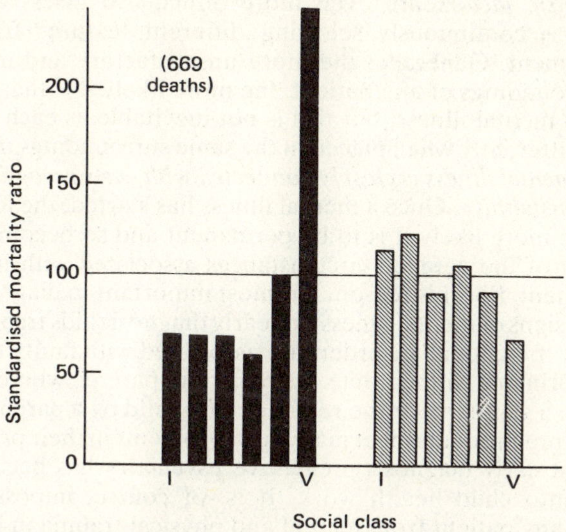

FIG. 19. Mortality from mental disorders by social class for men and married women aged 15–64, England and Wales, 1970–2. (From *Occupational Mortality*, 1970–2, OPCS)

The exact cause of most mental illness is not yet fully understood. However, a great deal is known of the factors related to the development of mental illness and these can be divided into:

1. intrinsic factors connected with the patient including (*a*) heredity and (*b*) phases of his development
2. extrinsic factors related to the patient's occupation, home and environment

Intrinsic factors are complicated. Hereditary ones are rather an inherited predisposition to develop mental illness than being born with a mental illness. This predisposition may or may not result in mental breakdown and the likelihood of such illness developing in any individual with such a predisposition depends on: (*a*) environmental (extrinsic) factors; (*b*) certain susceptible stages of his life—mental illness is most likely to develop at puberty, pregnancy, middle age (including menopause) or in retirement (old age).

Extrinsic factors are even more difficult to assess as each patient is continuously selecting different features from his environment. Generally, the more unsatisfactory and insecure the surroundings of any patient, the more likely it is that he will develop mental illness, but this is not inevitable as each person reacts differently when placed in the same surroundings. *Prevention of mental illness is closely connected with early recognition of mental instability.* Once a mental illness has started, the longer it lasts the more likely it is to be permanent and so become independent of the detailed circumstances associated with its commencement. For this reason, it is most important to diagnose the earliest signs of mental illness, for early diagnosis aids treatment.

Many 'functional' disorders are associated with faulty training and upbringing in the home, such as rigid parents who demand too high a standard, or the rejection of a child by a parent. Most general practitioners meet many such problems in their practices. To assist early diagnosis preventive psychiatry has been introduced into child health work. It is, of course, impossible to protect any patient from mental and physical trauma in life—in fact, attempts to do this may very well encourage mental breakdown. But it is usually practicable to alter a patient's environment in some way, and thus help to avoid an impending mental illness.

Balanced advice is always an important environmental factor. Health education of a personal nature can be most helpful in allaying many needless fears which may have been handed down by ignorant parents or relatives and which may otherwise precipitate a mental illness.

Occupation has an important effect on mental stability. Careful medical and psychological testing before persons are placed in various occupations can assist in avoiding subsequent mental breakdowns (personnel management).

Suicide

Suicide rates vary considerably throughout the world as shown by the WHO figures (Table 56).

There may, of course, be a recording error in any country which is predominantly Roman Catholic and the figures from Eire have often been questioned in this way. There is, however, a consistently greater number of suicides in men than in women and the variations shown in Table 56 are considerable. Apart from Eire, the figures for England and Wales are low and for Austria high.

In the UK, suicide is one of the causes of death which has shown a marked decrease during the past 10 years.

TABLE 56 Suicide rate per 100 000 population, 1973

	Males	*Females*	*Total*
Ireland	4·3	1·7	3·0
England and Wales	9·4	6·2	7·8
Netherlands	9·9	7·4	8·7
USA	17·7	6·5	12·0
Japan	20·1	14·7	17·3
Austria	31·6	13·6	22·1

(from the *Annual Epidemiological and Vital Statistics Report* of the World Health Organization Vol. **1** 1976)

Suicide is much commoner in certain occupations as shown by Table 57 below. In many cases, the high level is probably connected with the ease which certain occupations have in obtaining drugs—pharmacists, doctors and nurses.

TABLE 57 SMR from suicide, men aged 15–64, England and Wales, 1970–2

Pharmacists	464
Labourers	374
Doctors	335
Nurses	297
Deck and engine room ratings	275

(from *Occupational Mortality* OPCS 1970–2)

15 Preventive Medicine in Primary Health Care

The general practitioner accepts responsibility for dealing with the illness or disease from which his patient may suffer. Not only is treatment ordered, but advice should also be given on how disease may be prevented. Preventive medicine can be divided into two parts:

1. *Primary prevention* or complete avoidance of disease,
2. *Secondary prevention* concerned with preventing serious after-effects produced by chronic illness or disability. The general practitioner is concerned with both forms of prevention, but especially with secondary prevention.

The responsibility of a doctor for his patients never ends. It is quite wrong to consider that because a patient with a permanent handicap, such as hemiplegia, cannot be cured, the general practitioner cannot help further. Much can be done to prevent deterioration and to solve social difficulties. The majority of work in primary health care is, however, essentially curative, the problems of which are usually urgent, demanding the immediate attention of the doctor. But it is often as important for the general practitioner both to prevent disease and thus avoid unnecessary illness as to prevent deterioration in chronic diseases. The object of this chapter is to describe ways in which the general practitioner can do this.

TYPES OF PREVENTIVE MEDICINE SEEN IN GENERAL PRACTICE

Maternity Services

Obstetric care, including antenatal work, is an excellent example of a service carried out by general practitioners which is mainly preventive. The management of a pregnancy, already described in Chapter 4, is designed to prevent medical problems by checking on the health of the mother regularly and by giving constant health education advice on all topics. Minor abnormalities which may be the starting signs of a serious pre-eclamptic toxaemia can be recognized early and corrected before a more serious condition has developed. Success in this work depends on careful routine at regular antenatal examinations. Although the risk to the mother today is small (as shown by the maternal mortality rate of 0·13 or one death per 7700 confinements), *confidential inquiry into the* causation of *such deaths shows that 53% could have been prevented*. Apart from errors of maternity care, the fault may lie with the patient—for failing to attend when asked to do so. *All non-attenders must be followed up immediately to find the cause*. The simplest way for a busy general practitioner to do this is to ask the midwife to make an immediate investigation.

Health education, especially during a woman's first pregnancy, can be rewarding, for all mothers are eager to do everything necessary to ensure a healthy baby. The family doctor can help considerably in this respect and may find a patient who previously had been difficult to teach now very receptive.

Another aspect which is overlooked is *the importance of the postnatal* visit. Many mothers fail to attend—many more would come if the general practitioner asked the health visitor to help with non-attenders.

Child Health

More and more general practitioners are doing child health work in their practices. Many arrange special afternoon sessions and they are helped by health visitors working closely with them.

Others are employed on a sessional basis to conduct child health clinics for AHAs. Increasing numbers of health visitors are now attached full time to general practices and this development has resulted in family doctors becoming more interested in the preventive work for which the health visitor is responsible.

Non-accidental injury in young children (also called child abuse) can, in many instances, be prevented by exceptional vigilance on the part of the general practitioner and primary health care team. The condition and its diagnosis and management are discussed in detail in pp. 433 to 439. The general practitioner may be called to treat an injury in a young child and may, therefore, be in an excellent position to diagnose this syndrome. It is *particularly important that the early warning signs of this condition are recognized.*

Immunization

The prevention of disease by immunization is one of the most valuable examples of preventive medicine carried out by family doctors. A full schedule of immunizations for children is given on page 182. It is important that courses of immunizations are completed. If the mother is slack in bringing the child for second and third doses, the health visitor should be asked to call on the mother to ensure that the course is completed.

Another aspect with which general practitioners are increasingly concerned is the immunization of travellers and those going on holiday abroad (see p. 186). It is particularly important for the general practitioner to realize that *the majority of cases of typhoid are caused by holidaymakers neglecting to be immunized, especially those going to Italy, Yugoslavia, Spain and Portugal.*

Communicable Disease Control

As described in Chapters 9 to 12, much of the investigation of infectious diseases is carried out by AHAs. But early diagnosis is important and arrangements are made for community physicians to assist any general practitioner in the diagnosis of any rare infectious disease. A domiciliary visit will be made by the appropriate community physician (Area Specialist in Community Medicine (Environmental Health) or District Community

Physician). Assistance is also given with the collection of bacteriological or virological specimens from contacts within the same family.

The majority of infectious diseases should be notified immediately (see p. 176). Prompt notification in this way assists complete epidemiological investigation.

Contacts of serious infectious disease become eligible for sickness payment when certified by the Area Medical Officer that they should not attend work. This cannot be done by the general practitioner.

In tuberculosis, examination of close family or work contacts will be undertaken by AHA staff, but doctors may be asked at times by their patients whether such examinations are necessary. The value of contact tracing has already been fully discussed (see p. 195) and the general practitioner should do all he can to ensure that it is as complete as possible.

Occasionally difficulties arise in possible venereal infection, especially as the doctor may not wish to alarm his patient. It is essential that full investigation takes place and that this is undertaken before treatment to make certain that a serious double infection of syphilis and gonorrhoea is not masked. *If venereal disease is confirmed, it is important that the cohabiting partner be immediately examined*.

Prevention of Accidents in the Home

The majority of accidents in the home are preventable. Health visitors in their routine visiting of families are always attempting to teach how such accidents can be avoided and general practitioners have an excellent opportunity to do similar work while carrying out home visits.

All doctors prescribe potentially dangerous drugs in their practice. If these are carelessly left about, children can easily mistake them for sweets, with tragic consequences. Not all patients realize that any medicine or drug may be dangerous, especially if taken accidentally by a child. Patients should be warned of this hazard and posters for display in waiting-rooms will be supplied free to any general practitioner on request.

Home accidents in elderly people must be prevented for they are more liable to accidents and particularly to falls. Such a fall is always more serious than one in a younger person because (*a*) it is more likely to result in serious injury, especially fractures, and (*b*) so often a fall precipitates senile decay.

Women are more liable to falls than men and the tendency increases with age. Four types of home falls are described:

1. *Falls associated with attacks of vertigo*. A sudden attack of vertigo occurs in the course of movement and, unless there is a solid object to hand, the old person falls headlong.

2. *Falls associated with an increased liability to trip*. Old women seem particularly liable to trip over small objects or if there is a trivial unevenness of the floor.

3. *Falls due to difficulty in recovering balance*. Many old people find great difficulty in regaining their balance after a trivial false movement and this results in a greater tendency to fall.

4. *Falls due to sudden collapse or to their legs giving way*. In very old people over the age of 80. In such a fall, the elderly person may suddenly collapse and is often unable to move for some time afterwards even if he/she has not been injured by the fall.

The majority of such falls can be prevented by the old person being taught to take suitable precautions. The likelihood of an increased tendency to trip should always be remembered and care taken to ensure that floor fittings, carpets, rugs, linoleum are securely fastened. If the old person is living with a family, the children must not leave toys around on floors over which the old person is likely to walk. Loose electric flex across the floor is another hazard to avoid. If it is known that the old person has a tendency to fall or suffers from vertigo, she should learn to walk with some support from a solid object—banister, handrail, chair or table, so that if she suddenly feels giddy she can support herself.

Every old person depends increasingly on sight to maintain balance as his/her labyrinthine function is often faulty, and this dependence increases as age advances and is most important over the age of 80 years. Thus, an elderly person who is quite steady in daylight may be very liable to fall in the dark. This should always be explained to the old person and those looking after her, for it is essential that there is adequate light in any room or passage along which she walks. If the old person has to get up at night, a bedside lamp should be turned on before leaving the bed.

Hypothermia

This is a serious condition found mainly in elderly persons in which the body loses heat and cannot maintain a correct temperature control. It is discussed fully on pp. 494–5. It is important that the condition is recognized early as treatment is then much more satisfactory. It is not always understood that hypothermia can develop quickly in an old person who has suddenly been taken ill (such as an attack of pneumonia). General practitioners should therefore be on their guard in such circumstances.

Prevention of Blindness

It is particularly *important to watch for the early developing cataract* as so much can be done early in the disease. A history of rapidly failing sight, of seeing better in a dim room or of having to change spectacles frequently should always be fully investigated by an ophthalmic surgeon.

Some elderly persons will need help in making arrangements to obtain an eye test. The health visitor (or occasionally social worker) should be asked to help in making such arrangements which may involve taking the old person by car in certain instances. It is essential to assist in this way frail old people living alone.

Nutrition

As the level of nutrition today is usually very satisfactory, it is easy to ignore the important part it plays in maintaining health. With expectant and nursing mothers and young children, health visitors advise on nutrition and many welfare foods and vitamin additives are provided to assist in this work.

A number of elderly patients living alone at home fail to eat proper meals and recent investigations have shown that approximately 20% of those admitted to geriatric hospitals are suffering from 'latent' malnutrition. For this reason, it is wise for the general practitioner to assume that all elderly patients living alone, and especially those with limited mobility, may be borderline as regards satisfactory standards of nutrition. If further investigation confirms this, the doctor should arrange for a meals on wheels service or for a home help to be employed (see p. 499). Such social help should prevent serious degrees of malnutrition.

Cancer Education

General practitioners are constantly diagnosing and treating all types of cancer in their practices. In many instances, it is obvious that more could have been done for the patient if only advice had been sought at an earlier stage. The problem of cancer education is how to ensure early referral to doctors without unduly frightening patients. It is a difficult subject and one that becomes more important in middle-aged patients, as this age group is associated with an increased incidence of cancer. Schemes of cancer education are at present being introduced to help educate the general public in this subject and many general practitioners act as medical lecturers at public meetings. In this work, it is important to stress that many cancers can be treated successfully if only therapy is started early enough—examples include cancers of skin, breast and cervix uteri.

Screening Tests

Recently an effective screening test (exfoliative cytology) has been perfected to detect a precancerous condition in the cervix uteri. The technique of the test is simple. A vaginal speculum is passed and a direct smear is obtained from the cervix and examined histologically. If abnormal mitotic changes in the nuclei of the cells are found, further gynaecological investigation is necessary and a cone biopsy carried out to find whether a pre-invasive cancer *in situ* exists. This method of prevention is most promising for it enables treatment to be commenced before an invasive cancer has developed. All general practitioners should play an active part in collecting such material and persuading their patients to attend for examination.

Role of the General Practitioner in Mental Disorder

The general practitioner is usually concerned with the early diagnosis of all forms of mental disorder, and particularly with secondary prevention.

Mental handicap

The basis for determining whether a patient is mentally handicapped depends on: (*a*) an estimate of intelligence; (*b*) a social performance test to judge the ability of the individual to make use of that intelligence and whether or not the child is capable of benefiting from normal education including the special services for the educationally sub-normal. If the child is mentally handicapped, he should attend a special school for such children. (*c*) The emotional stability of the patient.

Most mentally handicapped persons are diagnosed in childhood. The general practitioner should seek the assistance of the school health service at an early stage so that an intelligence test, a period of observation and assessment can be arranged. A careful search should always be made for physical abnormalities such as deafness or cerebral palsy which may easily make the interpretation of tests more difficult.

A period of trial in a day nursery, nursery school or infant school is often invaluable to enable a highly trained teacher to observe the child.

One of the doctor's problems when dealing with a mentally handicapped young child is that most parents are very reticent to believe that their child is mentally handicapped and much patience is needed. Although a careful explanation is given, parents rarely accept the diagnosis and may seek further advice or even go to unscrupulous unqualified persons. In order to avoid this and to prevent greater difficulties later, it is important that the general practitioner realizes this attitude of non-acceptance is usual. Even among a well-defined group of mentally handicapped such as 'mongols', there is always wide variation in performance among the mentally handicapped and, with modern workshop training, this is increasing. It is helpful if a trained social worker takes the parents to see an adult training centre and workshops which helps them to realize that there is still plenty for the child to do after leaving special school.

Mental illness

In general practice, many of the problems associated with mentally ill patients arise from difficulties of admission to hospital. Full details of this procedure are given on p. 471. When in doubt, the general practitioner is advised to call in the social worker who has the responsibility of arranging most of such admissions. In cases in which there is a doubt about the diagnosis, domiciliary consultations with a local consultant psychiatrist are invaluable. Aftercare and follow-up treatments often take up a great deal of the general practitioner's time and much help can be given by the social services department with its teams of social workers.

Rehabilitation into a normal occupation is always important. It is best if the patient can return to his former occupation, but he may need to be found a new job. In both cases the doctor should discuss the case with the social worker, who then visits the employer to explain the position (see p. 477).

One important problem the general practitioner meets with mentally ill patients is the *prevention of suicide*. When taking a history from the patient inquiry must always be made into the possibility of suicide. To avoid the embarrassment of a direct question, it is helpful to ask if the patient has any morbid thoughts. Most will interpret this as a query about suicide and, if not, further direct questions can be posed. If the patient seems offended by the questions and resents any suggestion of suicide, it is relatively easy to explain that there are many other morbid ideas. This inquiry must be made as the majority of attempted suicides can be effectively helped and treated. Although suicide is a possible outcome in many mental illnesses, acute depression is the commonest mental disorder where it is a real hazard.

Anxiety not amounting to mental illness is occasionally present and it is difficult to treat. In all cases, it is essential to determine the cause of the anxiety; this inquiry may need lengthy investigations into the social circumstances of the home and occupation. This can be done by a health visitor or social worker.

Sex Education and Sexual Problems in Marriage

Although general practitioners are not usually involved in sex education, advice is occasionally sought from family doctors regarding sexual problems in marriage. Investigation of these problems usually shows a most unsatisfactory or even complete absence of sex education, and it is important that they are sympathetically and fully investigated for much stress and even neurosis may result if they are inadequately dealt with. Health visitors may be able to help with women patients.

In seriously disabled persons (such as paraplegics), much anxiety may be caused by uncertainty regarding sexual activity. General practitioners can help in many instances by raising the subject or by arranging for a health visitor or social worker to do so.

Abortion

Since the Abortion Act, 1967, general practitioners are consulted on many occasions by patients inquiring if they can have an abortion. The present law allows a pregnancy to be terminated by a doctor if two registered medical practitioners are of the opinion, formed in good faith:

a. that the continuance of the pregnancy would involve risk of the life of the pregnant woman or of injury to the physical or mental health of the pregnant woman or any existing children of her family, greater than if the pregnancy were terminated
b. that there is a substantial risk that if the child were born it would suffer from such physical or mental abnormalities as to be seriously handicapped

In assessing the question (*a*), account may be taken of the pregnant woman's actual or reasonable foreseeable environment.

It is clear that the responsibility of the doctor as set out in the Abortion Act is essentially a preventive medical one involving the likely result of the pregnancy on the health of the mother and child.

Family Planning

General practitioners have an important preventive medical function in relation to family planning and patients seeking such advice should either be dealt with directly (the doctor may prescribe for his patient), or be referred to a clinic run by the AHA. For full details of services available see p. 168.

COORDINATION BETWEEN GENERAL PRACTITIONERS, HEALTH VISITORS AND SOCIAL WORKERS

It will be obvious that a doctor can assist in the prevention of disease in his practice by working closely with health visitors and others, including social workers. In many areas of the country, health visitors are integral members of the primary health care team. In such cases much help and assistance can be given to the doctors and much time saved by health visitors carrying out investigations and health education.

Group practices and health centres are ideal units to facilitate health visitor/social worker/doctor cooperation. All such practices should have a health visitor attached and at least regular visits from the same social worker. It is possible for all doctors, even if working single-handed, to promote the 'health centre atmosphere' where ancillary nurses, and occupational therapists—are encouraged to meet him to discuss cases. Although this may take a little organizing, the advantage to the general practitioner is soon obvious—better services for his patients and more effective preventive medicine with a consequent reduction in disease within the practice. It is particularly important that full use is made of supporting social services provided to help patients in their own homes—home helps, meals services, occupational therapy, chiropody and the installation of various aids and adaptations.

REHABILITATION AND PREVENTION OF RELAPSES OF DISEASE

Effect of Social Circumstances

In many diseases, successful treatment is linked with the occupation or home conditions of the patient, e.g. peptic ulcers in which irregular meals or undue anxiety are contributory factors which obviously could effect the success of treatment.

Constancy of treatment by drugs

In many illnesses, for example tuberculosis and diabetes, the patient has to take regularly some drug or hormone and it is not always realized that many patients take their treatment irregularly. *A recent survey on tuberculosis patients* receiving domiciliary oral treatment with PAS and INH showed that 45% were taking their drugs inadequately. The reasons included slackness, forgetfulness and ignorance.

In diabetes, it is helpful for a health visitor to call and check that the patient understands the diet and can manage all the minutiae of treatment. This has proved so useful that a number of diabetic clinics now have attached to them a specially trained health visitor to do this work.

Housing conditions

Poor housing conditions not only predispose the individual to attacks of diseases (particularly *infectious diseases in children*, *bronchitis*, *rheumatic fever*, *level of accidents*) but may also be a most important factor in the correct management of illness. A patient with *angina of effort* or a chronic cardiac condition must avoid stairs. In a modern house it is usually possible to do this by turning a downstairs room into a temporary bedroom especially if there is a downstairs lavatory, but in a slum house this would be impossible and the management of such a case made difficult. A patient with *malignant disease* finds poor housing conditions a great handicap: for instance, it is difficult to look after a colostomy in the absence of a bathroom, internal lavatory and proper washing facilities. The majority of local authorities give special priority for urgent rehousing for important medical reasons. Doctors should acquaint themselves with these so that they can help their patients in this way—full details are available from the local Specialist in Community Medicine (Environmental Health) or District Community Physician.

Reference has already been made to the importance of living conditions in reducing problems in the elderly. The value of home helps, meals on wheels and soiled laundry services is described later in Chapter 26. It is not always realized that in the early senile dementia patient the rate of deterioration can often be checked by some form of occupational therapy.

Rehabilitation

The chronic patient should be encouraged to keep active even if the eventual prognosis is poor. It is useful to arrange attendance at either a handicapped persons' handicraft centre or an occupational therapy centre run by the social services department or by the AHA. Transport is a problem for many of these chronic cases, but most social service departments now provide special transport—personnel carrier vehicles and vehicles with mechanical lifts attached to carry patients in wheelchairs. Doctors requiring such facilities for their patients should contact the Director of Social Services.

Compulsory Removal of Elderly and Other Persons

The way in which such patients can be removed to hospital or hostel by section 47 of the National Assistance Act, 1948, is described on p. 506.

Rehabilitation and Help for the Chronically Handicapped at Home

Some chronically handicapped patients provide serious problems. Examples include hemiplegias, multiple sclerosis, chronic rheumatoid arthritis and osteoarthritis. When such patients are discharged from hospital, they need much nursing help at home and later assistance with rehabilitation and in many cases the provision of aids to daily living and special housing.

Home nursing

AHAs provide home nursing (including nursing aids) and social services department aids and adaptations. Each district nurse is a fully-trained State Registered Nurse having also undertaken a special course in district nursing. Special equipment such as hoists, special beds, wheelchairs, handrails, walking aids, etc. are usually lent by the AHA when needed. All forms of nursing are carried out, and in the most serious cases two visits a day are paid to the patient's home. The home nurse always works under the direction of the general practitioner. To assist the bathing of patients who are bedridden but do not need full nursing services, many authorities employ State Enrolled Nurses (SEN) and bathing attendants (see Chapter 8 for further details about home nursing and community hospitals).

Aids, Adaptations and Telephones

Aids, adaptations and telephones are available from all social services departments for the seriously disabled. Full descriptions of such services are given on pp. 448 and 451.

Links with Occupation and Disease

There are many special industrial health problems, and the general practitioner should always be aware of the main industrial processes in his area and their special hazards. Industrial medical officers, physicians in the local hospitals and the local Inspector of Factories will all help with information. It is important to realize that new problems in occupational health are continuously occurring. By keen clinical observation the doctor may discover a new relationship between an occupation and a disease.

Convalescent Care

There are two forms of convalescent care: (*a*) that carried out in special convalescent hospitals as a final part of a hospital treatment process, and (*b*) convalescent holidays.

Both are arranged by AHAs and full details will be provided to any general practitioner on inquiry to the Area Medical Officer.

16 Food and Nutrition

NUTRITION

Nutrition and public health are inseparable, as a well-balanced and adequate food supply is essential for complete health. In this brief survey, it is not intended to consider basic nutritional data which the student will have studied in physiology, but to concentrate upon the problems of applied nutrition and the methods used to control food supplies. Nutritional problems are (*a*) worldwide; (*b*) national; (*c*) individual.

Worldwide Problems

The task of providing an adequate food supply for the rapidly increasing world population is one of its major social problems. *Protein malnutrition* is one of the major public health hazards in developing countries. As food supplies are increased, a further complication is that this improvement in nutrition leads to an increase in population which, in turn, makes heavier demands upon the food supply. Indications show that food supplies are not keeping pace with the increase in world population. The solution lies both in controlling the growth of the world's population and in increasing its food supply by various improvements in agriculture, pest control and research to discover more suitable crops and animal stocks. Most of this is outside the scope of this book but is clearly connected with public health.

The National Problem

The national nutritional problems of the UK are complex, but for many years a national nutritional policy has been accepted which ensures the following conditions:

1. All essential foodstuffs are available to the whole population at reasonable cost, and present in variety.
2. Certain priority foods are provided for certain sections of the community. Examples include: (*a*) vitamins and subsidized dried milks for mothers and young infants; (*b*) subsidized school meals; (*c*) meals on wheels and lunch clubs for elderly (both services being subsidized).
3. Standards of milk production are controlled nationally—areas are designated where all herds must be free from tuberculosis and regulations introduced for the pasteurization of milk supplies.
4. Minimum standards are maintained for many foodstuffs and constant sampling ensures that these are reached.
5. Many foods are fortified to guarantee adequate supplies of vitamins.
6. Adulteration of foodstuffs is prevented by extensive legislation on such aspects as food preservatives or additives.
7. Foodstuffs are free from disease and this is achieved by meat and food inspection both at ports and at abattoirs and markets.
8. Food handlers are clean and do not contaminate the food—food hygiene.
9. Continuous health education is carried out to teach the public about nutrition.

The Individual Problem

The individual nutritional problems are directly related to the type, amount and variety of foodstuffs consumed. Foods must supply the energy needs of the body in the form of calories and the proteins necessary for growth and tissue replacement; hence the correct proportion of proteins, carbohydrates and fats must be present in the diet which should also contain adequate amounts of vitamins and minerals.

Proteins

Proteins may be of animal or vegetable origin and the best are obtained from milk, egg, meats, kidney or liver, for such foods contain large amounts of essential amino acids. The amount of protein required varies—the child uses about one-third of his protein requirements for growth, but the adult requires relatively little for replacement of tissue. Generally, it is accepted that a man requires a minimum of 70 g of protein daily, although this amount may often be exceeded. Unlike fats and carbohydrates, proteins cannot be stored in the human body. In adults, it is possible to obtain large quantities of proteins from vegetable sources, but for the child a high proportion of proteins should be of animal origin.

Fats

Fats are a concentrated form of energy and some of them are vehicles for the fat-soluble vitamins A and D. Fats are easily stored and form the main reserve of energy and large fat diets are taken by those doing heavy work in cold climates. The main sources of fat are butter, eggs, cream, cheese and fatty meats. Apart from the herring, salmon and trout, there is very little fat in fish.

Carbohydrates

These are the starches and sugars—bread, potatoes, cane sugar, glucose. They are the cheapest form of food and the body can metabolize them rapidly to produce energy. As family income diminishes, so the amount of carbohydrate in the diet increases and more bread and potatoes are eaten than fats and meat. Roughly half the energy requirements of the body are obtained from carbohydrates. Fats and carbohydrates are to some extent interchangeable, the latter being necessary for the proper metabolism of fats. Carbohydrates are stored in concentrated form—glycogen—in the liver and muscles and this can be rapidly broken down into glucose to provide energy in an emergency.

Mineral salts

Many different mineral salts are needed by the body including the following:

Calcium is required for ossification, clotting of the blood and for regulating muscular contraction, especially of the heart muscle and nerve excitability. The best sources of calcium are milk and cheese. Most vegetables and fruits contain satisfactory amounts. Note that meat, fish, sugars, fats and highly milled cereals are deficient in calcium.

Phosphorus is also required for ossification and for the proper metabolism of fat. With the exception of butter and sugar, most foods are excellent sources of phosphorus.

Iron is required to form the haemoglobin of the blood. Only a few foods—egg yolk, liver, whole grains, beans, kale and some fruits—are satisfactory sources of iron. It is absent in butter and present in only very small quantities in milk.

Iodine is necessary for the proper functioning of the thyroid gland and for preventing goitre. Fish, milk, and leaf vegetables are good sources.

In addition, potassium, copper, magnesium, manganese, zinc, boran, fluorine, selenium, molybdenum are also required in minute traces. The function of many of them is obscure and they are often referred to as 'trace elements'.

Vitamins

These are organic compounds whose presence in small quantities is necessary for correct growth and health. Many different vitamins have been isolated but the most important are:

Fat-soluble vitamins

Vitamin A is present in many animal fats in liver, eggs, fish-liver oils, and is introduced into most butters and margarines. The yellow plant pigment carotene, which is found in green vegetables and carrots, is transformed into the vitamin by the body. Vitamin A deficiency causes a degeneration of surface epithelium. This leads to (*a*) *night blindness* due to a deficiency of visual purple; (*b*) *xerophthalmia* which is a drying and thickening of the cornea; and later to (*c*) *keratomalacia* which is a softening and inflammation of the cornea leading to opacity and blindness; (*d*) *hyperkeratosis* of the skin.

These conditions are very rarely seen in the UK but are more commonly found in the Middle East.

Vitamin D is the vitamin which controls the deposition of

calcium and phosphorus in bones. The best natural sources of vitamin D are cod and halibut liver oils, but the vitamin can be produced by the action of ultraviolet rays upon ergosterol. Milk will contain vitamin D if the cow has been exposed to sunshine. Vitamin D deficiency in infants leads to *rickets* and in adults to *osteomalacia*, a disease where, due to inadequate utilization of calcium, there is a softening of the bones. This condition is endemic in underdeveloped countries and may affect pregnant and lactating women. It is extremely rare in European countries.

Rickets has been largely eliminated from this country by the introduction of vitamin D fortification of margarine and butter and by ensuring that all babies have cod-liver oil extract (see p. 116).

Vitamin K is necessary for maintaining the prothrombin level of the blood and therefore for promoting clotting. It is synthesized by bacteria in the intestinal tract and also is present in many vegetables (spinach, cauliflower, cabbage, kale). Vitamin K deficiency is seen as a hypoprothrombinaemia in haemorrhagic disease of the newborn produced by a deficiency of intestinal synthesis of the vitamin.

Water-soluble vitamins

The vitamin B complex contains at least four important factors: (1) vitamin B (thiamine), (2) riboflavin, (3) nicotinic acid, (4) vitamin B_{12} (cyanocobalamin).

Vitamin B (*thiamine*) is present in whole grain cereals and acute deficiency (*beri-beri*) is found in tropical countries. There are two forms, dry beri-beri characterized by a polyneuritis and wet beri-beri with a cardiac failure. In this country, *thiamine deficiency is usually seen in chronic alcoholics* who are taking a high carbohydrate diet with a very low intake of the vitamin. The symptoms usually are those of a peripheral neuritis. There is a slight risk of thiamine deficiency in patients on special diets for gastric ulcer, coeliac disease or obesity, but this risk is well known and vitamin B is invariably given to such patients.

Riboflavin is found in milk, eggs, liver and kidney. Deficiency of this vitamin shows itself as a dermatitis of the seborrhoeic type affecting the skin around the nose, mouth and ears. There may also be a sore tongue, an angular stomatitis and vascularization of the cornea which may eventually lead to a corneal opacity.

Nicotinic acid is found naturally in whole grain cereals excluding maize and deficiency produces the clinical syndrome of *pellagra* seen in the maize-eating communities of eastern Europe and Asia. Occasionally deficiency is seen in this country in conjunction with chronic alcoholism with steatorrhoea.

Vitamin B_{12} (cyanocobalamin) is found in whole grain cereals and deficiency causes pernicious anaemia as, in the absence of Castle's intrinsic factor from the gastric secretion, vitamin B_{12} in the diet is not absorbed.

Vitamin C (ascorbic acid) is present in green vegetables, fresh fruit, oranges, tomatoes and blackcurrants. *Note that milk, including human milk, is a very poor source.* Deficiency leads to scurvy, in which bleeding occurs in mucous membranes.

Today, in the UK, *vitamin C deficiency is mainly seen in old people living on their own* because often they neglect their diet especially during the winter. Spontaneous haemorrhages appear, teeth may become loose and skin purpura may be present from perifollicular haemorrhage. Preventive measures include arranging a varied diet for the elderly containing plenty of fresh vegetables and fruit.

Because of the deficiency of this vitamin in milk *it is essential to give all babies, whether breast or bottle fed, vitamin C additives.* Convenient forms include orange juice or rose hip syrup.

Calorie requirements of the diet

Every diet must contain a minimum quantity of protein (preferably first-class proteins) and a balance of carbohydrates and fats to give sufficient calories as well as adequate mineral salts and vitamins.

The calorie requirement of the body varies in men and women depending upon the energy needed for the performance of heavy work and to maintain body temperature, especially in cold climates. As a rough guide, a minimum daily calorie requirement for a person in bed at rest is approximately 1500 to 1750 calories. For light work about 2000 to 2750 calories are needed and for heavy work this is increased to approximately 3000 to 4500 calories. In pregnancy, women usually require about 2500 to 2750 calories daily and this must be increased to approximately 3000 calories during lactation.

About 300 calories come from the 70 g of protein in the diet.

The balance is made up from both fats and carbohydrates and it is always best to ensure a balance of these in varied foods. In old age, calorie requirements are less.

FOODS

Bread

Flour made from wheat grain is refined by using only a percentage of the original wheat grain. Ninety per cent extraction means that 90% of the original wheat grain is used—bread made from such flour is dark and brown and contains higher proportions of proteins, vitamin B_1 and nicotinic acid than 'whiter' flours of 70% extraction. Where bread forms a small proportion of the diet, a low extraction rate is of less importance nutritionally than in primitive communities, where bread forms a major part of the diet.

Milk and Diary Products

Milk is one of the most valuable foods and great stress has been laid on its nutritive value. It contains carbohydrates, fats and proteins in easily assimilated and balanced proportions and is also rich in calcium and phosphorus.

The composition of human and cow's milk differs as shown in Table 58.

TABLE 58 The composition of human and cow's milk

	Composition %					
	Specific gravity	Water	Fat	Lactose	Casein	Albumin
Cow	1·3	87·3	3·6	4·9	3·1	0·5
Human	1·03	87·3	3·3	6·2	1·0	1·3

By law, cow's milk must contain not less than 3% fat or 8·5% of milk solids other than fat. No colouring matter, water, dried or condensed milk, skimmed or separated milk or preservative may be added. The adding of water to milk is easily detected by the

Hortvet test on the freezing-point of milk. Genuine milk has a freezing-point of −0·53°C, but milk adulterated by the addition of water has a higher freezing-point. Heavy penalties are given to offenders.

The Milk and Dairies (General) Regulations, 1959, specify the conditions under which milk should be produced. The Ministry of Agriculture, Fisheries and Food is responsible for the registration of dairy farmers and for the enforcement of provisions affecting the standard of milk production on the farm. Attention is paid to cleanliness, ventilation and lighting of cowsheds, water supply to cows and the cleanliness of milk and cows at milking. Local Authorities register milk distributors and also have responsibilities when milk is infected or suspected of being infected with disease. Any person having access to milk in registered premises who is suffering from food poisoning, gastroenteritis or any notifiable disease, *must immediately notify the local 'proper officer'*—the Specialist in Community Medicine (Environmental Health) or District Community Physician.

The 'proper officer', after giving notice, also has powers to examine any employee who is suspected to be suffering from, or has been in recent contact with, a person suffering from a disease liable to cause infection in milk. If there is evidence or there are reasonable grounds for suspecting that a person is suffering from a disease caused by consumption of milk, the 'proper officer' may prohibit its use for human consumption unless it is heat treated.

At present there are four special designations, untreated, pasteurized, sterilized and ultra-heat-treated.

Untreated milk receives no heat treatment, but strict regulations are laid down as to its production. Any animal showing evidence of disease must be segregated and records of such animals must be carefully kept. Milk has to be placed directly into either retail containers or unventilated containers. Milk sent in unventilated containers to dealers must be pasteurized or sterilized or transferred immediately to retail containers.

Pasteurized milk has been subjected to heat treatment in one of the following ways: (a) the milk is raised to a temperature of 62·8° to 65·5° (145°F to 150°F) and maintained at such temperature for at least 30 minutes and then rapidly cooled to a temperature of not more than 10°C (50°F) ('Holder' process); or

(b) the milk is kept at a temperature of not less than 71·5°C (161°F) for at least 15 seconds and immediately cooled to not more than 10°C (50°F) (High Temperature Short Time process). In this method, there must be a device known as *a flow diversion valve* to divert for retreatment any milk which has fallen below the required temperature, and full records of temperatures and times must be kept for inspection. As the HTST process is usually a continuous flow method, it is more popular because of the small area needed for the apparatus.

The object of pasteurization is to destroy all pathogenic bacteria which may have gained access to milk including tuberculosis bacilli, *Brucella abortus*, streptococci, staphylococci, typhoid and paratyphoid bacilli and diphtheria bacilli.

Because of the widespread use of pasteurized milk it is very rare today to trace any infectious disease to the consumption of milk.

Sterilized milk is milk which has been filtered and homogenized and then maintained at a temperature of not less than 100°C (212°F) for such a period as to comply with the turbidity test. In practice the milk after filtering and homogenizing is poured into bottles and heated to 108·9°C (228°F) for 10 to 12 minutes.

Ultra-heat-treated milk has been retained at a temperature of not less than 132°C (270°F) for a period of not less than one second, and then immediately placed in sterile containers in which it is supplied to the consumer.

Ice cream must contain not less than 5% fat and not less than 7½% milk solids other than fat. If the ice cream contains any fruit, fruit pulp or fruit puree, it must either conform to the above standard or contain total fat and milk solids other than fat of 12½%.

All ice cream must be heat treated at either 65·5°C (150°F) for 30 minutes or not less than 71°C (160°F) for 10 minutes. After heat treatment the mixture must be reduced to a temperature of 7·3°C (45°F) or less within 1½ hours and kept at this temperature until freezing is carried out.

Butter is prepared by churning milk or cream until the globules of fat adhere together. Not more than 16% moisture is allowed in butter and no preservatives or colouring matter may be added.

Margarine is made from a mixture of vegetable and animal fats to which milk is added and must not contain more than 16%

water or 10% of butter fat. Today it is usual to fortify margarine by the addition of vitamins A and D.

Cheese is prepared by coagulating the caseinogen of milk with rennet. There are no legal standards and the composition varies with the locality. Cheese should be prepared from pasteurized milk because tubercle and typhoid bacilli are not destroyed in the cheese-making process.

Meat

All meat should be examined by an inspector prior to sale, and to facilitate this work notice of intended slaughter of animals must be sent to the local authority. In an emergency, notice must be sent to the local authority as soon as possible after slaughter.

A full examination of the carcase is made, including organs and glands. All serous membranes must be left on the animal for inspection. If there is generalized disease, the whole of the carcase may be seized and condemned, but if only part of the animal is affected, as indicated by diseased lymph glands, a portion only of the carcase may be condemned.

It is usual to condemn carcases of animals found to be seriously affected by the following diseases: tuberculosis, caseous lymphadenitis, actinomycosis, the cysticercal stages of *Taenia solium* or *T. saginata* and also *Trichinella spiralis*. Any condemned meat should be clearly stained with a green dye and subjected to heat treatment before it is removed from the abattoir. Careful legal standards are maintained for slaughterhouses, and all slaughtermen must be licensed.

Reference is made on p. 330 to the control of the importation of meat from overseas.

Shellfish are often infected with typhoid or paratyphoid bacteria if collected from areas liable to be contaminated with sewage. Many beaches are contaminated by neighbouring authorities discharging crude sewage into the sea or estuaries and *have been made prohibited areas for the collection of shellfish.* Oysters and mussels are cleansed by placing them for two weeks in sea water which has been sterilized with chlorine, but from which all traces of chlorine have been subsequently removed.

METHODS OF PRESERVING FOODS

The following are the more important methods of preserving foods.

1. *Use of low temperatures* either at temperatures below −4·4°C (24·F) (freezing), or at temperatures −3°C to −1°C (28°F to 30°F) (chilling). This principle relies on the inability of bacteria to multiply at low temperatures. Freezing is widely used for the transportation of meat and fish and provided it is rapidly carried out little alteration in the foodstuff occurs. Problems occasionally arise in the carriage of chilled meats because this temperature does not prevent mould growth.

Quick freezing, in individual retail packs, has become very popular in recent years. Freezing takes place at very low temperatures so that the food passes through the critical temperature range of 0°C to −5°C (32°F to 23°F) rapidly within 1½ to 2 hours. With all frozen foods it is essential to realize that *once they are thawed bacterial multiplication starts again.* The only safe way to use such foods is to cook and eat them as soon as the thawing process is complete.

2. *Exposure to high temperatures*—this principle is used in canning. The foodstuff is packed into cans, heated, cooked, sterilized and sealed. As the contents are then sterile, the food will remain sound provided the can is properly sealed to exclude air. Tins after sealing are cooled under water—*it is essential that pure water is used to prevent a repetition of the 1964 Aberdeen typhoid outbreak*, when a tin was probably contaminated by unclean water entering through a tiny pinhole.

3. *Curing or smoking* is used for bacon, ham and certain fish and is carried out by burning wood, when phenolic compounds in the smoke enter the flesh and inhibit the growth of organisms.

This method is mainly used to enhance flavour. Salting is occasionally used for food preservation.

4. *Drying* is applicable to many foods—eggs, milks, meat, fish, fruit and vegetables. In this process bacterial growth is inhibited by the absence of moisture. Vitamin loss in dried vegetables is not significant.

5. *Air conditioning* is used to enable fruit to be preserved commercially on a large scale. By careful regulation of the temperature, humidity, carbon dioxide and oxygen content of the air,

fruit such as apples and tomatoes can be kept in perfect condition. This method has also been successfully applied to meat.

FOOD CONTROL

Sampling to Prevent Adulteration of Foods

The adulteration of foods, drinks and drugs is prevented by the random sampling of these commodities by environmental health inspectors. Chemical analysis is made by public analysts to check that legal standards are maintained and this constant vigilance has raised standards and instances of adulteration are rare.

Preservatives are very carefully controlled and only limited amounts of either sulphur dioxide or benzoic acid may be used in certain foods—sausage meat, certain fruit drinks, coffee extract, pickles and jams. In the same way, many colouring substances are prohibited, including metallic compounds, gamboge and certain coal tar colours. Colouring matter may only be added to certain specified foods and never to milk and dairy produce.

Food Hygiene (General) Regulations, 1970

These regulations aim at the elimination of contamination of food in shops, restaurants and factories. Many different aspects are controlled including the following.

Hygiene of personnel (Reg. 10). Any person engaged in the handling of food must: (*a*) keep himself clean (especially hands); (*b*) keep his working clothes clean; (*c*) keep open cuts or abrasions covered by a waterproof dressing; (*d*) refrain from spitting; (*e*) refrain from smoking when handling food or when in a room where there is open food.

Cleanliness of food rooms (Reg. 25). The walls, floors, doors, ceiling, woodwork, windows and other parts of every room used for food must be kept clean and no refuse or filth is to be allowed to accumulate there.

Cleanliness of equipment (Reg. 7). Articles and equipment with which food comes into contact must be kept clean and in good condition so that they (*a*) can be thoroughly cleaned; (*b*) prevent them absorbing matter; (*c*) prevent risk of contamination of food. Food containers intended for food must be protected and kept free from contamination.

Protection of food (Reg. 9). Food handlers must take reasonable steps to protect food from contamination and (*a*) must not place food so as to involve such risk; (*b*) must not place food lower than 45 cm (18 in) from the ground.

(Reg. 12). Food shall not be carried in a vehicle with any article from which there is a risk of contamination.

Wrapping paper used must be clean. Printed papers (newspapers) must not come into contact with food other than uncooked vegetables.

Structure of premises (Regs 14 to 24). Insanitary premises must not be used for a food business. Sanitary conveniences must be kept clean and in good working order and must not communicate directly with a food room. A notice requesting users to wash their hands is to be affixed in a prominent position in each convenience. Wash hand basins shall be provided and be conveniently accessible to food handlers and there must be an adequate supply of hot and cold water. Lighting and ventilation must be suitable and sufficient. A food room must not be used for sleeping in and it shall not communicate directly with a sleeping place. First aid materials must be provided.

Facilities for washing food and equipment (Reg. 21). Where open food is handled, there shall be a sufficient number of suitable sinks and each must be provided with hot and cold water and kept clean and in efficient working order. Adequate supplies of soap and other detergents and towels must be maintained.

A good state of repair is required in every food room. The structure of walls, floors, doors, windows, ceilings, woodwork and other parts must be in such a condition as to: (*a*) enable them to be effectively cleansed (impervious surfaces if possible); (*b*) prevent risk of infestation by rats, mice, insects and entry of birds.

Precaution to prevent food infections (Reg. 13). Any food handler who becomes aware that he is suffering from *typhoid or paratyphoid fever, salmonella, amoebic or bacillary dysentery or staphylococcal infection likely to cause food poisoning* must notify the Specialist in Community Medicine (Environmental Health) or District Community Physician immediately.

Temperature at which certain foods are to be kept (Reg. 27).

This provision applies to all food consisting of meat, fish, gravy or imitation cream or containing any of those substances or any egg or milk (with certain clearly defined exceptions).

If such food is brought into any food premises on or from which a catering business is run, it must be brought to a temperature of 62·7°C (145°F) without delay. Likewise food which has been cooked or partly cooked must be kept at or above 62·7°C (145°F) or below 10°C (50°F).

Special similar regulations control the code and practice of handling food in ports—the Food Hygiene (Docks, Carriers, etc.) Regulations, 1960.

17 Environmental Health Control

Following the reorganization of the health services in 1974, most environmental health control problems remained with the new district councils—either metropolitan districts in the major conurbations or smaller districts in the 'shire' counties. These district councils do not employ doctors but obtain medical advice from their local AHA.

Each Local Authority has a named Medical Officer (a 'proper officer') seconded by the AHA from the health service who is their medical adviser. He will give medical advice when needed in other fields as well as environmental health, and help to control outbreaks of communicable disease or food poisoning.

Each district council employs a *Chief Environmental Health Officer* who is responsible for the environmental health control, and works closely with the named medical officer.

HOUSING

The house in which a person lives has an important influence upon his health and to be satisfactory should comply with the following standards: (*a*) be free from dampness; (*b*) have a sound stability; (*c*) be well ventilated and lighted (both natural and artificial light); (*d*) be adequately heated; (*e*) be in a good state of repair; (*f*) have a proper water system including hot water system and bath; (*g*) have an adequate internal water closet, sinks and drainage; (*h*) have proper means for the preparation and cooking of food; (*i*) be well maintained internally. Such physical standards are invariably found in newly built modern houses but are lacking in many older dwellings, especially in industrial areas.

There is, however, another very important aspect of housing—the planning of a town or neighbourhood. Many housing estates completed in the period 1920–39 were built without the essential community services such as shops. Modern planning insists that the following amenities be provided as houses are built—shops, churches, play spaces and parks, schools, doctors' houses, welfare centre, community centres, cinemas and libraries. Because industry is essential to the prosperity of a community, any new housing development should be within easy access of suitable industry. In new areas of development, it is usual to zone the industry to a few sectors so that its noise and traffic do not interfere with the residential areas. Planning aims at providing 'neighbourhood units' of 10 000 to 15 000 people within towns with 'green belts' of countryside preserved on the outskirts. When people who must be rehoused from the slums cannot be accommodated within the existing urban area (overspill population), new towns have been created. These are gradually developed into communities containing their own industry and have a population of 70 000 to 80 000. Examples include Cumbernauld in Scotland, Harlow in Essex, Skelmersdale in Lancashire and Dawley in the Midlands. Many of these are planned to segregate the motor car from pedestrians and make life quieter, safer and more comfortable for the residents. In the future, it is hoped that district heating for all the houses in an area will eventually be provided. This is already done in many parts of Scandinavia.

Effects of Bad Housing on Health

The health of people living in the slum areas of industrial towns is inferior to that of persons in good residential districts. Poor housing makes the individual more liable to disease or to the effects of illness. There is more infectious disease present and children who develop the usual childhood complaints have a higher incidence of complications. Overcrowding which is present in such areas leads to an increase in vermin and in the spread of air-borne diseases such as pulmonary tuberculosis. Dampness of many of the houses—caused by defective roofs, gutters or by rising dampness percolating upwards from the ground (no damp-proof course), or by condensation, leads to various rheumatic problems, a higher child mortality and an increase in chest conditions such as acute bronchitis especially in the elderly. The level of all types of accidents is higher in bad houses due to poor lighting, very steep unsuitable stairs and faulty floors. Many of these adverse factors are reflected *in the higher mortality in social class V* (see p. 88).

Poor housing is an important factor in the correct management of illness. A patient with angina or with chronic cardiac failure must be able to avoid stairs. In a modern house this is usually possible by turning a downstairs room into a temporary bedroom, especially if there is a downstairs lavatory, but in a slum house this is impossible and the case is more difficult to look after. Poor housing can be a contributory cause of mental illness and also makes rehabilitation from hospital difficult. In mental handicap bad housing is a great drawback, for the extra strain of looking after such a child in these conditions is considerable. It may become so difficult that the child has to be admitted to an institution, whereas had the house been suitable he could have stayed happily at home.

Poor housing conditions have a stultifying effect on the proper development of the family which consequently cannot reach its full potential. Children are unable to work properly and their progress at school suffers while individual preferences for reading, pastimes and cultural pursuits cannot be satisfied in damp, overcrowded, ill-ventilated, badly lighted and inadequately heated accommodation. Efforts to brighten the home with new decorations are ruined by dampness and other defects and parents eventually give up trying to cope with the overwhelming problems and low standards are accepted as normal.

On rehousing, encouragement and tactful education by health visitors, social workers, or environmental health inspectors are needed to assist the occupants to make full use of the new facilities. An effort should always be made to ensure that the rehoused person is brought actively into the community life of the neighbourhood so that new roots, so necessary to the security of the individual and his family, will be firmly made.

Methods of Dealing with Inadequate Houses Unfit for Human Habitation

Slight defects

Small defects of repair which, unless promptly dealt with, can lead to rapid deterioration of old property, are often not carried out by landlords. Under the Public Health Act, 1936, section 93, a local authority may, on being satisfied that a *statutory nuisance* exists, serve an *abatement notice* on the owner of the premises to do the necessary repairs. If the owner still does not do the repair, the authority may serve a summons requiring the owner to appear before a court of summary jurisdiction. This Court may then make a *nuisance order* requiring the owner to abate the nuisance within a specified time. In the case of some old 'slum' houses, this procedure may be difficult to enforce because the owner may have abandoned the property and cannot be traced. In this instance it is possible for the local authority to repair the house in default of the owner under either the Public Health Act, 1936, or local acts, and the cost of this repair may then be recovered from the rent. Where there is likely to be delay in dealing with urgent matters, a local authority may serve a notice under the Public Health Act, 1961, section 26 and, if the work is not done within nine days, the local authority may carry out the work in default. Such costs are always entered in the local Land Search Register and become a first charge on the property in the event of a sale. In practice, these powers are used widely for small urgent repairs—mending a leaking roof, repairing defective gutters and downspouts, renewing broken water closets, etc. If, however, there are many serious defects, it is more usual to deal with the house either as an individual unfit house or in a clearance area.

Individual unfit houses (s. 16, 17, 18 Housing Act, 1957)

These are houses which have become more unfit than neighbouring dwellings due to overcrowding, bad landlords neglecting the property, by excessive sub-letting or by general decay and the Local Authority may order either their closure or demolition. The standards mentioned in section 4 of the Housing Act, 1957 (see below), are used. The local authority must satisfy itself that the house is unfit for human habitation and cannot at reasonable cost be made fit. Although there is no legal definition of 'reasonable cost', it is generally accepted that if the cost of repairs is less than 50% of the value of the property *after* repair, this would be considered reasonable.

The procedure is for the 'proper officer' to make an official representation or for the Public Health Inspector to make a report to the local authority (usually to its Housing Committee), advising that the house is unfit for habitation. The local authority then acts in a judicial capacity and considers this representation or report, and the owner is invited to attend. If the local authority is satisfied that the house is unfit, it can make a *demolition order*. If an owner is willing to carry out all the necessary repairs the local authority may accept an undertaking to complete the repairs within a specified period (usually six months).

Closing orders and part-closing orders (s 18, Housing Act, 1957)

A closing order is made if the demolition of an unfit house would affect neighbouring houses or if the house is of special architectural or historic interest.

Where part of the house is unfit, i.e. cellars or attics, then part-closing orders may be placed on a portion of the premises.

Clearance areas

The replacement of most unfit houses (slum clearance) is carried out by action under section 42 of the Housing Act, 1957 by representation of a Clearance Area. Where any local authority is satisfied, after representation by the 'proper officer' or a report from the Environmental Health Inspector, that a number of the houses are unfit for human habitation, or by reason of their bad planning, narrowness or bad arrangement of streets are injurious to health, it may define them on a map as a Clearance Area ('pink land'). Under section 4 of the Housing Act, 1957 in determining whether any house is unfit, regard shall be paid to its condition in respect of: (i) repair, (ii) stability, (iii) freedom from dampness, (iv) internal arrangement, (v) natural lighting, (vi) ventilation, (vii) water supply, (viii) drainage and sanitary conveniences, (ix) facilities for the preparation and cooking of food and for the disposal of waste water.

Every unfit dwelling in a clearance area must connect directly with other unfit houses. Almost invariably, the local authority requires the land upon which the unfit houses stand for development and it is usual to make a Compulsory Purchase Order (CPO) covering both the clearance area and other neighbouring fit properties (usually referred to as 'grey land'). Wide publicity is given to the proposals and if there are any objections from owners, a *public inquiry* is invariably held. This is presided over by a Housing Inspector of the Department of the Environment (an architect or surveyor). Evidence is given by the Environmental Health Inspector and other officers substantiating their claims for the making of a clearance area and CPO. If medical evidence is needed, this would usually be provided by the Area Specialist in Community Medicine (Environmental Health) or by the District Community Physician. Objectors may cross-question and present evidence of their own. The inspector visits all properties about which an objection has been raised. After the inquiry, the Secretary of State for the Environment considers the evidence and publishes his decision usually a few months later. If the unfit properties are confirmed in a CPO, the *site value only* is usually paid to the owner, but in certain circumstances owner-occupiers will benefit from the enhanced compensation provisions contained in the Housing Act, 1969. *For fit properties (grey land), full market value is paid in compensation.* If an unfit house has been well looked after, a *small well-maintained grant may* be paid in addition to site value.

Persons resident in a clearance area, when the Council represents it, *must be rehoused by the local authority*. The whole procedure from the initial survey of inspection to the rehousing usually takes from 1½ to 2 years.

Houses in multiple occupation

Recently, many problems have been created by squalid living conditions produced by one house being occupied by many families. Each family may live in one room with many services shared and living conditions soon become most unsatisfactory. This is a special problem among immigrant coloured families and unscrupulous landlords (the worst of whom belong to the immigrants themselves) who charge high rents.

Under Part II of the Housing Act, 1961, powers have been given to local authorities to control this problem, including power, under section 12 (1) to apply a code of management to individual houses in which proper standards of management have not been maintained.

These give wide powers to insist on additional facilities, including adequate provision of natural and artificial lighting, ventilation, water supply, personal washing facilities, drainage and sanitary conveniences, facilities for storage, preparation and cooking of food and disposal of waste water, installations for space heating and adequate means of escape from fire.

In addition, powers have been given to local authorities (i) to carry out work in default and to recover the loss, (ii) to make a direction *limiting the number of persons who may live in a house, or part of a house, which is in multiple occupation.*

Improvement of houses

Although the ultimate aim is to replace all old out-dated property, in many industrial areas the size of the problem is so great that for many years only the worst slums can be tackled. Special provisions have been included in the Housing Acts, 1964–9, to encourage the upgrading and improvement of the better older property with an expected useful life exceeding 15 years. The Act differentiates the powers of local authorities in respect of: (1) dwellings in improvement areas, (2) dwellings outside improvement areas, and (3) dwellings in a tenement block.

Local authorities on receipt of a representation from a tenant can insist on a compulsory improvement to the Full Standard (including provision of fixed bath with hot and cold water, a water closet inside the dwelling or reasonably accessible to it, or to a Reduced Standard (as above but excluding fixed bath). (Section 19 of the Housing Act, 1964.)

Local authorities may specify areas of 300 to 500 houses as a General Improvement Area (GIA) and it is the duty of the local authority to bring to the attention of persons residing in the area or owning property therein the action they propose to take and the assistance available for the improvement of premises and amenities in the area. Consultations with owners and public participation are necessary to implement a successful improvement programme. It is intended that the improvement of dwellings in a GIA will be undertaken by voluntary action on the part of owners. The Act, however, empowers local authorities to acquire land compulsorily in the interest of the area as a whole where the unreasonableness of an owner threatens the success of a whole scheme.

Section 32 of the Housing Act, 1969, enables local authorities to carry out improvements of the amenities of a GIA. This may include tree planting, provision of play areas, parking spaces and garages.

ATMOSPHERIC POLLUTION

There are many impurities introduced artificially into the atmosphere by combustion, or by chemical and industrial processes which have a harmful effect upon health. These include various gases such as *ammonia*, *sulphur dioxide*, *hydrogen sulphide* and *carbon monoxide* as well as impurities such as *nitric acid*, *hydrochloric* acid and *sulphuric* acid and dust particles containing organic substances as well as carbon and soot. Many of these impurities are present in very small amounts but they cause much damage by their corrosive action. Dust and smoke also prevent the free passage of the ultraviolet rays in sunlight.

Changes in meteorological conditions tend to aggravate the effects of atmospheric pollution by trapping impurities within fogs so that their concentration rapidly builds up to reach toxic levels, when the health of many persons living in such areas will be affected. The worst effects occur in those who have some degree of chronic bronchitis and whose cardiac as well as respiratory function is impaired. In winter, damp foggy weather always makes such patients worse, but very serious problems arise when atmospheric pollution in the form of a smoky fog (smog) develops. The inhalation of smoke particles and sulphur dioxide probably produces acute irritation of the bronchial mucosa which aggravates the chronic bronchitis. For such patients, a major fog lasting two to three days brings them near collapse and many never recover. An example was the historic smog in London lasting five days in December 1952, when it was estimated that just under 4000 people with chronic bronchitis died.

Reference has already been made to the small but definite factor which atmospheric pollution plays in the production of lung cancer (see p. 245).

Control of Atmospheric Pollution

There are two main methods used to control atmospheric pollution:

1. Under the Alkali, etc. Works Regulation Act, 1906, pollution in certain scheduled chemical and industrial processes is dealt with by the Alkali Inspectorate of the Department of the Environment which works independently of local authorities. Various limits of pollution are laid down and any scheduled process may only be operated after a certificate of registration has been issued. Registration will only be granted if the plant is equipped with the best practicable means for minimizing the emission of any noxious or offensive gases.

2. Local Authorities are responsible under the Clean Air Acts, 1956, and 1968, for the reduction of atmospheric pollution in their area. This work can conveniently be divided into three groups:

a. Under the general powers no dark smoke should be emitted from any industrial premises apart from permitted short periods (see below). 'Dark smoke' is defined as smoke which is as dark as or darker than shade 2 on the Ringlemann Chart. The permitted short periods are defined under The Dark Smoke (Permitted Periods) Regulations, 1958, as a maximum of 10 minutes in any period of eight hours or, if soot-blowing is carried out, a maximum of 14 minutes and in *no case may dark smoke be emitted for more than four minutes continuously*.

In all old furnaces, every practicable means should be used to minimize the emission of grit or dust, but new furnaces must be fitted with efficient dust and grit arrestors.

b. Under the 'prior approval' section of the Clean Air Act (section 3), no furnace or boiler may be installed in industrial premises unless it is capable of being operated without making smoke. Local authority approval must be sought for each installation. The object of this clause is to enable the local authority to ensure that correct apparatus is used which will avoid atmospheric pollution, and local authority approval is necessary for each installation.

The local authority has similar powers to specify *the minimum height of any industrial chimneys to be built*, as it is important to secure adequate dispersal of dust and sulphur oxides in chimney gases. In deciding the minimum height of the chimney, special attention must be given to the position of neighbouring buildings and to the topography of the ground so that gases are safely carried away from the neighbouring population. In practice, recommended chimney heights vary with conditions from 20 m to 40 m or, in very large installations, either 40 m or 2½ times the height of adjacent buildings, whichever is the greater.

c. Under section 11 of the Clean Air Act, 1956, local authorities have power to establish *smoke control areas* in which the emission of smoke is prohibited. When a local authority decides on this action, a detailed survey of the area must first be undertaken and the authority then makes and submits the order to the Department of the Environment for confirmation. Wide publicity of the order follows and if there are objections put forward a local inquiry is invariably held at which evidence is submitted by the officers of the authority in support of the smoke control area. The Secretary of State for the Environment must be satisfied that adequate quantities of suitable recommended fuels are available before the order can be confirmed.

A substantial grant (up to 70% of recommended cost) will be paid to the householder to help with the alterations, *provided the work has been undertaken after the publication of the order*. Old firegrates have to be replaced with modern ones capable of burning smokeless fuel, or a change must be made to other forms of smokeless power—oil, gas or electricity. Conditions as to grants have varied recently as certain smokeless fuels are in short supply and there has been an increase in the range of appliances which will rank for a grant. All heating appliances must be maintained properly if they are to continue to function smokelessly and this is most important with oil-fired apparatus. Where smoke control areas have been widely established, there is a marked reduction in atmospheric pollution especially at times of mist and fog.

VENTILATION AND HEATING

Ventilation is concerned with the maintenance of satisfactory atmospheric conditions within rooms, factories and places of entertainment, including a regular interchange of air and the production of conditions that are healthy and comfortable. To achieve this, a careful balance must be maintained between heat gained or lost from the human body and this, in turn, depends on three factors: (1) temperature of the air, (2) movement of the air, (3) humidity of the air.

1. The cooler the air the greater the loss and *vice versa*. The temperature of the surrounding structures also plays a part—a cold wall will absorb heat and lower the temperature, while radiation of heat from warm walls helps to maintain the temperature.

2. The greater the movement of air the greater the cooling power as evaporation is increased.

3. The drier the air the more water vapour it can absorb and this means that evaporation is more effective and the cooling power increased. Likewise if the humidity of the air is high, there is a corresponding reduction in cooling power.

It used to be thought that stuffiness was caused by either a reduction in oxygen level or an increase in the amount of carbon dioxide present in the atmosphere. Neither plays a significant part, for experiments have shown that the level of oxygen can be reduced to 17% (a level at which a match will not burn) or the carbon dioxide content increased to 2·5% with no ill effects. In practice, such levels are never reached as the oxygen content of air never falls below 19% nor does the CO_2 content rise above 0·5%. It is now known that the main cause of discomfort felt in stuffy rooms is *heat stagnation*, due to inadequate heat loss brought on by a combination of increased temperature of the air, excess of moisture and a lack of air movement.

Heat can be lost from the body in three ways, *evaporation*, *convection* and *radiation*. The relative importance of these factors depends on the temperature of the surrounding air. In the temperature range 13° to 24°C radiation is responsible for 45%, convection 32% and evaporation 23% of heat lost. At temperatures above 24°C but under 37°C, heat loss by radiation and convection falls but evaporation loss increases. At air temperatures above 37°C evaporation is the only means of heat loss. The increasing role of evaporation in heat loss in high air temperatures explains why humidity is so important, for a low humidity will assist evaporation (and cooling by extraction of latent heat drawn from skin) while a high humidity will diminish heat loss.

Methods of Ventilation

For the efficient ventilation of any room there should be a steady inlet and exit for the air. The inlet should be large enough to allow the air to diffuse readily throughout the room but the rate of entry should be slow enough not to be noticed. A current of air that is noticeable is a draught. To avoid this it is best in cold weather to heat the air first by passing it over radiators.

Natural ventilation

Natural ventilation may be relied upon in most domestic dwellings. Air is introduced in the following ways.

1. *Action of winds.* Perflation—most building materials are porous and air will enter the room through the walls, especially on the windward side.

   Windows are valuable air inlets either by air entering an open window or by defusing around the edges. Doors also can be useful air inlets.

   Aspiration takes place by the action of the wind blowing across the top of a chimney and drawing air out of the room below.

2. *Movement of masses of air of unequal temperature.* Hot air being lighter rises and is replaced by a current of colder heavier air. In this way, there is a constant circular movement of air round a room (convection).

   Outlets for air include chimneys and, where there are no fireplaces, ventilators placed in outside walls near the ceiling.

Artificial methods of ventilation

In buildings where many persons congregate, e.g. cinemas and theatres, it is unsatisfactory to depend upon natural methods of ventilation, and fresh air must be forced into the building and foul air withdrawn. Two main methods are used.

1. *Plenum system* by which air is driven by powerful fans along ducts to the rooms. In this method it is possible to regulate

the temperature and water vapour of the entering air which adds considerably to its effectiveness. 'Air conditioning' is another term used for this system.

2. *Extraction method* in which air is forcibly removed from the building. Most frequently a combination of both methods is used and most large halls are ventilated in this way.

Heating

The type of heating used in dwellings will depend on many factors—the size of the room and whether heating should be continuous or intermittent or whether smokeless combustion must be used. Most heating depends on radiation and convection and to a limited extent by conduction. Because of the greater efficiency, more convection methods of heating are now used from some central source of heat; this may be a gas fire, a central heating system in which 'radiators' heat the air coming into contact with them and warm the room by convection. Constant central heating always leads to more efficient and equal heating of rooms. It also warms the structure of the house and reduces condensation and enables all the accommodation to be fully used in comfort. The aim should be to maintain the temperature of the main living-rooms of the house at approximately 18°C. The minimum temperature for all offices and shops under the Offices, Shops and Railway Premises Act, 1963, is 16°C.

Many different types of heating apparatus are used but, as smoke control areas spread, open coal fires are disappearing although the smokeless fuel grate is still widely used. Each year many people convert to more labour saving methods, including *gas fires*, *electric night storage heaters and various forms of full central heating* fired by oil, gas or electricity. Other new methods include the circulation of hot air through ducts from some central source of heat and underfloor heating.

It *is important to avoid heat loss from any house* and the roof space should be lagged with fibreglass. Double glazing, invariably used in cold climates, reduces heat loss by providing an air space between the two panes of glass which cuts down loss by conduction. In modern houses with large areas of glass, double windows have to be used as the potential heat loss is so great.

LIGHTING

Good natural and artificial lighting is important in all houses and workplaces. In houses, wherever possible, full use should be made of sunlight, for illumination from this source is best, and new houses should be sited so that large windows give maximum natural light. Electric light is invariably used to provide artificial lighting and a combination of many lamps usually produces the most restful results. In kitchens fluorescent electric lighting is often used as it produces a steady light with a minimum of shadow. The requirements for good artificial light include: (*a*) *sufficiency of light*—the important factor is the need to have good illumination on the *subject matter*; (*b*) *absence of glare*—this is best achieved by concentrating light on the subject matter and keeping the rest of the room in darkness or semi-darkness; (*c*) *constancy of light*—no flickering; (*d*) *absence of intense shadows*.

Really good lighting can be an important factor in reducing accidents in the home (see p. 266).

CONTROL OF WATER SUPPLIES

Sources of Water Supply

A constant supply of safe clean water is essential for domestic, industrial and agricultural purposes. In the UK, with its heavy rainfall, there are three main sources of supply: (1) underground water; (2) upland surface water; (3) river water.

Underground water

The level of underground water varies considerably, and is created by rain water sinking into the soil until it meets an impermeable stratum thus forming an underground lake. Occasionally, by sinking a shallow well, it is possible to tap such a source and this is the usual method of supplying isolated rural dwellings if they cannot be connected to the mains. Provided precautions are taken to ensure that sewage cannot pollute it, a shallow well can provide a clean safe water supply, but its main drawback is that it may run dry after a prolonged drought. More permanent supplies can be tapped by sinking a well which draws water from below the first impermeable stratum (a deep well), or one which is formed in a valley or basin by sinking a well to tap water under pressure from below the second impermeable stratum (an artesian well).

Purification of water in wells occurs by a biological process in the passage of the water through the soil. The deeper the well, the greater the purification, so that artesian wells provide very pure water which is, however, very hard as large quantities of minerals have been dissolved during this process.

Upland surface waters

The majority of artificial water supplies are provided by the construction of a dam enclosing a large volume of water, gathered from moorland districts, where the water is usually pure and very soft. From the impounding reservoirs, the water is normally carried to the town by aqueduct. Recently, a large scheme has been completed in which a natural river course, the Dee, has been used instead of an aqueduct—the water being fed into the head waters of the river and later extracted and purified downstream.

Rivers

Rivers are the source of the water needed by many towns and cities, the most striking example being London, which is mainly supplied by the Thames. River water is usually polluted, contains many dissolved minerals and is very hard. As modern methods of purification are very reliable, it is not difficult to convert a polluted river water into a satisfactory pure water supply.

Purification of Water Supplies

Before any water supply is safe for consumption, it must be completely purified. This entails three stages:

1. Storage

Storage is essential to provide the necessary reserve for a constant supply, particularly of upland surface waters. It also helps purification in three ways: (*a*) by sedimentation of impurities and suspended matter, (*b*) by the sterilizing effect of wind and sunshine, (*c*) by bacteria in the water outgrowing their food supply.

Filtration

Filtration is the next stage in purification and consists of either:

1. *Slow sand filters*—the sand acts as a filtering agent but its efficiency is due to the accumulation on its surface of a jelly-like mass of organic matter which holds up the impurities. In time, the thickness of this layer so impedes the flow of the water that it must be removed and the sand cleansed.

or

2. *Rapid chemical filters* in which powerful coagulants such as aluminium silicate form the jelly-like layer which acts as the filter. When the deposited impurities become too thick, compressed air is passed in the reverse direction through the filter and by agitation washes it clean.

Sterilization

Sterilization is the final stage in the purification process and is carried out by using chlorine which oxidizes the organic matter and kills microorganisms. There are many different methods of chlorination dependent upon the type of water, but all rely on the liberation within the water of free chlorine, so that after 20 minutes' contact there is a residue of at least 0·2 ppm of free chlorine. To ensure that sterilization is complete, the chlorination process should be introduced into the water supply at least one hour before the water reaches its first withdrawal point.

Other methods of sterilization are the use of ozone or ultraviolet rays.

Regular bacterial and chemical sampling of water is undertaken at various stages in the aqueducts and at the consumer end of the supply to check on the efficiency of the purification process.

Precautions for campers and travellers

The freedom from infection of water supplies in the UK is no indication of possible hazards in other countries. Most cases of typhoid are traced each year in travellers from Italy, Yugoslavia, Spain, North Africa, the Middle Eastern and Far Eastern countries especially when remote country areas have been visited on camping holidays. When such a holiday is undertaken *it is essential either to purify all water with a simple camp sterilization outfit*, or *to be protected with a course of TAB inoculations before starting.*

Fluoridation of water supplies

The variation in dental caries found in different areas is connected with the content of natural fluoride in the water drunk by people in that area. In localities where the natural fluoride content of the water supply is low, more can be added to bring the level to one part of fluoride per million parts of water. This has been done in many parts of the world and has always been followed by a substantial reduction in the amount of dental caries.

The DHSS strongly advises all water authorities to introduce fluoride artificially, and to help overcome opposition has agreed to indemnify any water authority from any civil action. A vociferous ill-informed minority of persons have campaigned forcibly against fluoridation on the grounds that it is 'mass medication and an intrusion into individual liberty'. There is ample evidence that fluoridation is a most valuable preventive medical factor, and it is encouraging that more authorities are introducing fluoride into their water supplies.

SEWAGE DISPOSAL

It is not intended to deal fully with this subject, which is more an engineering problem than a medical one. Water carriage systems should always be used to transfer sewage from domestic premises even in remote rural districts. The disposal of the sewage is carried out in modern plants or, in the case of rural dwellings, either by chemical closets or by septic tanks.

Chemical closets are the most satisfactory method for small isolated houses, caravans, etc. and consist of a closet containing a powerful disinfectant into which the excreta are passed. After a short period of time, sterilization of the excreta is complete and the contents may be safely buried in a trench.

Septic tanks are watertight structures with impervious linings into which sewage is admitted and retained in a quiescent state sufficiently long to permit the partial disintegration, digestion, or liquefaction of the solids by a biological process carried out by anaerobic bacteria and by enzymes (powerful digestive substances) secreted by these bacteria. The liquefied effluent is then discharged into subsoil drains or biological filters where it is purified by aerobic bacteria and the resulting effluent is discharged into a river, soakage pit, land drain, etc. The tank is desludged about once every 12 months.

Sewage disposal plants are usually sited on the outskirts of a town near a stream or river. The object is to dispose of the sewage in such a way that the end product is a clean safe liquid which can be passed into the stream without any danger of causing nuisance or contamination. The usual system contains the following stages.

1. The *separation process*—sewage entering the plant is passed into large concrete tanks where, by sedimentation, the solid matter of the sewage (sludge) is separated from the liquid. The sludge is then dried and mixed with refuse to form a compost, dumped at sea, mechanically dried or digested and dewatered for sale as a fertilizer.

2. The resultant liquid left after the separation process is then purified by passage through a *percolating filter* made of stones and chippings where a natural cleansing process occurs by bacterial action and oxidation. The final product is a clean liquid, free from pathogenic bacterial contamination, which can safely be discharged into a stream or river. Constant chemical and bacteriological sampling should be carried out and care taken not to cause pollution of streams or nuisances to neighbouring residents. Special arrangements have to be made for the disposal of various trade or radioactive effluents.

DRY REFUSE COLLECTION

Bins for the storage of dry refuse should be soundly constructed with lids that fit because this prevents vermin, such as rats, being attracted. Collection of the dry refuse should be undertaken in specially designed vehicles to reduce dust nuisances. There are two main methods of disposal of dry refuse:

Incineration and separation processes

First metal objects are separated from the refuse by the use of powerful electromagnets and pulverized and sold for scrap. The refuse is then burnt in a large incinerator which can provide steam power; the resultant clinker is useful for road construction.

Tipping

This is a common method and is useful to level uneven land or to fill in quarries. It is essential, however, that the tipping be controlled. This means depositing the refuse in layers not more than six feet thick and then sealing the layer on all sides with earth at least nine inches thick. Care should be taken to see that the refuse is left uncovered for as short a time as possible and never longer than 72 hours. Tips constructed in this way are safe but, if tipping is not carefully controlled, nuisances very soon follow. These include fire, which can be a serious danger, or infestations from vermin, especially rats, flies and crickets.

RATS

In the UK rats have been a constant menace to man during the last 800 years. The smaller black rat (*Rattus rattus*) first appeared in Europe in the 12th century and was soon responsible for devastating epidemics of plague (black death). In the early 18th century, the larger brown rat (*Rattus norvegicus*) was introduced from Chinese Mongolia; this pest rapidly drove out the black rats and other rodents which competed with it. The brown rat, living mainly in burrows and sewers, did not come into close contact with man and gave less opportunity for the passage of infected rat fleas to man, therefore rarely spreading plague. However, it is an unmitigated pest and nuisance and can live almost anywhere and eat anything.

Rats are very prolific breeders and are also cannibals. A single rat eats 40 to 50 lb of food per year. The following are the brief characteristics of the two common species.

1. *Rattus norvegicus*, the brown rat, is the larger, growing up to 330 g, and is the commonest rat found in the United Kingdom. It is dark greyish brown in colour, has a short thick tail and small hairy ears. It lives in burrows in banks, ditches, sewers and basements. It rarely climbs or is found in houses above the ground floor.

2. *Rattus rattus*, the black rat, grows to a weight of 250 g and is

a lighter-built creature. Its colour varies from a blackish grey to dark brown and it has a longer tail than the brown rat and has large translucent ears. It is a very active climber, spending most of its life above ground, and is the type of rat found in ships.

Diseases Spread by Rats

Rats carry the following diseases: plague, *Trichinella spiralis*, rat-bite fever, *Leptospira icterohaemorrhagiae*, salmonellosis and foot and mouth disease. Possibly they may be connected with the spread of typhus and trench fever.

Plague (see p. 236) is primarily a disease of rats and can be conveyed to man by the rat flea *Xenopsylla cheopis*. Because of their climbing habits, black rats are more likely to come into close contact with man and are, therefore, more liable to spread plague, especially in a country like India where this is endemic. Fortunately plague is rare in Western Europe and, unless an importation of infected black rats occurred, there is little danger of plague spreading in this country.

Rats are frequently infected with *Leptospira icterohaemorrhagiae*, a disease in which a chronic urinary carrier condition often develops in the rat. Spread occurs indirectly by persons paddling or bathing in ditches or ponds which are infested (see p. 225).

Rats are also often infected with *Trichinella spiralis*, and when dead may be eaten by pigs, which in their turn become infected. If this infected pork is not cooked sufficiently to kill the larvae of *Trichinella*, it may give rise to the disease in man.

Prevention of Rat Infestation

To avoid serious rat infestations, every possible method of destroying and denying them access to foodstuffs must be taken, including:

1. rat proofing of buildings and receptacles where food is stored
2. removal and destruction of refuse which would provide feeding materials and places for breeding

3. fumigation of ships (see p. 331)
4. prevention of migration of rats from ships by use of rat guards on all ropes
5. routine destruction of rats in sewers and drains
6. destruction of rats by 'block treatment' which involves thorough investigation and treatment over an area within a radius of 300 metres from the original infestation

The usual method of destroying rats is by poisoning, but, as the creatures are cunning and suspicious, great care must be taken in introducing poison by pre-baiting with unpoisoned food for at least five days, so that the rat's natural suspicion of new objects is overcome. Poisonous bait substituted after five days pre-baiting is usually successful. Poisons include fluoracetamide (mainly in sewers), Warfarin, zinc phosphide $2\frac{1}{2}$%, arsenious oxide 10%. Some poisons are more effective with the brown rat than the ship rat and it is best to identify which type is causing the infestation. Warfarin is usually the best poison for the ship rat and is also used at first for the brown rat and then a change is made to zinc phosphide and arsenious oxide.

In all instances it is essential to find the cause of the trouble, otherwise repetitive infestations will occur. This may be due to a faulty drain allowing rats to leave the sewers or it may be that they are attracted by food and warmth into a cellar, gaining entrance through a faulty door, window or opening. Trapping is used to identify rats but cannot control heavy infestations. On farms, cats and dogs are useful in controlling this menace.

FLEAS

There are many varieties. The common flea is known as *Pulex irritans* and does not carry disease, but its bite can be very irritating, leading to itching and lack of sleep.

Xenopsylla cheopis (rat flea) transmits plague from the rat to humans. When a rat already infected is bitten by this flea, the plague bacillus (*Pasteurella pestis*) is transmitted from the rat's blood to the proboscis of the flea, where it multiplies. If the flea then bites a human being, some of these bacilli are regurgitated into the bloodstream and infection results.

Control and Destruction of Fleas

The partially developed flea *may remain dormant in dust for long periods* and, if given suitable conditions, may then complete its life cycle. They are particularly sensitive to movement and this probably explains their sudden appearance in unoccupied free houses which seem to be vermin free.

For domestic animals, fleas may be prevented by dusting the animal's coat with insecticide powders containing 0·5% pyrethrum and 5·0% gamma BHC. Operatives cleansing dirty houses should wear rubber boots to reduce accidental infestation. Infested rooms should be sprinkled with powdered naphthalene and kept closed for 24 hours (2 kg powdered naphthalene per 100 m^2 of room). Furniture can be sprayed with liquid insecticide (pyrethrum and gamma BHC). Cleanliness of clothes and person does much to prevent problems but, if an accidental infestation occurs, a bath should be taken and be followed by a thorough dusting of the clothes with gamma BHC.

LICE

Lice have had a remarkable influence upon history. Through the devastations of *typhus*—a rickettsial disease which is spread by them—thousands died, and this determined the outcome of many of the battles in the Thirty Years' War and during the 18th century. In the same way, in 1812–13, Napoleon's retreat from Moscow was made almost a rout by the disease. However, the worst devastations from typhus were in Russia at the end of the First World War when in the years 1917–21 it is estimated that 25 million cases occurred resulting in 3 million deaths.

The head and body louse (*Pediculus capitis* and *P. corporis*) probably belong to the same species, while the crab louse (*P. pubis*) is a variant. The eggs (nits) are laid and cemented to the hairs or clothing and, under ideal conditions, the life cycle—egg→nymphal stages→adult—takes approximately four weeks. Nits will not hatch at temperatures below 24°C.

Lice are associated with lack of cleanliness and cause much discomfort and broken sleep. They are the vectors of typhus fever, trench fever and relapsing fever. Lousiness, once very common, is today rare, although about 3% of schoolchildren are found to have nits in their hair. During wars there is always a greater chance of lousiness in campaigns in cold climates as there is little opportunity of bathing or changing clothes regularly.

Control of Lice

There are three main methods of control.

1. *Prevention of infestation*—general hygiene should be of a high standard with frequent baths and regular changes of clothing and bed linen. It is also important to recognize infestations early so that prompt treatment can be arranged. For persons who are camping or are unable to change clothing, prophylactic dusting of clothing with 5% gamma BHC powder is useful.
2. *Cleansing of infested persons*. The person should have a bath and, when dry, dust his/her body with 5% gamma BHC powder and put on clean clothes. Where hair is infested this should be thoroughly washed with a solution of 5% Lethane. Later, nits should be removed by careful combing of the hair using a fine comb. It is essential to realize that reinfestation commonly occurs from other members of the same family. It is therefore, important to investigate the whole family when one member is found to be infested.
3. *Disinfection of clothing* is best carried out by moist heat (a temperature of 100°C is maintained for one hour to destroy lice and any rickettsia which have been deposited on the clothing). Ironing of underclothes will kill any nits deposited in seams.

MOSQUITO

Mosquitoes spread the following tropical diseases: malaria (*Anopheles* mosquitoes), filaria bancrofti (*Culex fatigans*), yellow fever and dengue fever (*Aedes aegypti*). The control of malaria is largely connected with the destruction and control of mosquitoes.

Control of Mosquitoes

Control of mosquitoes depends on destroying both adult and larval forms and includes:

1. removal of possible breeding places, e.g. stagnant water of any type—ponds, ditches, puddles or household water butts
2. spraying the surface of stagnant water which cannot be drained by diesel oil or kerosene
3. covering of static water tanks with wire gauze of at least a mesh of 18 to 1 inch
4. stocking of ponds with fish which feed upon mosquito larvae
5. mosquito proofing of houses with nets and residual gamma BHC sprays applied to walls and window frames
6. disinsectization of aircraft is most important to prevent spread of yellow fever by accidentally carrying within aircraft infested mosquitoes from a yellow fever zone. All mosquitoes which may be in the aircraft cabin or hold are destroyed just before take-off by using aerosol sprays containing both 'knockdown' insecticide (0·4% pyrethrum) and 3% gamma BHC

FLIES

Flies do not act as vectors of infectious disease, but may spread faecal-borne diseases by their legs becoming contaminated with faecal bacteria and then transferring infection to any human food on which they alight. The danger of flies is greater in primitive countries with old-fashioned methods of faecal disposal, where they can alight on human faeces. This rarely happens in the UK but flies may, however, easily reach animal faeces and so spread pathogenic bacteria from this source to man via food. In tropical countries, where fly contamination is greatest, gastrointestinal faecal-borne diseases which can be spread by flies include typhoid fever, cholera, dysentery, infantile gastroenteritis and poliomyelitis.

Control of Flies

1. *Prevention of breeding*—flies breed in rotting vegetable matter and care should be taken to see that manure or compost heaps are kept as far as possible from houses.
2. Covering of refuse bins to ensure they are fly-proof.
3. Controlled tipping (see p. 308).
4. Treatment of manure heaps with chemical insecticides.

5. Destruction of adult flies by insecticides including pyrethrum and gamma BHC starting early in the summer.
6. Tangle foot traps for adult flies.
7. Fly-proofing of larders, meat safes and the use of refrigerators to store perishable foods and prevent contamination.

BED BUGS

Fortunately infestations with bed bugs are becoming rare. Although it has never been demonstrated that bed bugs carry disease, they cause much discomfort and have a very unpleasant smell. Bed bugs migrate from their hiding places in walls, furniture, crevices, books, picture frames, behind skirting boards and mattresses, at night, and cause much irritation by their bites to humans sleeping in the house. On feeding, the adult usually is gorged with blood in five to ten minutes and then may show no inclination to feed again for many days. Eggs are laid in their hiding-places and the minimum development period from egg to adult through five nymphal stages takes seven weeks. Adult bed bugs live from six to eight months, and are most active in hot weather.

Bed bugs are disseminated and spread in the following ways:

1. Removal of infested furniture—this is an important method and includes new furniture sold on hire purchase which has had to be reclaimed.
2. Removal of secondhand furniture in vans.
3. Sale of secondhand furniture.
4. Migration of bed bugs from one house to a neighbouring one. The bugs cannot fly but move rapidly by crawling.
5. The use of old infested timber in new buildings.

Control of Bed Bugs

If there is a heavy infestation, it will probably be difficult to eradicate and it is best to call in the local authority disinfestation service. It may even be necessary to evacuate the building and to fumigate with HCN gas. Hard furniture can be fumigated at special centres using HCN or SO_2 or gamma BHC. Steam disinfestation is used for bedding.

COCKROACHES

There are two common species of cockroach—black beetle (*Blatta orientalis*) and the German cockroach (*Blatella germanica*). The first is about 2·5 cm long and *Blatella* half that size. The black beetle is uniformly mahogany-brown in colour, while *Blatella* is yellowish-brown with darker patches. Cockroaches are mainly found in houses, bakehouses, hospitals and institution kitchens. They are nocturnal in habit and usually live behind stoves, cupboards and in crevices. In *Blatella*, eggs are laid in batches of 12 to 20 in a sealed oblong case attached to the abdomen, but the eggs of *Blatella* are deposited in dark corners. Incubation takes approximately 10 weeks and the cockroaches do not reach maturity for a further six months. There is no direct evidence that cockroaches can transmit disease, but they have an unpleasant appearance and smell and are indicative of dirty conditions.

Control of Cockroaches

Infested sites should be treated weekly with an insecticide containing 5% gamma BHC dust. It is also possible to use sodium fluoride (50%) in kaolin. As a prophylactic, a 5% water emulsion spray of gamma BHC can be used.

SCABIES MITE *(Sarcoptes scabiei)*

In scabies minute burrows are made in the skin by the gravid female mite and intense irritation is caused, this being worse at night. In chronic cases, the scratching usually causes secondary infection of the skin and an infected impetigo follows. The mite is spread by close contact—often from sleeping with an infected person—and, for this reason, it is not unusual to find more than one member of the same household infested.

Control of Scabies Mite

Treatment of scabies is simple provided the following instructions are carried out. After a bath, the patient should be painted with a 25% solution of benzyl benzoate covering the whole body from the neck down. It is best applied with a shaving brush and when dry a second application should be given. It is not essential to cleanse the clothing, although this is often done. It is most important *not* to repeat the treatment for at least a week as benzyl benzoate, if applied repetitively, soon causes a skin rash. If the above instructions are carried out, all cases of scabies—even those with impetigo—will rapidly clear up. It is most important to prevent reinfection and therefore other infected members of the family should be treated at the same time.

INSECTICIDES

There are two main types of insecticide widely used:

Gamma benzene hexachloride (gamma BHC)

This is undoubtedly one of the most valuable insecticides available. It has the great advantage (*a*) of a high residual toxicity (its effect lasts a long time); (*b*) its application is easy; (*c*) it is lethal to most common insect pests.

It is primarily a contact poison and is absorbed through the tarsi of the insect. After a few hours, paralysis of the nervous system develops leading to a lack of muscular coordination and finally death of the insect. Gamma BHC may be used as:

1. a spray 0·3% gamma BHC mixed with pyrethrum (0·05%); it has an immediate insecticidal effect
2. a residual spray of 5% gamma BHC in kerosene. When applied on walls of unpainted wood, plaster or cement, its effect lasts some weeks
3. an insecticide powder containing 5% gamma BHC mixed with chalk

Pyrethrum

Pyrethrum is used because of its extemely rapid immediate effect—a spray containing it will result in an immediate 'knock down' of flying insects. Therefore it is mainly used in combination with gamma BHC in sprays, to rid a small area quickly of flying insects. Pyrethrum is comparatively innocuous against vertebrate insects (cockroaches or crickets).

PARASITOLOGY

Taenia solium (Pork Tapeworm)

This tapeworm, which is rarely found in the UK usually has the pig as its intermediate host, and small cysts containing the embryo worm may be found in its flesh ('measly pork'). If such meat is insufficiently cooked and is eaten by man, the adult worm develops in the human intestine, and eventually reaches a metre or more in length and contains up to 1000 segments. The ova are discharged from the terminal segment and pass out into the faeces. The life cycle will be completed if these eggs are ingested by a pig. Occasionally, man may ingest ova and act as the intermediate host; in this case, the embryo hatches, penetrates the gut wall, invading the brain and muscles of man.

Control depends on (*a*) adequate meat inspection; (*b*) safe disposal of sewage, and (*c*) thorough cooking of all pork products.

Taenia saginata (Beef Tapeworm)

This worm is also rarely found in the UK. The intermediate host is the cow or bullock, otherwise the life cycle is essentially the same as in the pork tapeworm. The head is larger than *T. solium* and has no hooklets.

Control is by (*a*) meat inspection; (*b*) thorough cooking of meat, and (*c*) safe disposal of sewage.

Taenia echinococcus (Hydatid Cyst)

This worm, measuring 6 mm in length, usually inhabits the gut of canine animals but man may act as the cystic intermediate host. Where man is infected a cyst containing the embryo worm (a hydatid cyst) will be found. The Cassoni test for a hypersensitivity skin reaction is a useful diagnostic aid for it is positive only in persons harbouring a hydatid cyst. *Persons who associate with dogs are liable to become infected* and the disease is not uncommon in Australia, South America and the Middle East. Care in handling dogs, particularly when there is a possibility of faecal contamination, will reduce the chance of infection.

Oxyuris vermicularis (Threadworm)

This worm measures 0·5 to 1 cm in length, inhabits the caecum and rectum of man and is commonly found in children. At night, some worms migrate out of the anus, causing irritation. In all cases, large numbers of eggs are passed in the faeces and hands may become contaminated leading to family infestations.

Control depends on prompt treatment of patients and any other infested members of the same family. The drug of choice is piperazine phosphate—500 mg daily for one week for a child and 1000 mg twice daily for a week for an adult.

Ascaris lumbricoides (Common Roundworm)

The female adult worm is about 10 in long and the male 4 in and is white or yellow in colour; the worm inhabits the small intestine of man. The eggs are passed out in the faeces and owing to their thick shell are resistant to heat and cold. If man swallows eggs of this worm, they change in the upper intestines to larval forms which then penetrate the intestinal wall and gain access to the venous system. Entering the liver, they develop further and finally are carried by the bloodstream to the lungs, where they may produce an area of pneumonitis. The larvae then enter the sputum, are swallowed and, in the small intestine, develop into adult worms.

Control is by effective treatment with piperazine phosphate (see above). Frequently no symptoms are found and the diagnosis is made by finding the worm in the stools. Occasionally worms in the intestine can give rise to intestinal colic or to biliary obstruction.

Trichinella spiralis

The adult worm is usually found attached to the intestinal wall of the pig or rat. Embryo worms are then deposited in the intestinal wall and later migrate, via the bloodstream, to the muscles where they develop into small cysts, 1 mm long—the dormant stage. Occasionally man becomes infected by eating partially cooked pork which contains such cysts, and the same cycle then occurs in man with the adult worm developing in the intestine and embryo worms migrating to various muscles. Symptoms are produced during this migration—fever, muscular pains, tenderness and oedema of eyelids. If cardiac muscle is invaded, sudden heart failure may occur at this stage.

Control is maintained by careful meat inspection, including regular sampling of pig muscles by microscopic examination. Snippets of muscle from the diaphragm, flanks and cheeks are cut from the pig carcases after final inspection has been completed. Particular attention should be paid to sow carcases which are often used in sausage manufacture. Recently it has been shown that low doses of gamma radiation to carcases will kill any parasites. Probably the most certain method of avoiding this disease is to ensure that all pork products are properly cooked. Many recent outbreaks have been traced to the ingestion of infested partly cooked sausage meat. The disease is more common among the Germans, probably due to the habit of eating under-cooked pork.

18 International Health Control

The international controlling body for health in the world is the World Health Organization (WHO) which has 142 member states including all the major powers in the world. The headquarters of WHO are in Geneva and regional offices have been set up in Africa (Brazzaville), USA (Washington DC), India (New Delhi), Denmark (Copenhagen), Egypt (Alexandria) and the Philippines (Manila). The main principle constantly followed by the organization is that 'health is now a world responsibility—for health, like peace, is one and indivisible'.

There is an annual World Health Assembly at which delegates from member states discuss the future programmes of WHO. These have generally been concerned with:

1. the training and interchange of medical personnel, particularly from the underdeveloped countries
2. preventive work aimed at controlling the spread of communicable disease throughout the world including expanded immunization programmes
3. advising on national health service developments in the poorer countries of the world
4. research work into preventive health, health education and therapeutic services
5. standardization of procedures in statistics and drugs

At the World Health Assembly in 1976, agreement was reached on the General Programme of Work for WHO for the period 1978–83. Apart from its usual programmes, WHO will concentrate especially on initiating or increasing work in relation to:

1. smoking and health
2. surveillance of congenital defects
3. rheumatic diseases
4. occupational health
5. leprosy
6. prevention of blindness
7. primary health care

Much emphasis in WHO studies is concerned with helping the underdeveloped countries and the contribution of Europe to WHO is very considerable—approximately 50% of the budget of WHO comes from European countries who only receive back about 5% for their own health service development.

In addition to WHO, there are two other European international organizations which assist with international health matters:

The European Health Committee of the Council of Europe which deals with current medical problems of the nine member states of the EEC, and Austria and Switzerland and with participation in certain activities from Spain, Norway, Sweden, Iceland and Greece. Recently the Committee has considered:

1. the setting up of a European Bank of frozen blood of rare groups
2. general practitioner training
3. modern management methods in health institutions
4. the causes of ageing
5. methods of treating alcoholism
6. the reasons for failure of some family planning programmes
7. the organization of public health laboratories
8. the problem of prevention of drug dependence
9. the methods to be used in handling cases of Lassa fever and Marburg disease

The European Economic Community (EEC) also has a health responsibility and has been particularly concerned with encouraging the freedom of movement of doctors and health personnel throughout the EEC. In December 1976, the EEC issued a directive establishing freedom of movement of doctors and working groups have been set up to look into a similar arrangement for nurses and dentists.

Reciprocal health agreements

There are now a number of agreements whereby health care for UK residents travelling temporarily in other countries is provided. As far as possible, arrangements are made in line with the provision of the national health service in the UK but considerable variations exist. In return, health care in this country is provided on a reciprocal basis. Current details are available in a leaflet entitled *Medical Treatment Overseas* and should be studied by intending travellers. Most European countries have *some* type of reciprocal arrangements except Switzerland, Spain and Greece.

DETAILED INTERNATIONAL HEALTH CONTROL WORK

Training

As far as possible the main concern of WHO is to induce self-help by sending small teams of experts to the underdeveloped countries to study their methods and suggest ways in which their health services can be improved. Key medical workers are given travelling fellowships to visit other countries for postgraduate study. It is hoped by this method to train a nucleus of experts in each country who later can arrange for the training of many other medical workers and raise the standards of medical care. Some of the most dramatic improvements have been in the child health field to reduce infant mortality, in the environmental field to improve water supplies, in many aspects of the communicable disease field (see below), and special work to assist in the control of trachoma which leads to so much blindness in many tropical countries. It is important to realize that only 20% of mankind live in the highly developed countries; the remaining 80% of the world's population are still mainly threatened by biological pollution, unsafe water supplies, poor sanitation, poverty and malnutrition.

Communicable Disease Control

The WHO runs a reporting service on the worldwide incidence of serious communicable diseases. A weekly bulletin is published on the world distribution of cholera, plague, yellow fever and smallpox. In addition, a daily epidemiological radio-telegraphic bulletin is broadcast by WHO from Geneva, Saigon, Keelung, Manila and once or twice weekly from Tokyo, Hong Kong, Singapore, Karachi, Madras and Mauritius. As well as giving full details of existing infections of the above four diseases, any unusual distribution of other infectious diseases is mentioned including influenza and rabies.

Malaria eradication

Malaria eradication has been one of the main aims of the WHO. Its schemes have been so successful, in the past, that the annual number of malaria deaths has dropped significantly. In 1945, 1800 million people lived in malarious areas of the world. The malaria eradication programme was started in 1956 and, by 1972, 721 million persons had been freed from this threat. However in the last four years there has been a setback in this programme and this has resulted in an increasing number of imported cases of malaria into the UK (over 1100 in 1976) and other European countries. These setbacks are mainly due to political unrest, administrative and financial difficulties in the countries concerned.

Malaria eradication schemes have three main phases:

1. The *initial or attack phase* which is concerned with active treatment of faulty environmental factors which encourage mosquito multiplication. This includes the drainage of swamps, ditches and other stagnant water and the widespread spraying with insecticides.
2. The *consolidation phase* is next reached in which officers visit all houses monthly to find out if any of the inhabitants have suffered from fever and, if so, take blood slides and, when necessary, give treatment to malaria cases.
3. Finally, the *maintenance phase* is reached where very few attacks of malaria are found but in which the preventive measures are continued for some years to ensure that the

improvement is permanent. In a few instances, widespread preventive treatment is given by arranging for whole populations to have prophylactic drugs.

In addition, much research into the problems of malaria is assisted and financed by WHO including work on the susceptibility of mosquitoes to new insecticides, drug resistance and the effect of new antimalarial drugs.

Smallpox

Smallpox eradication programmes have also been one of the major aims of WHO and these efforts have been so successful that the disease is on the brink of extinction.

By 1975, smallpox had been controlled so that it was only present in Ethiopia and neighbouring Somalia. The last case of smallpox (one of variola minor) was reported on 26 October 1977 from Somalia. WHO are now supervising the final stage in the world eradication programme of smallpox. This will include the reduction of stocks of variola virus in laboratories to a minimum, held for global, not national, reasons. Then WHO will supervise the dismantling of the restrictive national regulations on travellers.

In August, 1978, a laboratory outbreak of smallpox affecting one case occurred in Birmingham, England, and illustrates the potential hazards which the retention of smallpox virus in laboratories poses.

The eradication of smallpox has been an excellent example of the success of WHO. Because smallpox is a disease attacking only man, its extinction was always a possibility but it has required coordinated action of all countries especially those whose medical services are largely underdeveloped and WHO has acted in this role.

Cholera

WHO has been very active in the prevention of cholera especially in India and the East. In 1971, there was the threat of a cholera pandemic with the spread of the Eltor vibrio which has almost completely replaced the classical cholera. A total of 171 329 cases were traced by WHO in 38 countries but by 1976 the numbers reported had fallen to 67 000. Much of the recent control has depended upon better diagnosis and hygiene and, only to a limited extent, upon immunization whose effects are relatively short lived.

The international surveillance of cholera has been one of the major tasks of WHO. It constantly receives, consolidates and disseminates epidemiological information. As many of the countries at greatest risk of cholera have limited health resources, much of the work of WHO has been to help research into finding suitable methods for cholera surveillance. Specialized cholera teams have been developed by WHO for this purpose. In addition, WHO continues to carry out research into an improved vaccine and oral immunizing agents.

Tuberculosis

Tuberculosis has been an important subject in the preventive medical campaigns launched by WHO and many surveys have been carried out into the incidence of the disease and widespread immunization campaigns have been undertaken with BCG. Treatment campaigns have also been planned and assisted financially by WHO. The high cost of certain antituberculosis drugs, including PAS, has been prohibitive for some of the developing countries and research has been promoted to discover cheaper alternative drugs. An outstanding problem has been the widespread indifference of patients in the self-administration of antituberculosis drugs. Because of this difficulty, research at the WHO assisted Tuberculosis Chemotherapy Centre in Madras into the value of intermittent (twice weekly) supervised treatment of tuberculosis with isoniazid and streptomycin has shown that the results are as good as unsupervised daily self-administration. Once weekly supervised treatment was found to be unsatisfactory.

The WHO Expert Committee on Tuberculosis recommend that all infectious cases diagnosed should be provided with *drugs free of cost.* Experiments with direct BCG (without prior tuberculin testing) have shown no problems such as local reactions or reactivation of old lesions and this method is now used in developing countries. International quality control of BCG vaccine has been achieved by the adoption of the WHO Requirements for Dried BCG Vaccine and the establishment of an international reference preparation (avoiding any danger of mutation).

Further WHO research work into tuberculosis has shown:

1. that domiciliary treatment is as effective as that in a sanatorium or hospital
2. that a cheap and effective combination of drugs is isoniazid and thioacetazone
3. the need for a standardized methodology for the determination of drug resistance

Sexually transmitted (venereal) diseases

Many studies into the levels of sexually transmitted (venereal) disease throughout the world have been carried out and these have shown a rising trend in the level of early syphilis and gonorrhoea. In many areas the incidence of early syphilis has approached, or even exceeded, the maximum of the first few years following the Second World War, and in particular levels have been very striking in the younger age groups. A number of special teams from WHO have studied these trends and special worldwide conferences have been held. The last of these was organized in Vienna by WHO Regional Office for Europe in 1976. Topics covered included a study of trends, case finding by both screening and contact tracing, economic aspects, health education and training of personnel.

Leprosy

WHO has always been very active in developing services for the diagnosis and effective treatment of leprosy. Many prevalence surveys have been undertaken in a number of countries, the most recent in Burma and Thailand, and these have been followed by special treatment campaigns. Trials into the efficacy of antileprosy drugs have been undertaken and much stress has been laid on the early treatment of cases in children to prevent them becoming open cases, and thus reduce the contagiousness of this disease. Many WHO advisory teams have visited affected countries to train local medical workers and to undertake surveys and give advice on antileprosy programmes. Leprosy has been chosen as one of the major areas for the work of WHO in the period 1978–83.

Trachoma

Trachoma, a virus disease, is a constant grave medical problem in tropical countries because it is responsible for so much blindness. WHO has continuously assisted in two main ways: (*a*) by arranging large-scale surveys to discover cases followed by treatment programmes; (*b*) by supporting work in the search for an effective trachoma vaccine. Many different strains of virus have been traced and there is much further work needed before it will be possible to predict the ultimate value of mass vaccination against this disease.

At present WHO is assisting 15 member states in the development of trachoma control programmes and this work will increase with the present efforts being made by WHO to prevent blindness (see p. 328).

Influenza

A network of 68 national centres to collect information on the viruses responsible for outbreaks has been established. In London there is a WHO Influenza Centre, while in Atlanta, USA, there is an International Influenza Centre for the Americas. By the use of this network an accurate record is kept of the spread of epidemics throughout the world and this information is published regularly in the WHO weekly epidemiological bulletin.

Parasitic diseases

Extensive preventive work is carried out by WHO into various tropical parasitic diseases such as bilharziasis, filarial infections, trypanosomaisis, leishmaniasis, and the helminthiases. The pattern of work is similar to other preventive work—survey, treatment and training of local health workers to encourage extension of local preventive campaigns.

Veterinary public health

WHO carries out much research and preventive work into the zoonoses—diseases of animals which may also infect man. Recently much of this work has concentrated upon brucellosis, rabies, leptospirosis, hydatidosis and toxoplasmosis.

Advising on National Health Service Developments

The UK has been particularly concerned with this important work of WHO especially in the encouragement of appropriate primary health care systems.

Research Work into Preventive Health, Health Education and Therapeutic Services

The list of preventive and research work assisted by WHO includes:

1. many vaccine trials
2. promotion of maternity and child health services
3. research into causation of accidents
4. research in mental health
5. studies in environmental health problems
6. research into cardiovascular diseases
7. research into social and occupational health
8. research into human genetics
9. studies to improve the level of nutrition
10. promotion of dental health
11. health education
12. improvement of nursing services
13. prevention of radiation hazards
14. promotion of health laboratory services
15. problems of drug addiction and its prevention

Prevention of blindness

A good example of the detailed preventive work undertaken by WHO is given by the current campaign on 'Prevention of Blindness' which is being promoted. A world wide study has revealed that an estimated 40 million people suffer from blindness in the world (1% of its global population). Probably between 15–25 million of these suffer from preventable blindness caused by such disease as trachoma, onchocerciasis and xerophthalia. In addition, easily curable blindness from cataract is also a large problem.

The campaign will concentrate upon identifying those communities with the greatest risks so that the highest priority can be given to them in making available advisory, training and health education services. WHO is stressing that primary eye care should be provided as *part of general primary health care* with the development then of specialized local and central eye care services in each country. Intensive care programmes should be mainly used not only to treat blindness but to train local health personnel in the prevention of blindness as part of their normal duties.

Standardization of Statistics and Pharmaceutical Products and Drugs

WHO is continuously helping with the standardization of statistics for it is obviously essential that there should be complete agreement in the world about the classification of diseases and the ways health statistics are collected.

WHO has also played an important part in the international standardization of pharmaceutical products and drugs.

PORT AND AIRPORT PREVENTIVE MEDICAL WORK

Every international port and airport has a medical staff on constant duty to assist in international disease control. Full up-to-date records from WHO are available so that the exact level of disease is known in the country from which the plane (or ship) has travelled. The means by which this service prevents disease from entering this country will now be discussed. Airports are now much more important than seaports and procedures at both are now similar: pilots (or masters of ships) must report by radio in advance of their arrival the occurrence of any illness in *terms of signs and symptoms rather than specific disease.* Where necessary a doctor then visits and sees the patient. In addition, random samples may be submitted to medical inspection.

Medical Inspection of Aliens and Commonwealth Immigrants

Under the Aliens Order, 1953, and the Commonwealth Immigrants Act, 1962, special medical examinations are carried out at air and seaports. The airport/port medical officers are specially appointed by the Home Office as medical inspectors of aliens and Commonwealth immigrants. Only a small percentage of immigrants landing are medically examined. Those on holiday with independent means, members of diplomatic staffs and students, are exempt from inspection. However, aliens coming to the country on a working permit and all Commonwealth immigrants entering the country on an employment voucher are medically examined. The port/airport medical officer carries out a clinical examination but may order further special tests such as X-rays if these are indicated. In cases of serious doubt, temporary admission to a local hospital may be arranged. If as a result of the medical examination, it is found that the immigrant is unlikely to be able to support himself due to medical illness or disability, entry into the country is refused.

These medical arrangements have been criticized by many doctors as not being stringent enough. Many countries in the world have stricter medical examinations before entry is allowed and there is a sound case for introducing a compulsory chest X-ray examination for all immigrants.

Food Inspection

Stringent regulations are laid down for all food imports as many bacterial and parasitic diseases could be introduced into the country in this way and a large staff of food inspectors is available for the inspection of imported foodstuffs. If signs of disease are found in meat, it is condemned and must be either re-exported or used for commercial purposes (e.g. glue manufacture).

All imported meat must bear the recognized official certificate of the country of origin. This must show (1) that the meat came from animals which had been inspected *ante*- and *post-mortem* and passed as fit, and (2) that all necessary precautions for the prevention of danger to public health were taken in the preparation and packing of the meat.

Certain meats are 'prohibited meats' and are not imported, including: (*a*) scrap meat which cannot be identified; (*b*) meat comprising parts of the wall of the thorax or abdomen from which any part of pleura or peritoneum has been detached; (*c*) meat, except mutton and lamb, from which a lymphatic gland has been taken out; (*d*) the head of an animal without a submaxillary gland.

All tinned products are examined and tested to make certain that tins are sound. A small proportion are sent to a bacteriologist for further tests to ensure that the tins have been correctly processed and the contents sterilized.

Under the Liquid Egg (Pasteurization) Regulations, 1963, all imported liquid eggs have to be pasteurized by being retained at a temperature not lower than 64·4°C (148°F) for at least 2½ minutes and immediately thereafter cooled to a temperature of 3·3°C (38°F), and pass the alpha-amylase test. This is necessary because investigations and sampling have shown that such imports can be infected with salmonella and paratyphoid bacteria.

Desiccated coconut is another imported foodstuff shown to be infected with salmonella bacteria. Most imports came from Sri Lanka and, new regulations improving the standard of production have been introduced by that country.

All imports of fruit and vegetables are inspected and checks are made to ensure they do not contain poisonous chemicals. Various arsenical insecticide sprays can lead to a residual amount of arsenic on apples. The maximum permitted level is one part per million. Where higher levels are found it may be necessary to unpack the fruit, wash it and repack it.

Much work has been done on a toxic mould (*Aspergillus*) which may grow on groundnuts and causes a disease of turkeys. A standard has now been fixed—the permitted amount being 0·05 part per million aflatoxin, the toxin produced by the fungus.

Control of Rats in Ships

Because of the connection between rats and plague, strict regulations are enforced at all ports to reduce rats. Every ship from foreign ports must hold a valid *Deratting or Deratting Exemption Certificate* (valid for six months). At the end of this period, a complete inspection is undertaken by the port health inspectors. If there is no evidence of rats, an exemption certificate is issued, but if rats are present, fumigation of the ship is carried out using hydrogen cyanide, and a new deratting certificate issued.

In addition, any rats trapped are sent for examination to a

public health laboratory to test whether they are infected with the plague bacteria (*Pasteurella pestis*).

Further Control Work by Government Staff

Visits are regularly paid by staff from the DHSS and the Ministry of Agriculture, Fisheries and Food to foreign countries supplying foods to this country. The conditions at food and canning factories are inspected to ensure that satisfactory standards are maintained.

Whenever poor standards are found either abroad or on importation, the staff immediately contact health staff of the exporting country to investigate the matter further. Usually this method results in a rapid improvement, although occasionally new legislation is necessary to improve standards.

PART II

Community Health and Social Services

19 History of Community Health, Preventive Medicine and Social Services

The history of public and preventive medicine and social services in Britain is an integral part of the social history of the last 200 years. Before the middle of the 18th century, medicine had been intensely individual and almost completely curative in character. Although there had been repeated epidemics of serious infectious disease, little had been achieved in preventing illness. The first preventive measure came with Jenner's discovery in 1790 that an infection with cowpox protected the individual against smallpox, but the mechanism of this protection was incompletely and imperfectly understood. This was not surprising as Jenner made his discovery 90 years before the first pathogenic bacteria were demonstrated by Koch.

To understand how our system of public preventive medicine and social services developed, it is important to sketch the social conditions in the 18th and 19th centuries. In this country, the one outstanding feature of these times was the tremendous change which occurred in the pattern of life. It was the time of the great interrelated agricultural and industrial revolutions. In the early part of the 18th century (1720–50), England was essentially a rural community in which farming was the main industry and was carried out in many small-holdings. The village was self-supporting and industry as such was mainly centred in the home, for it was the time of the home craftsman. Spinning of wool served as an occupation for the wife and children of the struggling peasant farmer. There was, however, considerable stability within the village community. Roads were poor and consequently the ordinary villager rarely travelled beyond the town which served as a market centre for the countryside around. This was the pattern of life in England which had hardly altered for many centuries.

Seventy years later (1820), the picture was quite different—the pattern of life and mode of farming in the country areas had changed completely and there had been a great forced migration of country folk to the new, ugly, industrial towns which had mushroomed up in the North, the Midlands and South Wales. This remarkable change commenced with advances in farming. The enclosure of open fields developed, forming a system of hedged fields so characteristic of our countryside, allowing for more efficient farming methods with proper scientific rotation of crops. This proved so successful that more and more pressure was brought on Parliament to accelerate this change, which it did by introducing various Enclosure Acts. Small farms amalgamated and the size of holdings greatly increased. However, the significant result on the social conditions of the people was the great reduction in the numbers of independent peasants who could farm. At the same time, important discoveries by Arkwright in 1769 had soon resulted in all spinning being undertaken in workshops or factories and the profitable work of the peasant's wife and children (spinning at home) was removed.

Industrial Revolution

The independence of the country peasant had disappeared and the drift from the countryside began—many seeking a new way of life in the rapidly expanding industrial towns. Very soon it became obvious that these changes in the pattern of agricultural life which had led to much greater efficiency of cultivation were unfortunately producing social problems. There was a great increase in the number of agricultural labourers without any land, who became more and more dependent upon the new class of landlord farmers. Soon there was more and more poverty among the peasants and the living conditions of many of them deteriorated.

These changes coincided with a rapid rise in the population which aggravated the position, for the market price of labour fell. More peasants left the country villages for the new industrial towns. New well-designed roads assisted this exodus and the drift from the countryside became a flood. No longer were the young people content to live all their lives in the village—their ambition was to go to the new industrial towns. The villages, now connected to the towns by better roads, no longer needed to be self-sufficient and many village craftsmen, carpenters and tailors lost their livelihood and had to leave the villages. By 1820–30 the character of social life in England had been completely altered.

The rapid and uncontrolled growth of the new industrial towns in the 19th century produced even more problems and reforms became necessary and urgent. Alterations in franchise in the Reform Bill of 1832 and other Acts extended the vote. In the industrial towns a new ruling class emerged—those in charge of the new factories—and this class soon showed itself to be harsher and more exacting than the traditional country squire who still ruled supreme in the country areas. Conditions in the new industrial towns were appalling. The migration from the country, which the Industrial Revolution had started, made essential the provision of accommodation for the newly arrived workers as close as possible to the new factories. This was done by large-scale building of overcrowded and ill-designed houses. Every possible expedient was used to crowd in the dwellings, and back to back houses (joined at the back as well as sides) were introduced together with many other unsatisfactory devices. Within a few years, vast areas of slums were created in many towns. It is difficult today to understand how such deplorable development was allowed, but there were no effective local authorities or any other form of local control.

The rapidly developing factories demanded large-scale finance from the owners, and a very competitive industrial age had started. It commenced with the ordinary workers of the factories being very ill organized—later the Trade Union movement slowly developed in the face of acute opposition. It is easy to be highly critical of many of the factory owners, but it is important to remember that these changes followed closely on the dreadful atrocities of the French Revolution. This was the image always in the minds of those in charge and, although changes were slowly accepted, any signs of organized labour were always looked upon as possibly highly dangerous. This meant that, during this period (1830–60), changes came slowly and hesitantly.

Problems of Poverty

The large-scale migration of peasants from the countryside to the new industrial towns not only produced much overcrowding but also much poverty. It soon became apparent that the Poor Laws, which had virtually been unchanged since the time of Elizabeth I, were quite inadequate to deal with this problem. These laws had given to the parish the responsibility of relieving poverty, and under the stable self-sufficient village community before the 18th century they had worked satisfactorily, but under the new conditions of mass movement of populations they soon proved inadequate. In 1834 a completely new Poor Law was created by the Poor Law Amendment Act. Although introduced to improve the conditions of those in poverty, it soon produced exactly the opposite effect. Wages at this time were very low—there was no accepted minimum wage—and there was an excess of labour. Hours of work were very long and conditions in industry generally very bad. The new Act created a national Poor Law Commissioner and Boards of Guardians to administer the Poor Law locally over a number of parishes. The overriding principle behind the new Poor Law was to provide an adequate system, but to avoid at all costs making unemployment and the consequent poverty at all attractive. No direct financial help was given, but in its place was created the workhouse system, whereby those in poverty were housed and occupied. Conditions in the new workhouses built in all the new towns soon became much worse than in industry, so that no one in the workhouse could ever be in doubt that he was living in less attractive circumstances than outside.

These workhouses were grim indeed—families were split up, men to one part, women to another and children to a third. Discipline was harsh and food bad. Inmates included those who were ill, crippled, mentally disabled or aged and who could not work, and all were badly looked after. It created a loathing of Poor Law by the ordinary person which still exists today in the minds of the oldest inhabitants of our community.

Much discussion developed regarding the best way to mitigate the obvious social problems of this period. Two main schools of thought developed—the *humanist* and *humanitarian* views. Both were agreed that reforms were urgent but for different reasons.

The humanitarian school advocated reform because it was considered to be immoral to leave unchanged the appalling social conditions of the working populations of the industrial towns. Lord Shaftesbury, who spent so long working to improve conditions, was a leading figure of this group. It is interesting and revealing to see how little help he obtained from the church or the medical profession. It has been a regular feature of social and preventive medical history that reforms are usually vigorously opposed, particularly by the medical profession, and this trend has continued into the 20th century.

But the other view—that of the humanist—proved to be more telling in producing reforms. This school argued that it was unwise to force such a harsh system on the poor and ill because, by doing so, it was more likely that the pauperism would be made permanent. Illness was shown to be a greater cause of poverty as laziness. In this case, to deal harshly with a person was to make it much more difficult and perhaps impossible for him to overcome his poverty; in fact the humanists preached that the new system of Poor Law and harsh treatment only tended to produce a vicious circle and increase poverty. Slowly the views of the reformers were having an effect. The first changes were shown in the new laws concerning the employment of children and women. In a very halting way, the hours both were permitted to work were reduced, but often the new laws were ignored by unscrupulous factory owners.

Start of Medical Statistics

In this stormy period of social change, many other important developments were first recorded. In 1837, a great step forward was taken by the appointment of a medical statistician, William Farr. As will be explained later, the very essence of preventive medicine is connected with the assessment of the changing problems of health and social conditions of any community. The only way to do this is by careful collection and analysis of records of illness and various vicissitudes of life—births, marriages and deaths. William Farr was the first person to tackle this problem efficiently and his value in this age of social change was considerable. For the first time *it became possible to estimate the extent of disease* and this emphasized the deficiencies of the medical services. Farr's careful analysis did a great deal to measure the mortality problems in the country and his remarkable administrative ability laid the foundation for one of the most efficient government departments—that of the Registrar General. It also soon resulted in a close connection being demonstrated between poor social conditions and ill health.

Establishment of the Board of Health

In the period 1839–43, Edwin Chadwick, a lawyer who had been very much concerned with Poor Law reform, and a London general practitioner, Dr Southwood Smith, instigated various inquiries into living conditions of the poor. The results were published and contained graphic descriptions of the dreadful plight of many people, and stressed the connection between chronic sickness and poverty. These reports did much to arouse the members of both Houses of Parliament and a Royal Commission to inquire into the Health of Towns was set up in 1843. Its reports advocated many reforms, including the establishment of adequate local control over various sanitary conditions in the towns. A few towns acted quickly; these included Liverpool, where in 1847 a doctor to be responsible for the health of the community was appointed—the first Medical Officer of Health.

In this atmosphere of impending change, the sudden appearance in 1847 of another outbreak of cholera had the immediate effect of forcing the Government to act swiftly. The first Public Health Act was passed in 1848, setting up a central national body—a General Board of Health—for a period of five years. It had three original members including Lord Shaftesbury and Edwin Chadwick, and soon Dr Southwood Smith was also appointed. The Board was given widespread powers to remove public health nuisances and functioned quite separately from Parliament. Chadwick, the salaried officer of the Board, although efficient had the unfortunate habit of making himself extremely unpopular. Although the Board strove hard, it had the great disadvantage of having no well-organized local body to put its recommendations into immediate effect. It was also advising without adequate medical understanding on the method of spread of cholera (this was only worked out by Snow in 1854).

Criticism of the Board of Health mounted and when its first five-year period came to be renewed, Chadwick and Southwood Smith were dismissed and the Board itself was renewed on an annual basis.

Demonstration of method of spread of cholera

Cholera again broke out in 1854 and in this epidemic Dr (later Sir) John Snow demonstrated epidemiologically that cholera was spread by water. This, coming at least 30 years before the first discovery of cholera vibrio, was to prove highly significant. Before, there had been no general agreement about the method of spread of this disease. Many fanciful and extravagant theories were advanced, but Snow showed that water contaminated with faeces could lead to the spread of cholera. At about the same time, Budd in Bristol also showed that typhoid fever, a much commoner disease in this country than cholera, was also usually spread by water. It so happens that these are the only two infectious bacterial diseases spread in this way, but the effect was very marked. Immediately interest and effort was directed to improve the standards of water supplies and methods of disposal of sewage. In fact, the main efforts to improve the conditions affecting the health of the public were directed to define and set up a minimum standard for such environmental factors.

Development of Central and District Health Authorities

In the meantime, the Board of Health had managed to drag on annually until 1858 when it was finally disbanded and its functions transferred to the Privy Council. In 1855 a young doctor, John Simon, had been appointed to the Board and he was later transferred to the Privy Council. He worked steadily and tirelessly towards improving environmental sanitary matters. In 1871 a new body, the Local Government Board, was created and took over the health functions of the Privy Council. The Local Government Board also became responsible for the national functions of the Poor Law. This amalgamation of Poor Law and health functions nationally was an advantage although locally the Poor Law was administered separately. Shortly afterwards a national minimum standard of hygiene was laid down in the

Public Health Act of 1875 and the basic standards Simon had worked so hard to achieve were created.

Slowly during the 19th century local bodies were given the responsibility for the health of the local community. The ancient boroughs had this function given to them in 1835, but the absence of effective local authorities in other parts of the country hampered efforts. In 1872 Sanitary Districts were created in both urban and rural areas and it became obligatory for each to appoint a Medical Officer of Health. Local authorities were created in 1886 consisting of County Councils and County Borough Councils. Urban and Rural District Councils were instituted in 1894 and assumed the public health responsibilities formerly undertaken by the sanitary districts.

The development of community (public) health in the 19th century can conveniently be divided into a period of uncertainty and change until 1875 and then into a period of consolidation until the end of the century. But the emphasis of all development at this time was on the establishment of *basic minimum standards of environmental conditions*—good water supplies, good sewage systems, adequate roads, etc. It is, however, essential to realize that this stage in the development of the preventive health services had been reached by the end of the 19th century.

Care of Children

Public conscience was slowly changing and, towards the end of the 19th century, there was a gradual improvement in the way in which children were treated. Lord Shaftesbury had worked ceaselessly to improve working conditions with little immediate success. In many ways the great writers, Charles Dickens and Kingsley, achieved more by their novels. *Oliver Twist*, *Nicholas Nickleby* and *The Water Babies* are good examples of novels which did much to emphasize the plight of children. Other reformers were having their effect too and the Ragged School movement grew up to help educate the destitute child. A young London doctor, Thomas Barnardo, was so impressed with the plight of abandoned London children that he set up the first of the homes for destitute children that were later to become famous as models of their kind throughout the world. The extent of the problem can be understood when it is recalled that one night in 1870 Barnardo found 73 homeless boys sheltering among empty boxes and under tarpaulins in Billingsgate Fish Market. It is interesting to note the pioneering work in the care of children by individuals and voluntary bodies. Statutory responsibility for children came much later—in the 20th century. The strong influence of voluntary bodies such as Barnardos, NSPCC, Shaftesbury Society and National Children's Homes has been very obvious, and various other church-based social services are still most active in helping with the care of children.

By 1870 education was accepted as an essential public service and elective school boards were established at this time. By 1891 education had been made compulsory and free for every child in the country.

Personal Preventive Health Services

At the start of the 20th century a completely different stage in preventive medical history commenced—*the development of the personal preventive health services.* The reasons for this included the many great medical discoveries which took place towards the end of the 19th century. In particular, the discovery by Koch of pathogenic bacteria led to an understanding of the mechanism of infection of many diseases including pulmonary tuberculosis, typhoid fever and streptococcal infections. For the first time, the medical profession knew the nature of the infective agents they were trying to avoid and prevent. Very soon remarkable advances were made—Lister produced his antiseptic techniques in surgery. These attempted to reduce infection by operating in a spray of carbolic. Although now replaced by the aseptic technique, the results were startling. From a position of almost universal infection of all surgical wounds, Lister soon had results where infection was the exception rather than the rule. As with so many reformers before and after, Lister's efforts were first ridiculed, but his outstanding results finally convinced the profession. The age of elective surgery had started with all its great benefits.

Development of immunization

Bacteriology soon became of the greatest importance in diagnosis and, in the Boer War, Almroth Wright showed for the first time that it was possible to prevent typhoid fever by previously injecting a mixture of dead typhoid bacilli into the body. Many thousands of soldiers were immunized and so prevented from developing and probably dying of typhoid in South Africa. Another significant stage in the history of preventive medicine had been reached—*mass immunization*. What had been started quite empirically by Jenner 100 years previously with smallpox was now beginning to be understood and applied. The first advance had been made which 50 to 60 years later was to play such an important part in the eradication of diphtheria and poliomyelitis.

Start of School Health Service

The Boer War was an important turning-point in another type of preventive health development—that of *the medical care of the school child.* For the first time in war, it had been decided to examine medically all those young men who had volunteered to fight. On a simple clinical examination, over 50% had to be rejected because of some serious medical defect. This finding that over half the young men of the country were unfit for military service shocked the Government and a special investigating committee—an Interdepartmental Committee on Physical Deterioration—was appointed. Its report in 1904 was a remarkable document and suggested among other recommendations that there should be: (*a*) periodic anthropometrical surveys in schools and factories; (*b*) a system of registration of sickness; (*c*) special inquiries into the cause and effects of over fatigue; (*d*) a systematic medical inspection of children in schools and of young persons in mines, factories and workshops; (*e*) registration of stillbirths; (*f*) a special inquiry into the problems of syphilis.

At the same time, the committee recommended that there should be: (i) a central advisory council to help give prominence to public health; (ii) full-time medical officers of health appointed to all districts above a certain population; (iii) proper reports issued locally and nationally covering public health problems; (iv) more coordination between medical officers of health and factory inspectors to consider insanitary conditions in factories.

This report marked the starting-point of important reforms including *the introduction of the school health service.* By 1907 education authorities were given power to provide a medical service, and from this starting-point the school health service grew.

Child Welfare and Health Visiting

These changes coincided with many similar ones in child welfare. At the end of the 19th century many different authorities had been experimenting with a new kind of visiting service in which trained nurses went into the infant's home to advise and help the mother to care for her child. Manchester, Liverpool, Birmingham and Huddersfield were all pioneering this work —the beginning of the *health visiting* services which was to prove so valuable in the next few decades.

Quite suddenly, research started into the problems of child welfare and child health. The Chief Medical Officer to the Local Government Board (Sir Arthur Newsholme) was a leader in this respect and was responsible for three reports on *child mortality*. The first analysed the geographical distribution of infant mortality in England and Wales for 1908 and demonstrated that enormous variations occurred. The second made a special study of urban areas and showed that the worst mortality occurred in the industrial areas of North England, the Midlands and South Wales. The third report showed that the causes of infant mortality in Lancashire were complicated, but the most important were the *living conditions within the home and especially the standards of the mother.* It further demonstrated that the most dangerous period was the first month after birth. These investigations encouraged the development of the child welfare services. A further advance was the introduction of the *system of notification of the birth of a newly born child* which enabled the preventive health services to give immediate help. By 1907, authorities could insist on notification of births in their area and many did so. In 1915, notification of births became compulsory throughout the country.

The demonstration that poor living conditions had such a serious effect on infant mortality centred attention on: (*a*) the importance of improving housing conditions especially in the industrial areas—slowly it was realized that uncontrolled building had produced serious problems and that future development must not make the same mistakes, and (*b*) the length of time it would take to demolish all the unsatisfactory slum houses. Even today in the industrial areas of this country some still remain. It was, therefore, essential that personal advisory services were introduced to help mothers who had to live in poor conditions; *health visiting and child welfare clinics* did this by concentrating upon preventive rather than curative medicine.

Midwifery Services

In many other fields similar changes were occurring. Much criticism was aimed at the domiciliary midwifery services. It had become quite common for untrained women to attend confinements, often with most unsatisfactory results. Dalrymple-Champneys demanded reforms, but his suggestions that only trained and qualified midwives or doctors be allowed to attend women in childbirth were ridiculed by the medical profession! (Yet another example of how reforms, no matter how necessary, are so often rejected initially.) He persisted in his demands and in 1902 the Midwives Act was passed which insisted on all midwives being qualified and made it illegal for unqualified persons to attend women in childbirth.

Social Reforms 1906–14

With so much consideration being given to personal health services, it is not surprising that new social reforms in other fields were introduced. The Liberal government of 1906–14 passed many outstanding reforms including:

1. Education Act (1906)
2. introduction of the first old age pensions (1908)
3. start of the Borstal system dealing with child offenders and of probation (1908)
4. control of hours of work and the introduction of a statutory half day weekly holiday—Shops Act (1911)
5. introduction of the first national scheme of health insurance (1911)

The one outstanding omission was that the poor law system was left unchanged. This was surprising as many doubts had been expressed about the workhouse system. A Poor Law Commission was set up in 1905 and its report four years later showed opinion was widely divided. The majority view advocated no change but the minority view of Beatrice and Sidney Webb was a powerful indictment of the injustices of the Boards of Guardians. The Webbs recommended that the administration should pass to large local authorities but this was not accepted by the government (such a change finally occurred in 1929).

Lloyd George had a major influence in the introduction in 1908 of the first *non-contributory old age pensions.* By modern standards the pension was very modest, 5 shillings per week for those over 70 years of age whose income was less than 10 shillings per week. Yet it was a major reform and resulted in a classic struggle between the House of Commons and Lords which resulted eventually in the Parliament Bill which restricted severely the powers of the House of Lords.

The Borstal system of dealing with child offenders meant that no child under 14 years of age could be imprisoned. The recognition of the importance of prevention of crime was emphasized in the introduction of probation for first offenders.

The minority report of Beatrice and Sidney Webb did result in further active considerations of the health problems of the poor. In 1911 Lloyd George introduced a national scheme of health insurance supported by compulsory contributions from both employers and employees which provided domiciliary medical care. *Only the very lowest paid employees were included and their families were not covered by the scheme.* But it was the first official recognition that health is too important in any community to leave to the chance arrangements of individuals. The 'panel' system was to remain an important, if limited, part of the medical services of this country for the next 37 years.

Other treatment arrangements were introduced for *tuberculosis*, *venereal disease* and *ophthalmia neonatorum*. It also became obligatory for the Medical Officer of Health to be notified of all serious infectious diseases which occurred in his area. Effective preventive health schemes in all parts of the country were rapidly being introduced.

Ministry of Health

The next landmark in preventive medical history was the establishment in 1919 of the Ministry of Health which took over the functions of the Local Government Board. The new Ministry soon published its policy for the future which included developments in: (*a*) maternity services and a reduction in maternal mortality; (*b*) child health services and a reduction in infant mortality; (*c*) school medical services; (*d*) sanitation in the community; (*e*) industrial health; (*f*) prevention of infectious diseases; (*g*) prevention of non-infectious diseases (rheumatism, heart disease); (*h*) promotion of health education; (*i*) research projects; (*j*) international health control.

The Social Problems of 1920–39

In the next 20 years (1919–39), the housing problems of the country became acute and the first steps in *slum clearance* were undertaken. Following this lead, many thousands of slum houses were cleared between the two world wars and replaced by vast new housing estates. Many old unsatisfactory living conditions were abolished, but the improvement in the health of many persons moved from the slums was disappointing. One survey in Stockton on Tees in 1932 actually showed that the health of the persons rehoused deteriorated on moving to new housing estates. The reason for this was that the move meant that those rehoused were worse off financially because of higher rents and fares and, with their very low wages, could not afford adequate food and nutrition. This finding demonstrated that the factors affecting the health of any community were multiple and complicated and that soundly built houses are only one factor in good living conditions.

In 1929, the Local Government Act transferred the Poor Law to large local authorities, but in the atmosphere of economic depression which was present in many of the industrial areas at this time, few marked improvements were seen in the local administration of the Poor Law, and the hideous workhouses with their regimes of bureaucratic tyranny remained. All they achieved was to impress on the next generation the need for complete reform of the system. Then followed an unhappy period of development in which much unemployment in the depressed industrial areas created appalling living conditions for the majority of workers, with many associated social and physical ills.

These difficult economic conditions of the 1930s emphasized that *nutrition is a major public health factor in any community*. Many of those living in the depressed industrial areas of the North, and in South Wales, showed too clearly the effects of malnutrition.

By 1934 the *maternal mortality rate* had risen to 4·41 and was causing great concern at that time. A special committee of the British Medical Association carried out a survey on maternal mortality, and discovered that many of the maternal deaths were due to factors which could have been avoided, resulting from mistakes either by the mother herself or her attendants. This study coined the phrase *'primary avoidable factor'* to describe these preventable problems, which even today are present in 53% of maternal deaths. A dramatic improvement in maternal mortality occurred in 1937 with the introduction of chemotherapy which reduced the dangers of puerperal infection. The establishment of a blood transfusion service later, further reduced the hazards of postpartum haemorrhage.

The 1939–45 War Period

The problem of nutrition was not forgotten in the Second World War that followed in 1939. Although the housing conditions in the war deteriorated with the destruction of many houses, great care was taken to safeguard the nutrition of the country with special *welfare food rationing schemes*. As a result, the level of nutrition of the population actually improved. Full employment with the resultant higher wages also greatly assisted and when the war ended in 1945 there was ample evidence that the health of the country as a whole was better than in 1939. Two further spectacular advances were seen in preventive medicine during the war: in immunization and in social security.

Advances in immunization. A large-scale scheme for diphtheria immunization was started in 1942. Within eight years the annual number of new cases of diphtheria had fallen from over 41 000 to 962. This serious disease which had been responsible for 2700 deaths each year was already becoming rare by 1950. This successful campaign not only virtually wiped out *diphtheria* but stimulated a series of further successful immunization efforts which have now almost eliminated *poliomyelitis* and reduced whooping cough, tetanus and tuberculosis. The diphtheria immunization campaign also showed for the first time the value of *mass health education* which was later used widely to popularize immunization.

Social security. In 1943, well before the war was ended, Beveridge published his famous report on social security which was later adopted almost unchanged. This concept was to mark the final stage in the development of the social and health services which had started at the beginning of the century. An essential part of the scheme was the introduction of Family Allowances in 1945 and in 1948 of a comprehensive National Health Service in which a full medical service was made available to all people in the country without any payment at the time of need. The finance necessary is provided by an insurance scheme paid for by a special weekly contribution and general taxation.

Children Act, 1948

At the same time, a new Children Act was passed setting up an independent child care service under the central control of the Home Office and locally run by the large local authorities. This followed the Curtis report which investigated the deaths of children boarded out and which emphasized the need to have locally an independent committee (Children's Committee) responsible. During the next 23 years, excellent child care services were developed throughout the country and remained independent of other local services until amalgamated in 1971 into the work of the new social service departments.

National Health Service Act, 1946

This Act introduced the National Health Service. The new services, which remained unchanged until 1974, were divided into three parts.

1. *The hospital and specialist services* run by 20 new Regional

Hospital Boards (15 in England and Wales and five in Scotland). Local hospital administration was run by Hospital Management Committees. The large teaching hospitals in England and Wales (but not in Scotland) were run by separate Boards of Governors. Treatment in all hospitals was free although amenity beds (for greater privacy) were introduced.

2. *The general practitioner service* was run by Local Executive Councils which also looked after the pharmaceutical services, the dental service and the ophthalmic service. Special professional committees were set up locally, Local Medical Committee (for doctors) Local Pharmaceutical Committee (for Chemists), etc. and special procedures were laid down by which smaller committees of professionals and laymen dealt with complaints, over-prescribing, etc. Special machinery was set up to assist in the more equal distribution of doctors throughout the country (it still exists, see p. 29).

3. *The preventive or community health services* remained (until 1974) with the larger local authorities—County Councils and County Borough Councils. These included:

a. health centres
b. the care of expectant and nursing mothers and young children under five years of age (day nurseries transferred to social services, 1971)
c. domiciliary midwifery services
d. health visiting
e. home nursing
f. vaccination and immunization
g. ambulances
h. home helps (transferred to social service departments, 1971)
i. Prevention of illness, care and aftercare. Under this heading many different functions were included:

i. services to prevent tuberculosis and assist in the rehabilitation from this disease
ii. the provision of convalescent care
iii. the provision of domiciliary occupational therapy to help the disabled to live with their disabilities and prevent further breakdown

iv. chiropody services to help old and disabled people
v. wide health education services

The first most obvious improvement after introduction of the new National Health Service was *the upgrading of many hospital and specialist services*. This was achieved by the training and appointment of consultants, the extension of services and eventually the establishment of regional centres where specialized treatments could be concentrated; neurosurgery, chest surgery, cardiac units and radiotherapy to mention a few examples.

General practice did not improve as expected in the first 17 years of the new National Health Service because of shortages of general practitioners and very few new health centres. But since 1966 there has been rapid improvement with the emergence of the primary health care team and many more health centres. There has also been a marked upgrading of the status of general practice.

Many people expressed doubts about the wisdom of keeping the preventive health service with local authorities in 1948. However the level of the preventive medical services of local authorities was widened with emphasis on maternity and child health, home nursing, ambulance, immunization and home help service. The role of health visitors was extended so that the advantages they had brought to young children were made available to all age groups. Stress was particularly laid on health education and much wider use was made of modern methods of teaching health matters, including radio and television.

Much very effective work has been carried out in improving medical and social services for the aged and handicapped. Services such as *meals on wheels*, *chiropody* and *domiciliary occupational therapy* have been developed to a marked degree. In fact, in all fields of health the emphasis has been on *developing services within the community* wherever possible. This has resulted in the length of inpatient stays in hospital becoming shorter. More serious diseases are being fully investigated in outpatient departments. Geriatric services have developed rapidly for the elderly (see p. 495) and many special problems in the elderly demonstrated, such as hypothermia.

Improvements in the Level of Infectious Diseases

A national *Public Health Laboratory Service* (run by the Public Health Laboratory Board) was also introduced in 1948 which brought bacteriological and virological investigations to all areas of the country. Diagnostic facilities have been improved and have hastened the reduction of infectious diseases. Successful trials have led to the *introduction of effective vaccines against whooping cough and poliomyelitis* and the numbers of cases of both diseases have now fallen to very low levels. The improved treatment facilities made possible by the discovery of chemotherapy and antibiotics have continued to prevent disease. The reduction of pulmonary tuberculosis has been most satisfactory; from an average of 52 000 cases with 21 983 deaths in 1948, the level has fallen to 7712 cases with 575 deaths in 1976 in England and Wales. Many new methods of control have assisted in this improvement; mass X-ray services have been used in many ways. From 1957 to 1959 there were a number of very successful mass X-ray campaigns in Glasgow, Edinburgh and other Scottish cities and in Liverpool in which about 80% of the adult population were X-rayed and many latent cases of tuberculosis discovered especially in men over 45 years of age. Although campaigns are no longer worthwhile, mass X-rays still are of value (see p. 195). The introduction of BCG vaccination has further assisted in the reduction of tuberculosis and is still used especially for vulnerable family groups including certain immigrants in whom tuberculosis is still fairly common.

One of the most encouraging features of preventive medicine in the last 26 years has been the improvements in international health control. The WHO has developed into a powerful international preventive health service. Indeed, smallpox is on the verge of extinction from the world—a remarkable achievement which would have been impossible without worldwide coordination (see p. 320). Many successful campaigns to reduce tuberculosis, leprosy, malaria, yaws and various other diseases have been undertaken. WHO has also organized a worldwide system of collecting and disseminating information about the serious infectious diseases in the world (see p. 323).

In the field of food control, numerous improvements have taken place. Tuberculosis has been virtually eradicated from the cattle of the country and, as a consequence, infections of bovine tuberculosis in humans have disappeared. New stringent control methods of handling foodstuffs have reduced the danger of other diseases.

Maternity and Child Health

Further advances in the early recognition and treatment of toxaemia of pregnancy and in the treatment of haemorrhage in pregnancy have resulted in a further steady reduction in maternal mortality to a figure of 0·13 per 1000 in 1976 (representing one maternal death per approximately 7700 deliveries). This compares with one maternal death per 900 deliveries in 1948.

Infant mortality continued to fall helped by the improved general standard of living. From a figure of 33·9 deaths in the first year of life per 1000 born alive in 1948, the infant mortality rate fell to 13·8 in 1977 (see p. 66).

During the past ten years, there has been considerable interest shown into the problem of *non-accidental injury to babies and young children* (child abuse). Recent research has shown that the incidence is greatest in the youngest parents and those living in poor housing conditions (see p. 434). This problem is a perfect example of the integration between health and social problems. The recognition, prevention and treatment of this distressing problem is for general practitioners, paediatricians, surgeons, social workers and voluntary workers to tackle in a coordinated team approach.

Environmental Health

The Clean Air Act, 1956, set out to reduce the dangerous problem of atmospheric pollution and, after 22 years, more than half its target has been achieved.

Slum clearance has accelerated in the large cities and other methods of improving houses have been tried. Measures designed to improve the conditions of houses let as lodgings, in which large numbers of poor families including immigrants are accommodated, have only been partially successful.

In 1963, the Offices, Shops and Railway Premises Act was introduced and improved the working conditions of many clerical and office workers, a group which had been neglected in the past.

Mental Health

The National Health Service Act, 1946, did not alter the out-of-date law relating to mental illness. In 1959 a new Mental Health Act was passed to modernize the approach to mental illness and subnormality (now renamed mental handicap) with special reference to the prevention of chronic hospitalization of patients by introducing new and extended community mental services. It is hoped that this will lead eventually to a marked reduction in the size and scope of mental hospitals as more and more of the mentally disordered are looked after in the community.

In the 18 years since the introduction of the Mental Health Act, many excellent schemes have been started, especially in the field of employment. But these changes have also demonstrated the urgent need to develop social services for the mentally ill or disordered within the community and especially to develop adequate day care facilities. In 1971, the education of the mentally handicapped was transferred from health to education departments and junior training centres became special schools. This meant that no longer were the mentally handicapped children segregated from other disabled children and their education was integrated into the normal education system.

A review of the Mental Health Act was started by the DHSS in 1977 and much debate and criticism centred around the slow development of certain services.

Social Services Development

During the past decade, there have been large-scale developments in the field of social services culminating in 1970 with the passing of the Local Authority Social Services Act. This produced a new unified social service (introduced in April 1971), which deals with all the elderly, handicapped, homeless and mentally disordered, with child care protection, day nurseries and home help services. The growth of the new social service departments meant that, for the first time, it was possible to uniformly develop social services. Social workers are able at last to deal with all types of social problems rather than be divided into child care officers, welfare officers or mental welfare officers. The development of new 'generic' social workers in this way did much to prevent overlap of functions.

The new profession of social work is rapidly developing and will have a very important function in the prevention of adverse social conditions which can lead to illness and disease. In their way, these changes are as significant as those seen at the end of the 19th century when the emphasis suddenly changed from environmental health to personal health control.

In 1977, the care of the homeless was transferred to housing authorities with social service departments still remaining responsible for social work advice.

It is important that every doctor, whether working in hospital or general practice, understands how social work can assist him in his work. For these reasons, there is likely to be an increasing link forged between social workers and doctors in the future.

Community Problems

In the period 1960–70, many community problems became more serious. Much interest has been focused on the difficulties of *immigrants and community relations* and new laws have been introduced in an attempt to reduce problems. A Community Relations Council was set up in 1968 and it is steadily extending its scope and usefulness.

Various types of *social malaise* have been identified. Problems of drug dependence and addiction have led to new legislation to tighten the rules regulating the prescribing of *addictive drugs*. At the same time, new centres of treatment and prevention have been developed in an attempt to reduce this evil. There has been an increase in crime and especially in vandalism in many cities. Social malaise has shown itself in other ways including an increase in the rate of illegitimate births (from 6% in 1960 to 9·2% in 1976).

Much research has been carried out to find the factors influencing social malaise and it has shown that the lack of interest by ordinary persons in the conditions in which they live is a contributory factor. A new movement called *Community Develop-*

ment has emerged to encourage more active participation by ordinary people in all types of problems. The movement has grown rapidly and in 1969 the Home Office and government departments set up five-year research programmes into community development in certain large cities.

Special programmes called *Urban Aid* were introduced in the late 1960s to assist towns and cities suffering from urban deprivation. In 1977–8, a further *Inner Area Partnership* was introduced to attempt to halt the decline of certain parts of London and other cities.

Chronically Sick and Disabled Persons Act, 1970

This Act coming into operation in 1971 emphasized and extended the responsibilities of local authorities in relation to disabled persons. Its aim is to improve information services, direct services to the public especially within their own homes, to improve housing for the disabled and to ensure that access to public buildings is improved (see p. 442). The Act has resulted in many excellent schemes being developed and in particular many severely disabled people living alone at home have been provided with a telephone. It has also emphasized the inequality of services as a few local authorities have been very slow to respond. In 1974, the Member of Parliament, Alfred Morris, who had introduced this Act became the first *Minister for the Disabled.*

Control of Population Growth

Throughout the world during the sixties, one of the most discussed problems has been the population explosion. In the UK there has been a rapid growth in family planning with the extension of the powers of local authorities to help in cases of both medical and social need (National Health Service (Family Planning) Act, 1967). In 1972, these services were extended to include vasectomy and also all female contraceptive methods were made free.

The Abortion Act, 1967, for the first time introduced legal abortion in the UK where it can be shown by two doctors that the mental or physical health of the mother or children would be seriously affected by the birth of the child. Much controversy has followed, and after an initial peak in 1973, the number of abortions performed are now falling. It is, of course, hoped that this Act will reduce markedly the serious problem of illegal back street abortions.

Recent Advances in Preventive Medicine

Immunization

In the last 12 years, immunizations for measles and rubella have been introduced. The latter is an example of an attempt being made by immunization to *prevent damage to the next generation by ensuring that all future mothers will have developed an immunity to rubella* and that consequently the accident of infection during the first three months of a pregnancy will rarely occur.

Screening

Much work has recently been undertaken to perfect simple tests which can discover early abnormalities which may later lead to serious disease. The *cytology test for cervical cancer* is a simple example (see p. 268). In the field of paediatrics, *congenital dislocation of the hip and phenylketonuria* are two diseases in which serious after effects can be prevented by early recognition using screening tests.

Such new methods have been welcomed by some as representing a very important advance, but others have pointed out that, in many instances, screening tests are disappointing as they require complicated investigations and it may be impossible to treat the early stages effectively. Controversy of this kind has surrounded screening efforts for various cancers, for diabetes, for ischeaemic heart disease and for glaucoma. Although screening tests represent promising new methods of preventing disease, caution is needed before making extravagant claims of their value.

Study of congenital deformities

Much work has been carried out in the last decade into the problem of diagnosis and the causes of congenital deformities. Careful records have been collected of all congenital deformities discovered so that epidemiological studies can take place. Interest has centred increasingly on intrauterine development and the factors in pregnancy which may adversely affect the child. This has also led to a new speciality being identified—*Developmental Paediatrics.*

Child health and education

In 1976, a special government committee set up to review the health services for children (the Court Committee) reported and its findings are discussed in Chapter 4. Much of the report concentrated upon the continuing problem of perinatal morbidity and particularly was concerned with the need for the development of an integrated service.

Another special government committee set up to review the educational provision for handicapped children (the Warnock Committee) reported in 1978 and its findings pointed out the need to consider that group of children, estimated at 20%, disadvantaged by learning difficulties of all types (including social deprivation). Integration was emphasized but the report also recommended the need for certain special school provisions to be continued.

Health service changes

Primary health care has received much emphasis in the last eight years with the secondment of health visitors and home nurses to the team based on general practice.

Special training schemes for general practitioners have been developed including a three-year course of special experience in hospitals and in nearby general practices. In the near future, it is hoped that all new principals in general practice will have to take such a training.

Health centres have been rapidly developed in this period—by the end of 1978, approximately 22% of all principals in general practice work from health centres. Social workers also have become identified as essential members of the primary health care team.

In 1974, the massive reorganization of the health services took place as well as the reorganization of local government. All the health services were unified in AHAs (see p. 17) which, in the majority of instances, were made contiguous with the majority of new major local authorities who were responsible for social service (and education)—the new counties and the new metropolitan districts.

Many difficulties in the new arrangements have been highlighted and in 1976 a Royal Commission was appointed 'to consider in the interests of both patients and those who work in the National Health Service the best use and management of the financial and manpower resources of the National Health Service'. Debate has ranged over all aspects such as considering how good the service is, how it should develop in the future, an assessment of the services to patients, the management and financial resources of the NHS. Their report is expected early in 1979.

20 Management Techniques, Measurement of Need and Determination of Priorities

The control or management of health and social services involves many different features. The larger the range of services controlled, the more important it is for the various stages of management to be carefully organized. In any medical or social service organization it is possible to recognize certain essentials which have to be undertaken to ensure an efficient delivery of service to the patient. There are six steps:

1. *definition of the aims or objectives* of the service
2. *consideration of various alternative methods* of achieving these objectives and then the selection of the *best method.* (This is often referred to as 'issue analysis')
3. *planning various actions* which will enable the chosen method to be carried out effectively
4. *directing and controlling* the actual implementation of the methods chosen
5. *assessing results* (evaluating the relative success or failure)
6. *adjusting the methods* if the results obtained are not as good as expected

Input and Output Measurement

In the above list, the first four items deal with the planning and operating of services. In management terms, they are often referred to as *'the input'*—in other words they refer to services that are introduced or planned in an attempt to improve health or social services. The 'assessment of results', is quite different—this is often referred to as *'the output'* as it indicates the effect on the patients and clients of the services. Another way of describing 'the output' is that it measures the impact or results of these services on the people they are designed to help.

A very simple example from preventive medicine in the immunization field illustrates the differences between input and output measurements. The planning of any immunization campaign—who should be immunized, method of administration, timing of the campaign and the actual immunization methods used are examples of 'input' measurements. In England 79%, 81% and 80% of the under two-year-olds are protected by immunization against whooping cough, diphtheria and poliomyelitis respectively. These are all *'input' figures* and represent much hard work but, on their own, *give no indications of the value of these immunizations.* This can only be shown by considering the number of cases of these diseases (and therefore indirectly the numbers prevented). In this example, the number of cases of these diseases in 1972 is given in Table 59, where the percentage immunized is an 'input' figure and the second line, representing the number of cases, is an 'output' figure.

TABLE 59 Immunization and number of cases of specific diseases, 1972, England

		Whooping cough	*Diphtheria*	*Poliomyelitis*
Input	Percentage of population immunized (in first two years of life)	79	81	80
Output	Number of cases (all ages)	1988	4	5

(from *On the State of the Public Health*, 1974, DHSS)

This simple example illustrates how *much more useful are 'output' figures in assessing the usefulness of any procedure.* In this case, the 'input' figures indicate that in all instances almost the same proportion of the population are immunized (approximately 80%), but the results obtained are clearly quite different. In diphtheria and poliomyelitis almost complete eradication of these diseases was obtained and therefore the results were excellent, but in whooping cough although the proportion of the population protected was similar, 1988 cases were reported.

If a decision had to be made that one of these three immunization procedures had to be stopped or curtailed because financial or health resources were inadequate, it is quite obvious from the 'output' figures that everyone would choose to drop whooping cough immunization. But *it would be impossible to tell this from the 'input' figures of 79%, 81% and 80%.* This illustrates why 'output' measurement figures are becoming so important in the control or management of health and social services.

Unfortunately in the past, little emphasis has been given to developing effective techniques of 'output' measurement or methods of evaluating results (unless the results are very dramatic). The surgeon operating on various cancers is obviously an exception. In carrying out a careful follow up and later expressing his results as 'five year cure rates' a perfect example of 'output' measurement is provided (Table 60). Clearly many operative procedures have been stopped because the 'output' results were bad.

TABLE 60 Survival after cancer treatment, England and Wales, 1970

Cancer site	*Patients surviving five years* (%)
Skin (excluding melanoma)	59
Uterus (other than cervix)	56
Uterine cervix	44
Breast (female)	44
Breast (male)	28
Rectum	22
Ovary	20
Colon	20
Prostate	17
Stomach	5
Lung	5

It is apparent from the table that hysterectomy and mastectomy in women are obviously much more valuable operations than pneumonectomy or gastrectomy.

Monitoring the Health and Social Services

Monitoring the health and social services is a new phrase often used in documents describing the reorganized services. This phrase means that there should be a *continuous process of assessing the results of both services* so that adjustments can be made to make them more efficient. Monitoring should include all forms of output or input measurement and these should be analysed in *both financial and manpower terms* as both are in short supply. If this is done, then the most effective services will be those developed to help the largest number of patients or clients by using the smallest number of staff and by spending the least money.

Many different types of methods are being developed including individual assessment and professional judgement which have always been the most widely accepted. However as financial or manpower resources become scarcer, more detailed and sophisticated studies will be required.

In social services, it is difficult to develop effective and fair methods of comparing the results of different services. One of the more important questions now being considered is whether *residential care or community care* should be developed for the *elderly*. Should new services for the elderly be linked to building more hostels, or should they be concentrated on helping more old people to stay in their own homes by providing more home helps, meals services, day centres, etc? How can management techniques be used to answer that sort of question? Once again the six points mentioned at the start of this chapter should be used starting with the definition of the main objective. In this case, probably the *main aim is to keep the elderly person independent for as long as possible*. Having defined that objective and having considered various alternatives, the plan will probably include:

1. attempting to keep the elderly person for as long as possible living a reasonably normal life in his or her home
2. supporting the elderly person at times of crisis—after illness or after perhaps the death of a spouse by introducing home helps, meals services, good neighbours, social work support, rehabilitation and many similar schemes

All these would seem likely to support the view that *community services* rather than residential hostels would be better. But many old people become very frail and may, in the end, be unable to look after themselves and will need to be admitted to a hospital or hostel. Even in this instance, the main aim should be to retain independence. After a period of residential care, it may be possible to return the old person to his own home provided special rehabilitation arrangements are made—including a part time home help, meals-on-wheels or special home nursing care, etc. In such a case, *success could be measured by how quickly the old person regains his or her independence.*

If no attempt is made to rehabilitate an elderly person admitted to a hospital or a hostel and, particularly if everything is done for that old person, very soon that old person becomes more and more dependent.

It would not be difficult to devise a *scale of independence* with 15 points on it. Point 1 represents complete independence with the old person looking after him/herself; point 14 is equivalent to complete dependence (a bedfast person unable to do anything for him/herself). Point 15 equals death. On each visit by a social worker, an assessment could be made on such a scale indicating the degree of independence of that old person. After receiving care, a further visit could be made to assess whether an improvement or deterioration had occurred or whether his/her condition had remained unchanged. Many critics have pointed out that such a method of assessing results (or 'output' measurement) would be inaccurate as different social workers would not necessarily choose the same point on such a scale. This criticism is valid if different social workers were used for the same case, but *if the same social worker always visits* and if only the *degree of change is measured* the results are likely to be roughly comparable.

Take the case of an old person who is struggling at home with difficulty; on such a scale of dependence, one social worker might call the level 8, another 9 and another 10. Assume the elderly person is getting frailer (and therefore more dependent) the first social worker at a later visit, who called the original level 8 would record a worse level say 9 or 10, the second social worker who assessed the condition originally as 9, now records the level as 10 or 11 and the third 11 or 12. *In all instances, the degree of change* as measured on the 1–15 points scale of dependence is the same (a deterioration of 1–2 points). If such estimations were made in all routine casework with the elderly at home and the results analysed by computer, a large scale process of continuous output or impact measurement could be introduced.

The introduction of such measurement systems is currently being carefully investigated in a research project at York University and results have shown that such a system would be practicable. However the introduction would need more staff and resources.

Unit costs

A further method used is to assess *'unit costs'* in which the costs of delivering any service—whether it be a hospital, hostel or day professional service—are measured in terms of daily or weekly costs. These should be estimated both in *financial* and *manpower* terms for both are constraints: either can be limiting factors. Unit cost measurements can be even more valuable in judging the effectiveness and efficiency of various alternative services. When such an exercise is carried out comparing residential and community services for the elderly, *many of the advantages of the community services become more obvious*. This is because it is much more costly to look after an old person in any residential unit than to do so at home. It is also far less satisfactory for the old person concerned. A further point in favour of community services is that it is much easier to employ staff to work in the community than those who have to reside in old people's homes.

In practice the choice is not between residential or community services, because both will always be required but to find the most efficient combination of these two forms of service.

Occupancy measurements

When scarce resources are used, such as hospital or hostel beds, it is most important that a continuous process of measuring occupancy is undertaken if the most efficient usage is to be made of the places available.

Hospital occupancy analysis must always take regard of four important aspects:

1. length of stay in hospital of the patient
2. the speed of turnover—the time which it takes to fill the bed
3. the type of case admitted
4. the type of home the patient has come from and must return to

Comparisons must indicate the type of case and the type of home the patient must return to otherwise it is easy to assume that different results may be caused by more 'efficient practice' when all they might indicate is a different standard of selection of patients or a different standard of social class (and home) of the patients. It is therefore important when comparing occupancy figures to consider other alternatives which may be developing in some areas such as day surgery and its effects.

Occupancy in old people's homes

A major difficulty with occupancy occurs if an elderly person living in the home is admitted to hospital. Although there may be a number of persons on the waiting list for entry into the home, this place cannot be filled until *it is certain that the elderly person in hospital is not returning*. Unless the illness is very serious and short, the eventual outcome may not be certain until four to six weeks after admission. This means that once an old person goes into hospital it is not possible to fill the vacancy until four to six weeks later. This is on the assumption that no elderly person living permanently in an old persons hostel should be denied the opportunity of returning there when better. As most hostels are constantly dealing with some illness in their residents, few hostels ever achieve higher rates of occupancy than 94–6%.

This means that approximately three to four persons in a 50 bed hostel are never in that hostel, which then virtually becomes a 47 bed hostel. Therefore in an authority with, say, 1000 places (20 hostels) about 60 places are wasted at any one time, this is equivalent to more than one very large hostel costing about £700 000 to build. The designing of two large utility rooms which can act as emergency bedrooms in such a hostel would seem to suggest an answer, i.e. the 50 places would be increased theoretically to 54. There could then be an 8% under-occupancy and the average figures would rarely fall below 50, the true figure.

Occupancy in day nurseries

These are notoriously difficult units in which to avoid serious under-occupancy. This is because young children often develop minor illnesses preventing them from attending, or the family circumstances are unstable which often means irregular attendances of the child. Many day nursery matrons in the past have been worried by the dangers of infection which might occur if they allow the numbers of children to rise, but in practice, this danger is insignificant.

In Liverpool it has been possible to improve occupancy in day nurseries from 80% to 95% *by accepting up to 15 more children on the register of each nursery than its true capacity*. Assuming the nursery is planned to take 50, then up to 65 children are accepted on the register. Experience has shown that only rarely does this lead to the ideal numbers ever being exceeded on any one day and then only by an insignificant one or two. The advantage can be judged when it is realized that with 14 day nurseries with 825 places, an 80% occupancy means an average daily figure of 660 children but a 95% occupancy means 784 children attending—a difference of 124 children. This is equivalent to building three nurseries each accommodating 41 children; capital cost (1979) would be about £180 000 per nursery. By accepting more children on the register, running costs go up very little as the same staff are needed, the same overheads, the same heating and the only extra cost for these additional children is the cost of feeding them.

Issue Analysis

Efficient management always involves *constant consideration of alternative methods*. In some cases alternative methods are sought because it is obvious that the results are ineffective. The clinician seeking new ways of treating disease is always involved with issue analysis although he may not realize it.

It is when alternative methods are not obviously sought out, because no one really critically questions the results, that issue analysis becomes really important. Because so many actions in managing or controlling health and social services come into this latter category, it is most important to carry out periodic analysis, as part of any evaluation or monitoring process.

Continuous issue analysis

Ideally this should be carried out for every activity annually but if this is beyond the scope of the manager, then some annual issue analysis should be undertaken but different subjects should be studied each year so that *each subject is analysed once every three or four years.*

To be effective, the *analytical process must be as complete as possible* and should involve not just an examination of the way things can be done but what is being attempted. The following eight questions should be carefully answered about each activity:

1. What is the essence of the problem being faced?
2. What does the activity hope to accomplish?
3. What alternative methods are available?
4. How effective is each likely to be?
5. What is the cost of each method? 'Costs' should be estimated in terms of both *money* and *manpower.*
6. What are the costs and relative effectiveness of different methods when measured over a lengthy period of time? The advantage of some alternatives will only become obvious after some years.
7. What other factors are relevant? In particular what other services might be influenced by new actions? For instance, it might be possible to improve some part of the services but only at the expense of another and perhaps more important section of the work.
8. Having considered all the above questions, what is likely to be the best answer?

In many instances, the appraisal of current methods (those used at present) will be most effective when carried out by persons coming new to the local tasks for then it is less likely that they will be prejudiced in favour of traditional methods or by custom and practice. For this reason, outside *management consultants* have often been used for major issue analysis. Such persons have great freedom of action and are often more readily accepted by staff without too much resentment. Even if the staff do resent their work, good personal relationships within the normal services are not disturbed.

In the *reorganized health services it is planned to undertake more 'issue analysis'* at both AHA and RHA and also at national levels. Much of this analytical work will pass under the general heading of 'monitoring and future planning of the services'. Such work is even more important at a time of restricted growth as it is then essential to consider possible redistribution of resources between different services.

The emphasis now being placed on *Joint Care Planning* between the health and social services (see p. 22) will also be concerned with practical issue analysis. In addition the *Health Advisory Service* and the *Social Work Service* are both concerned with issue analysis in the health and social services.

Health Advisory Service (formerly Hospital Advisory Service)

A special unit was set up in 1967 called the Hospital Advisory Service which was directly answerable to the Secretary of State for Social Services to examine the management of patients in various types of hospitals. Early in its career, it concentrated upon geriatric and psychiatric hospitals and set out to help the hospitals to analyse their problems independently. The aim was to improve hospital patient care and in many ways, it is an example of using continuous issue analysis to check standards of care by introducing into a national service a small and relatively independent body to carry it out. Since reorganization of the health services the Hospital Advisory Service has been renamed *Health Advisory Service* and it is intended to extend the range of its activities to cover all types of health activities.

Social Work Service

The *Social Work Service* is part of the DHSS and operates both centrally at the Department in London and through a series of regional offices (see p. 386). One of its most important functions is to assess, monitor and advise on the delivery of social services locally and in specialized fields. In this way, it is continuously carrying out important issue analysis.

Estimation of Needs and Priorities

When planning services, the first action should always be to make an accurate assessment of the needs and requirements. As any health and social service must cover hundreds of different tasks, it will eventually be necessary to determine priorities between services so that the best possible use can be made of all the resources available.

The simplest way to determine priorities must be to compare on the same basis the needs of all services and particularly to judge each service on what it actually achieves, i.e. on its results.

Calculation of needs

The simplest method of calculating needs is:

1. to state clearly the aims of the service, and then
2. to estimate: (*a*) the number of persons who require that service (*the clientele or patient figures*) and (*b*) *the standard of service* (carefully defined in terms of time) that is required to ensure that the 'service' is effective and satisfactory.

Then a simple multiplication of (*a*) by (*b*) will give an *estimate of total need.* A few simple examples will help explain this.

1. Assume one is attempting to calculate the numbers of *home helps* required to satisfy the needs of very frail old people living on their own at home in any community. First estimate the number of such frail old people living alone who need this help. Assume it is 3500. Then find out the amount of service each requires (expressed in hours per week); assume that local research and analysis has shown that a satisfactory result can be achieved when about 6 hours home help per week on average is given. This is the standard of service required. Then the total need is 3500 × 6 hours per week or 21 000 hours per week. This represents approximately 1050 part-time home helps each undertaking 20 hours per week.

Now two further headings are added to the calculation—the *number of home helps who are already available* in the social services for this task and whether there are enough, too many (*surplus*) or too few (*gap*). Assume there are 550 part-time home helps available to do this work, then obviously there is a gap of 500 home helps (part-time). This gap can then be costed in terms of extra money and staff required annually (Table 61).

TABLE 61 Estimation of home helps

Clientele (i.e number of frail elderly people needing home help) (*a*)	Standard of help needed in hours/week (*b*)	Total need (*a*)×(*b*)	Present provision	Gap/surplus	Cost of filling gap (1978)
3500	6	21 000 hours/week or 1050 part time home helps	11 000 hours/week or 550 part time home helps	Gap of 10 000 hours/week or 500 part time helps	Annual revenue cost £800 000

2. A second example could be concerned with the estimation of the number of *health visitors* required to carry out an effective preventive child care service for young children under five years of age. This is of course only one function of health visitors. In this example the need will be influenced by:

a. the number of children who require the service (clientele)
b. the length of time needed by health visitors to carry out their main tasks including: (i) home visiting; (ii) immunization; (iii) health education; and (iv) tasks at clinics

In Table 62 the breakdown of the figures of an area of approximately 600 000 persons is used for this health visitor function. There are 62 880 children under the age of five years living in the area. Assume locally it is agreed that an ideal service would provide eight visits per year for children under the age of 12 months and two visits per year for children aged one to five years. This means 196 260 visits per year (94 000 for children under 12 months and 102 260 for children aged one to five years). At present 80 health visitors are able to make 174 914 visits a child (2185 visits/health visitor/year). There is therefore a gap of 21 346 visits which is equivalent to 10 health visitors.

TABLE 62 Estimation of health visitor needs for home visits to children aged 0 to 5 years

Objective	*Clientele*	*Standard of service*	*Total need*	*Present provision*	*Gap*	*Costs of filling gap*
To provide home visits to children under 5 years of age	11 750 children under 12 months of age	8 visits a year	94 000 visits per year	174 914 visits/year =80 health visitors (assuming each health visitor undertakes 2185 visits/year	21 346 visits per year=10 health visitors	£52 700
	51 130 children aged 1–5 years	2 visits a year	102 260 visits/year			
			(Total = 196 260 visits per year)			

Calculations on such a basis provide a useful check on the staffing of any service and the cost of filling this gap is approximately £52 700. It may however be impossible to fill such a gap without increasing the training facilities for health visitors for there will also be a *manpower gap*. The cost of such training should also be included in 'costs of filling the gap'.

3. A third example could be provided by assessing the need for *hospital social workers* in a paediatric unit. First it would be necessary to assess how many children who are admitted to the unit (or attend outpatients) require the services of a hospital social worker. Assume that 2000 children come into such a category and a staff of four hospital social workers is already provided. It is next necessary to calculate a 'standard of service'. Recently in a survey undertaken, it was found that on

average approximately five hours of time was spent by a hospital social worker dealing with each paediatric case and that this was divided as follows:

Initial assessment	¾ hour
Liaison with social workers on health visitors in the community	1 hour
Mobilizing community resources	2½ hours
Liaison with medical and nursing staff	¾ hour
Total	5 hours

If such a standard is accepted, the need and gap in such a unit would be two social workers calculated as in Table 63.

TABLE 63 Need for Hospital Social Workers

Clientele	*Standard of service*	*Total need*	*Present provision*	*Gap*	*Cost* (1978)
2000	5 hours each	10 000 hours= 6 social workers	4 social workers	2 social workers	£9000

Estimation of social worker needs

It is possible to calculate (using the methods already described) the requirements for social workers within a large community. In Liverpool, this has been done and the results indicate a need for 382 staff (at basic grade, i.e. excluding any supervisory staff); at present 237 are provided. *This could be expressed crudely by saying just over 62% of the staff required are now provided.* But such a figure is misleading for there is unequal provision for different services. This is best indicated in Table 64 where needs are shown in three age groups: children, adults (23 to 60 years) and elderly (60 years plus).

TABLE 64 Social workers: needs and provision by client group (based on apportionment of social work support time)

Client group	*Need*	*Present provision*	*Percentage provision*
Children	139	106	(76)
Adults (23 to 59 yr)			
Homeless	28	21	(75)
Physically handicapped	22	18	(82)
Mentally ill	36	7	(19)
Mentally handicapped	19	3	(16)
	—	—	—
Total adults	105	49	(47)
Elderly (60 yr)			
Active	18	3	(17)
Physically handicapped	68	51	(77)
*Mentally disordered	44	26	(59)
In residential accommodation	8	2	(25)
	—	—	—
Total elderly	138	82	(59)
Total numbers of Social Work staff	382	237	(62)

* Mentally ill mainly but also including some work done for mentally handicapped.

When it is realized that many social problems which occur in children are in the emergency category (i.e. a child left without parental support) the relative provision of social work support for children (76%) is not excessive compared with adults (47%) and the elderly (59%). However, there are very clear differences between the standard of provision for different types of needs. The best provided services are the child care services and those for the physically handicapped while the worst are the mentally handicapped and mentally ill.

It is clear from this table that the mentally ill and mentally handicapped are both likely priorities—they are *implied priorities.*

Determination of priorities

Whenever the needs of the health and social services are calculated in this way, certain *implied priorities* are defined.

Although such indications are always important in the determination of priorities, it must be realized that there will always be certain acute emergencies which must be dealt with. In management terms, these are referred to as *'constraints'*. Obvious examples include the need to admit to hospital immediately (as a top priority) *any acutely ill patient who would die if not immediately operated upon (perforated gastric ulcer, ectopic gestation)* or to *admit to a children's home a young child abandoned by his parents.* There may also be 'political' or 'legal' constraints. Priority may be given to a service because Parliament has decided to give priority to certain groups of patients or clients (such as the mentally ill) or because the law has been changed and a new statutory duty has been imposed on a local authority (the Children and Young Persons Act 1969 or the Chronically Sick and Disabled Persons Act 1970).

Apart from those types of constraints, most priorities will be determined by needs and the levels of services already provided and particularly upon the likely impact of various services. Where there is an obvious need for a particular service and the provision is well below average, there is always an implied priority.

The actual *determination of the order of priorities* will depend on certain other factors including the following:

1. Priority should be given to *services which are likely to give excellent results* (as judged by output measurements described above).
2. Wherever possible, *the effects on the population as a whole should be considered.* Health and social services designed to help large numbers of chronically ill or handicapped persons (such as hemiplegic patients) will achieve more than dramatic new operations for only a small proportion of the population.
3. Priority should be given to *those services which have evolved to meet new trends*. An example is the development of new health and social services within the community to aid patients and clients in their own homes. This means that the improvement of primary health care is a priority as well as the encouragement of health centres. This includes hospital services development but this should ideally be

designed to meet this trend. Therefore *early discharge from hospital, day surgery* and the *rehabilitation services* also become priorities although based in hospitals.

4. Services which may *prevent future health and social services problems should always have a high priority.* Generally all preventive health and social services for children come into this category. Some may think it is sentimental to insist on high quality services for children but the reason for doing so is logical, for failure with children may result in a life of chronic disease (with consequential heavy demands on the health services). Likewise a child with serious social deprivation will be more likely to develop into a socially deprived adult and, in this way, make very heavy demands on the social services all his life. Hence successes with children in health and social services will avoid many future permanent difficulties.
5. Priorities must always be developed so that *the best possible use is made of available finance and manpower.* Further constraints always arise where priorities require new buildings (capital) for national financial priorities have to be taken into consideration as well as the time schedule. The construction of *large capital projects* (i.e. a new hospital) takes many years to complete and means that such a priority cannot come into effect for about eight years. In the same way, certain *manpower shortages* will be an important determining factor in the decisions on priorities. It is no use giving high priority to a very desirable service if it requires large numbers of skilled professional staff (such as doctors, health visitors or social workers) who are not available. If such a priority is to be realistic, it should include an educational programme to train such staff.

When assessing priorities between different services all of whom are urgently required, *the 'unit-cost' of the service* may be most important. Obviously it is desirable to introduce cheap and effective services and therefore unit cost output measurements (as explained earlier in this chapter) are most relevant.

It is important *in developing health and social services never to be too rigid.* There should always be ways to encourage new developments and to carry out pilot experiments. Initiative by doctors and other professionals originally was the only method of determining priorities and, although this can lead to the wrong services being developed first, it is important that doctors and other professionals should be able to influence local priorities.

In the field of social services, in which the revenue finance needed for developments is voted by local politicians, it is important to realize that *elected representatives are keen to develop services whose success is self-evident.* Services such as meals-on-wheels, luncheon clubs, home helps, aids and adaptations, telephones, special transport, bus passes, special sheltered housing, home alarm systems and schemes of self-help involving more community participation are popular. All these can be developed without new capital or an increase in the numbers of professional staff and also are useful services to bring the problems of the under-privileged to the attention of the population as a whole.

Corporate Management

It is usual for many documents on the planning of health and social services to speak of the importance of 'corporate management' and it is important to explain exactly what is meant by this term. Corporate management really means *accepting that no one service or part of any service is ever likely to be self-sufficient* particularly if looked at from the viewpoint of the patient (or client) who is being helped. Action (or lack of action) by one service is bound to have an influence upon the other. Three simple examples will help to illustrate this principle.

1. With young children (under the age of five years) day care facilities in the form of day nurseries or playgroups can do much to alleviate deprivation. Certain families are otherwise at a disadvantage because they live in poor circumstances or perhaps because the family is a one parent family. Both day nurseries and playgroups are mainly under the control of the social services and therefore it would be easy to assume that the Social Services Committee alone is in a position to solve this problem. But the Education Committee is responsible for all nursery schools which takes children of three to five years and it is often pure chance whether a child of this age group goes to a nursery school, playgroup or day nursery.

To achieve a satisfactory answer to such a problem, *it is essen-*

tial that both social and education services realize that they should be contributing to the same end and that to develop one without considering the consequences of the other would be stupid. Therefore the *future planning of such services should be carried out together or in a 'corporate' manner* recognizing that both have an important integral contribution.

2. A second example could be provided by the mental health services. The aim of modern treatment (as indicated by the Mental Health Act, 1959) is to encourage shorter stays in mental hospitals so that patients can return home to a more normal life as quickly as possible. This would seem to be a simple decision for the hospital psychiatrist who is responsible for determining the time of discharge of any mentally ill patient in hospital. But, in practice, *the ability to discharge any patient depends not only on his mental condition but on the services which are available in the community to help him.* These include satisfactory medical care based on the family doctor to ensure that proper treatment is continued and three types of social services:

a. the provision of day care services (see p. 477)
b. suitably trained social workers to assist with the after care of the patient at home
c. suitable residential accommodation for those who have no suitable homes to return to

This means that the development of any ideal modern mental health service needs very careful planning so that *the psychiatric hospital, the general practitioner services and the social services are balanced* and work together (in a corporate way) towards the same end.

3. A third example could be given by the case of a seriously handicapped person suffering from a permanently disabling condition such as paraplegia (see p. 479). The successful treatment and management of such a patient will involve many different services including:

a *hospital services* during the initial treatment period and during the treatment of any complications later
b. the *primary health care team* and especially the family doctor and home nurse
c. the *local social services* for various *aids* and *appliances* and

for any structural alterations which are necessary—this department will also be concerned in many instances with *industrial therapy* and *retraining* (in conjunction with the Disablement Resettlement Officer (DRO)

d. the local *Artificial Limb and Appliance Centre of the Department of Health and Social Security* may have to supply the correct invalid vehicle or car (if the patient can manage such a vehicle) or the patient needs to be advised about other alternatives concerning mobility (see p. 450)

e. the local DRO of the Employment Service Agency will advise and may arrange for the patient to go for industrial retraining at an Industrial Rehabilitation Unit

Most professionals working in those fields—doctors, nurses, social workers, physiotherapists, occupational therapists, resettlement officers realize that it is important that all of them plan together the future care of the patient. What is not so obvious is that if one service fails to provide a crucial piece of equipment or service, this cooperation will be made very difficult. If for instance, the local authority fails to provide the various aids or structural alterations necessary, it may be impossible for the patient to return home from hospital. In County areas two different local authorities may be involved as the County Council provides the social services but the smaller District Council the housing needs. So if any disabled person requires special housing (and a number do), the successful answer will only be provided by careful corporate management between the health, social, housing and employment services.

This aspect of corporate management is so important that care has to be taken in the reorganization of the health services to make it easier by setting up statutory *Joint Consultative Committees* whose task will be to ensure everything is done to improve joint planning and management (see p. 23).

PART III

Social Services

21 Administration of the Social Services

The 'social services' cover three main groups:

1. Social services provided by *local authority social services departments* which include a wide range of statutory, community and residential services for the elderly, children, physically disabled, mentally disabled and homeless. The hospital social work services are also provided in this way although working entirely within a hospital setting. Centrally these services are the responsibility of the DHSS.

2. *The probation and after care service* which is attached to the courts and works mainly with adult offenders who, as part of their sentence, are placed on probation. In addition, much of the aftercare work for discharged prisoners is undertaken by this service. The probation service is quite separate from the services in paragraph 1 above and, like the Prison Service, is centrally the responsibility of the Home Office. This book is not intended to deal with this service.

3. *Voluntary bodies*. There are many well established voluntary bodies providing social services both on a national and local basis. They include Family Service Units, Women's Royal Voluntary Service, the various bodies working for children, NSPCC, Barnardos, National Children's Homes, the Family Welfare Association, Age Concern, the various bodies working in the field of the disabled, The Royal Association for Disability and Rehabilitation, and locally through Councils of Social Service and Rural Community Councils. These local voluntary bodies often undertake a coordinating function in respect of smaller local voluntary bodies or local branches of the large national bodies already mentioned.

As many of these voluntary bodies are undertaking responsibilities which could also be covered by social services departments, *it is essential that very close working arrangements are made.* In many instances, much of the local finance necessary for their functions is provided by the Social Services Committee of the Local Authority.

The government minister who works most closely with these voluntary bodies is the *Secretary of State for Social Services.* In some instances, special financial grants are paid by the Department of Health and Social Security to large voluntary bodies to promote research (e.g. in *alcoholism*) and develop certain specialized social services (e.g. *work with deprived children*).

A final group of voluntary bodies is the *Citizens' Advice Bureaux.* These bodies were first developed in the 1939–45 war to help with various queries about rationing, missing relatives, etc. Their role has widened recently especially in the field of *consumer protection*, the provision of *legal advice* and the explanation of various *pension rights.* They are particularly valuable in helping families who may be unwilling to seek statutory assistance from social service departments or social security offices because they feel aggrieved for some reason—they may have been evicted for rent arrears or generally are resentful of the way they have been treated by local authorities and other statutory services. For this reason, many Social Services Committees provide financial grants to the Citizens' Advice Bureaux to enable them to help such clients who otherwise would be unlikely to seek help. Centrally there is a National Association of Citizens' Advice Bureaux linked to local bureaux by a regional committee.

FUNCTIONS OF THE SECRETARY OF STATE FOR SOCIAL SERVICES

The Secretary of State for Social Services has overall responsibility for the wide range of social services run by Social Services Committees of local authorities and also for helping to promote similar services by the voluntary bodies mentioned above. The Secretary of State is a member of the Cabinet and, of course, is also responsible for the health and social security services and is therefore in an ideal position to coordinate all these services nationally and to ensure that their individual developments are balanced. The overall cost of the personal social services in 1975/6 was £1021 million.

In 1973 a *Personal Social Services Council* was established as an advisory body to advise the Secretary of State on policy issues and to provide information and guidance on development and research projects. Its chairman is appointed by the Secretary of State but the majority of the other members represent statutory or voluntary organizations working in the social services. It therefore includes representatives from the Local Authority Associations, the Association of Directors of Social Services, British Association of Social Workers, teaching bodies and from various voluntary bodies—Age Concern, National Children's Bureau, etc. It has established special groups to study research requirements, children and family life, consumer protection, people with handicaps and residential care. It publishes various reports and arranges seminars and conferences on important relevant social service topics.

Method of Control exercised by the Department of Health and Social Security on the Development of Social Services by Local Authorities

There are three main ways in which the DHSS exercises control of local social services:

1. In an *advisory* capacity—important advisory memoranda are issued giving advice in detail on the development of certain services. Sometimes such memoranda deal with the need to develop services in a coordinating way with other services—a recent example was the circular on *non-accidental injury to children* and in the development of services for the *elderly*. In some cases advisory memoranda deal only with items of immediate concern to social services departments.

Occasionally joint memoranda are issued by both the DHSS and another ministry such as the Department of Environment—a recent example was the memorandum on *homelessness*.

2. *Planning and policy*—this is an essential function of the DHSS and is becoming more important with the trend towards developing more services for people within the community, for

this means that these services can only succeed if balanced provision is made by social and health services. The development of services for the mentally ill is a very good example of the need for the planning and policy to be carefully balanced and coordinated so that the needs of those mentally ill persons are provided by social services departments to enable the health and hospital services to discharge their patients from hospitals. Recently the central structure of the DHSS has been completely reorganized to improve the integration of planning between the social and health services. A central planning division has been established alongside a central regional division and in both social service and health service professional officers are closely working with their linked administrative officers. There is also a *Social Work Service* based centrally and within the 10 regions of the DHSS (see Fig. 20). The function of this service is mainly advisory and to assist in developing better social services. Its regional staff assist, advise and help the social services departments in their areas. These staff carefully study suggested capital developments and advise the Central Department. They also act as the local adviser to Directors of Social Services and their staffs in the region. These are also the regions for the Regional Planning Committees which are involved in ensuring a balanced development of various forms of residential accommodation for children.

3. *Financial* This is an important method by which the DHSS can control the development of social services. It is more apparent as regards new capital development than revenue expenditure because local authorities must obtain loan sanction from the Department of Health and Social Security in respect of all new buildings (capital). This means that all new residential accommodation (unless it is sheltered housing provided separately), i.e. day centres, day nurseries, workshops, can only be built with government permission *(key sector finance)*. Office accommodation is not covered by this as it is provided from a block grant called the *locally determined schemes*.

Revenue (or costs of running day-to-day services) is financed by means of the *rate support grant* from the government and from the local rates. The rate support grant is the large block grant of money made from the government to local authorities to assist them with their services. It has a population element in it and a 'needs' element which reflects the social problems and social services provided by that authority. The actual division of the block grant is the responsibility of each local authority (and therefore it decides what proportion of revenue expenditure goes to education or social services or other services). But the larger the rate support grant provided by the government, the greater the likelihood of social services being developed locally.

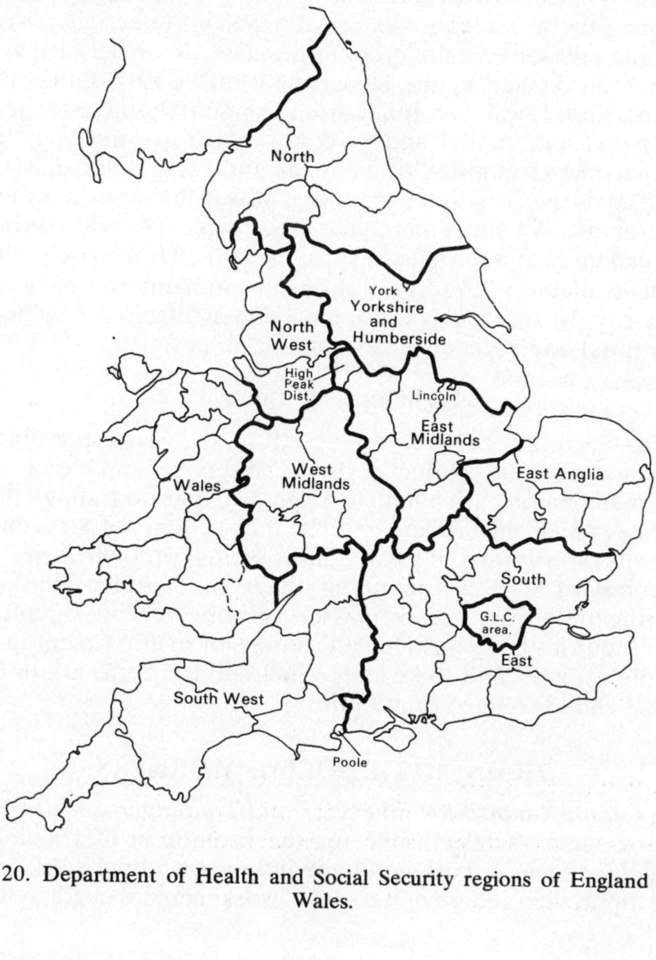

FIG. 20. Department of Health and Social Security regions of England and Wales.

During the last few years, certain special financial schemes have been introduced to help either deprived urban areas or to promote special schemes. The *Urban Aid Scheme* provides, from government sources, 75% of the cost and the local authority 25% Schemes are mainly chosen in education, social services and housing areas and include grants to voluntary bodies, and direct services provided by the local authority. However, this Urban Aid help is now being reduced and a new concept introduced—*Inner Area* or *'Partnership'* help. This aid is aimed at assisting the worst inner city social problems in certain parts of London and some of the other large cities. So far 15 such areas have been defined by the Department of the Environment for Partnership. Locally an Inner Area Committee suggests special schemes (both capital and revenue) which are then put to a Partnership Committee of national and local politicians plus their advisers. It is this Committee which finally decides each programme. An initial three-year programme 1979–81 has been decided upon and the necessary finance (like Urban Aid) will be made available—75% from central government and 25% local authority. In Liverpool, the annual sum available for 1979–81 for capital and revenue is £10 million.

Parliamentary Control

The Secretary of State for Social Services is responsible to Parliament for the conduct of the social services and it is open to any member of parliament to raise any question about these services which must be answered by the Secretary of State either verbally or in writing. If a particularly serious problem arises, the Secretary of State can set up an inquiry to consider all aspects relating to the question and to issue a report. Recent examples of such inquiries have included allegations of maltreatment in old people's homes and the events which led up to the death of a young child (non-accidental injury).

TRAINING OF SOCIAL WORKERS

The Central Council for Education and Training in Social Work. This Council is responsible for the promotion of training in all fields of social work—in field and in residential work—and also approves and reviews social work courses leading to a professional qualification in social work. Most courses of training are held at Polytechnics and Universities and last usually from one to two years depending upon the qualification and the standard of the candidates. At present there are two main ways to train to become a social worker:

1. by obtaining a relevant degree in Social Sciences and then taking a one year course
2. by taking a two year course (with or without any other type of degree)

Most candidates are either sponsored or seconded to training courses from social services departments.

LOCAL AUTHORITY SOCIAL SERVICES

Comprehensive social services are provided by all major Local Authorities (county councils and metropolitan districts and London boroughs) under the Local Authority Social Services Act, 1970. Fig. 21 shows the local authorities in England and Wales and social services including the names of local authorities in metropolitan counties and in Greater London.

Each authority has a Social Services Committee which controls services and in each authority there is a *Director of Social Services* who is the chief officer in charge of the social services department administering all these social services.

Types of social services provided by the social services department

The following are the services provided by the social services department:

1. Care of the elderly.
2. Care of the physically handicapped, including blind, deaf, spastic, epileptic and paraplegic cases.
3. Care of the homeless.

All these services are provided under the National Assistance Act, 1948.

4. Child care protection including child care supervision, acceptance of parental rights of children committed into the care of the local authority, control of children's homes, admission units, reception centres, boarding out arrangements, community homes (approved schools and

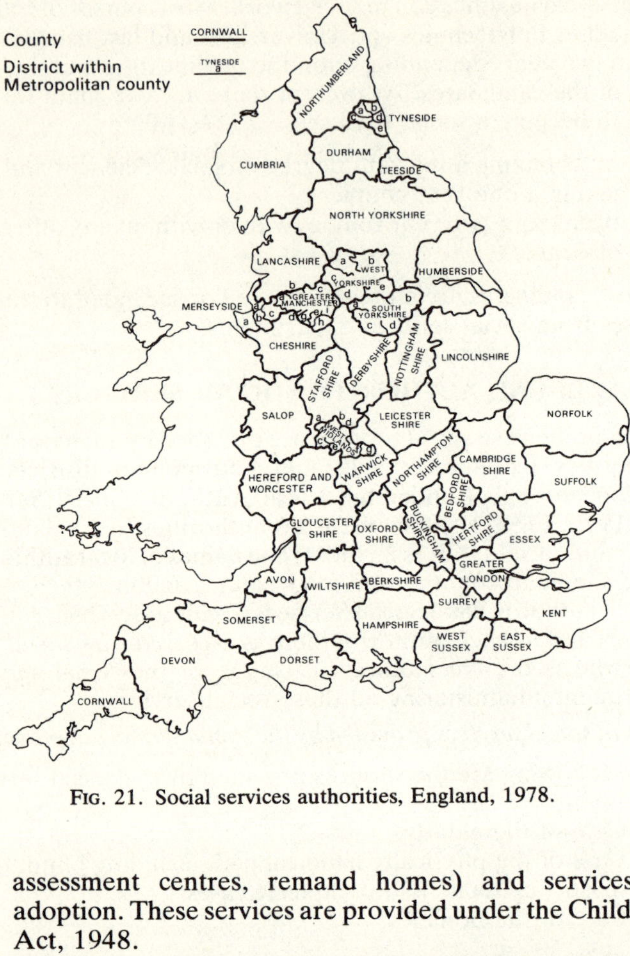

FIG. 21. Social services authorities, England, 1978.

assessment centres, remand homes) and services for adoption. These services are provided under the Children's Act, 1948.

5. Social work and family casework with the mentally disordered including provision of social workers (formerly mental welfare officers). Also included are day centres, adult training centres, workshops and residential accommodation (hostels) for the mentally disordered.
6. Day care of children under five years of age, day nurseries and child minding.

7. The provision of home helps.
8. Care of unsupported mothers including residential care.

Social service departments

A typical layout of the social service department is given in Fig. 22. It will be noted that there are four main parts of the department:

1. that dealing with residential services
2. that dealing with field work services
3. that providing training facilities for practical social work training
4. that providing the hospital social work services

Residential services are provided for:

a. the elderly (see p. 505)
b. physically and mentally handicapped (see p. 457 and 485)
c. children. There are many different types of accommodation for children including residential admission units, residential nurseries, reception centres, and large and small children's homes. Full details are given in Chapter 23 together with descriptions of the specialist units of approved schools, classifying centres and remand homes.

Field work services look after facilities within the community and provide social work services for:

a. family and child care (Chapter 23)
b. disabled (Chapter 24)
c. homeless (Chapter 27)
d. elderly (Chapter 26)
e. mentally ill or subnormal (Chapter 25)
f. adoption services (Chapter 23)
g. transport facilities especially for handicapped (Chapter 24)
h. home helps (Chapter 27)
i. meals on wheels or lunch clubs (Chapter 26)
j. day nursery accommodation (Chapter 23)

Training facilities are provided by all social services departments and include all types of training from induction courses for new recruits and in-service training courses for trained staff, to providing field placements and supervision for students on the

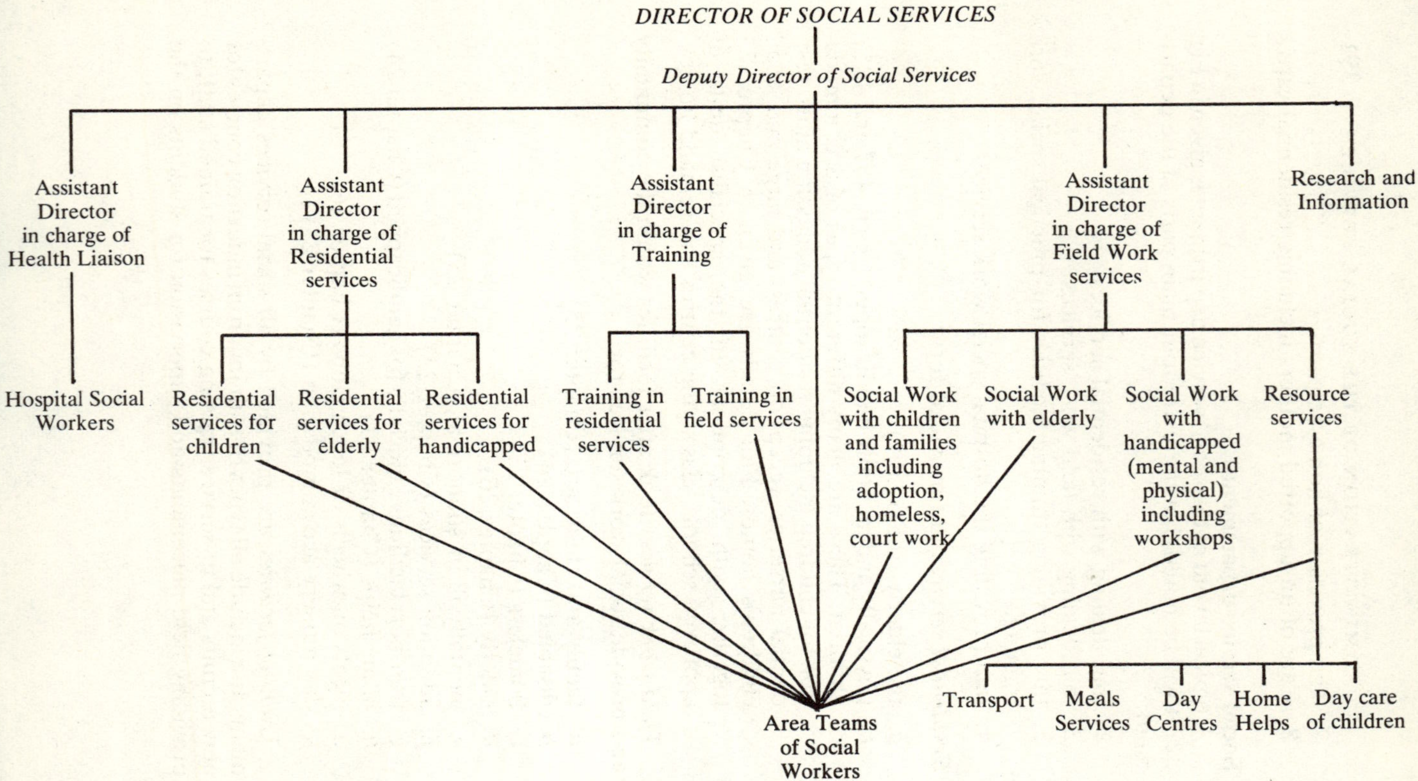

FIG. 22. Structure of a social services department.

one and two year courses at Polytechnics and Universities. Training is also provided for other staff employed by social service departments such as home help staff.

Hospital social work services have been taken into social service departments in the reorganization and are briefly described in Chapter 28.

Area Teams

An important innovation in the social services is *the team method of deploying the main forces of social workers*. The size of the area covered by each team varies considerably in different authorities and ranges from 40 000 to 100 000 depending upon the social problems present and the geographical area. Ideally each area should cover approximately 50 000 population. The aim is to have 10 to 30 social workers working closely together so that the various types of social problem can be dealt with quickly and without overlap. In each of these teams social workers who specialize in either child care, welfare work with the elderly and handicapped, or mentally disabled, all work closely together under the leadership of a senior officer. The aim is that most types of social problems will eventually be dealt with by each social worker although a certain amount of specialization is inevitable and desirable. But the main object of these teams is to provide a balanced social service which can quickly deal with any problem. Therefore the doctor whether in general or hospital practice should refer any social problem direct to the senior officer in charge of the area. The Director of Social Services will be able to tell each doctor who this individual is and how he can be located.

It is usual in the social work field to refer to persons requiring help from the social services as *clients* and this term will be used by social workers when discussing their patients with doctors.

Because social workers need to use many different specialist services to resolve problems with their clients, most area teams will have attached to them the main community resources. Examples of area team responsibility include the allocation of home helps to clients or the ordering of meals on wheels to elderly or handicapped people requiring them. The doctor, needing this sort of help can obtain it through the senior officer in charge of the area team. For this reason, it has become increasingly usual to arrange for a social worker from the area team to attend regularly a large health centre or hospital to ensure direct and easy communication with the medical staff working there.

LIAISON BETWEEN COMMUNITY HEALTH SERVICES AND SOCIAL SERVICES

The reorganization of the health services and local government has been undertaken as far as possible to ensure that the areas used by the health services as their main units—the AHAs, are contiguous with the new county councils and metropolitan district councils which administer the local social services. In this way, it is expected that both services will be able to cooperate and help each other more easily. The health services provide medical advice to the social services and the local social services provide the hospital social work services and any social work advice and help required by doctors working within the community. It is, however, very important that liaison between the two services is good. On the health side, a community physician is appointed with responsibility for liaison—the area Specialist in Community Medicine (Social Services)—and on the social services side a senior officer is appointed (usually an Assistant Director of Social Services) to take charge of the hospital social work service and be responsible for integration.

Whenever possible there should be similarity between the District Management Team areas of the AHA and a number of social services areas so that officers from both services work in similar geographical divisions (there will often be two to four social service area teams to each District Management Team). It is also important that close working relationships should be built up between general practitioners and social workers from the local social services department. This can best be achieved by social workers being attached part-time to the primary health care teams. Eventually it is hoped that such an arrangement will be general and that whenever the hospital admission is arranged of an individual who is 'at risk' of social deprivation (perhaps because he/she is elderly and living alone) the team in hospital will be alerted by the social worker.

Close liaison between the two services is important in all

problems, but particularly in the case of children, the severely physically or mentally disabled and the elderly. Many individual examples illustrate the need for such arrangements, especially the instances of non-accidental injury in babies. More details of the way such coordinated arrangements are ensured are given on p. 435 where joint Area Review Committees are described.

Joint Consultative Committee (JCC)

The Joint Consultative Committee provides a permanent statutory committee between the local authority providing social services and the matching AHA. The constitution and role of such committees have been described on p. 23. They play an increasingly important part in assisting coordination between the social and health services through *Joint Financing* arrangements (see p. 24) and *Joint Care Planning Teams* (see p. 22).

22 Measurement of Social Problems

OBJECTIVE SOCIAL INDICATORS

Social problems in a community can be assessed by various statistics which point to serious social difficulties, and these are often referred to as *social indicators.* It is possible to measure the objective conditions known to be associated with the development of social difficulties and to show how such conditions have contributed to the problem. For instance, very poor housing conditions are known to be associated throughout the world with high levels of crime and social deprivation. Thus, the measurement of the number of unfit slum houses could be said to be an indirect measure of social problems. *Objective* social indicators are usually measurements of this sort, but many different examples occur including the following:

Age and sex structure of any community
Marital status and especially one parent families, widowhood and divorce
Migration levels
Type of house occupied and whether owned or rented
Household amenities
Social grouping (social class)
Household size and density of occupation of the house
Levels of crime
Levels of disease
Dependence of family upon social security benefits
Unemployment and job stability.

In attempting to build up the background picture (or profile) of a community, information on all these factors could be obtained. This has been carried out in various research projects and one of the more interesting examples was the *Social Malaise Study in Liverpool*, 1968–9, which was published in 1970. In that study, 36 different indices were used including:

Children in care
School absenteeism
Physically handicapped children
Educationally subnormal children
Adults who were mentally ill
Adults who were mentally subnormal
Illegitimacy
Dysentery levels
Children deloused
Dwellings disinfested
Adults in receipt of free meals on wheels
Education grants for clothing
Job instability
Unemployment
Possession orders
Debtors
Homeless families case conferences
Higher education grants
Electricity Board entry warrants
Crime, mainly assault, sexual morality, burglary
  theft, fraud and malicious damage
Infant mortality.

In this study, correlation analysis was used to test the likely levels of connection between two of the various indices, and the results were published as a matrix of correlation.

There was a very high association between unemployment and assault, a high association between unemployment and debtors, homeless family cases, electricity board entry warrants, burglary, theft, but a low association between unemployment and higher education grants.

Such a table gives a complicated picture of the interrelationships and in many instances only states the obvious, but such studies do attempt to measure the spread of social problems and to indicate the great differences between the various causative factors.

Illegitimacy has a high connection with the number of children coming into care, a moderate connection with school absenteeism and children who are educationally subnormal, but less obvious connections with most of the other indicators.

This Social Malaise Study also analysed the levels of social problem or malaise in different parts of the city. The result showed a greater degree of variation than might have been expected merely from studying the statistics for the whole city—*there was a much greater degree of spread of social problems than expected.*

For instance, *illegitimacy varied between 3·4% and 23·2% (mean for city 11·4%)*, and children classified as educationally subnormal from 0·6% to 4·7% in different wards of the city. The exact figures are not as important as the range of social problems they represent.

This type of information has been used by the social services department to identify areas in the city with a profusion of problems. Many social service departments in the UK have set up *Research and Information Units* to collect similar data to enable such problems to be identified, which then assists in the determination of priorities. In this way, an estimate is built up of the *groups of any population that are at special risk of further* deprivation. Resources (staff, playgroups, day centre facilities, etc.) can then be concentrated in those areas which have the greatest problems. If such studies are to be really effective, they must be repeated, if possible, annually or biennially, to enable the results of introducing services to be measured.

National Objective Social Indicators

The collection and analysis of various social statistical data from different areas will enable a national picture to be built up. Many of the Tables giving details about population, migration, employment, education, housing, crime, in the publication 'Social Trends', published annually by the Central Statistical Office, deal with this type of indicator. This chapter should be studied together with Chapter 3 for *there is much overlap between health and social problems.* For convenience, examples already mentioned in Chapter 3 are not repeated although in many instances (Infant Mortality Rate, Social Class, etc.), the measurements relate to both health and social problems. A few further examples are given below:

Population

The age structure of a population, especially as regards the elderly, can have a marked effect on the social problems likely to be encountered. Table 65 shows the *sex ratio* for different ages of the population in 1971.

TABLE 65 Sex ratio for different ages of population UK, 1971

Age group	*Males per 100 females*	*Age group*	*Males per 100 females*
0–9	105	60–4	88
10–19	106	65–9	79
20–9	101	70–4	63
30–9	102	75–9	53
40–9	98	80–4	44
50–9	93	85+	37

Note that the proportion of males in the population steadily falls as the age rises, *but only becomes marked after 60 years.* In the oldest age group (over 85 years) *there were only 37 men for every 100 women.* In addition, further studies have shown that there is a greater proportion of such elderly women with special social and medical problems: it is not just a simple relationship between numbers of very old women and men in the country.

Family building and size

There are many ways the family size distribution can be demonstrated. One of the more useful ways is illustrated in Fig. 23. This figure considers family size distribution after 10 years of marriage over the last 14 years (1961–75). It will be seen that approximately 10% of marriages have no children at all after 10

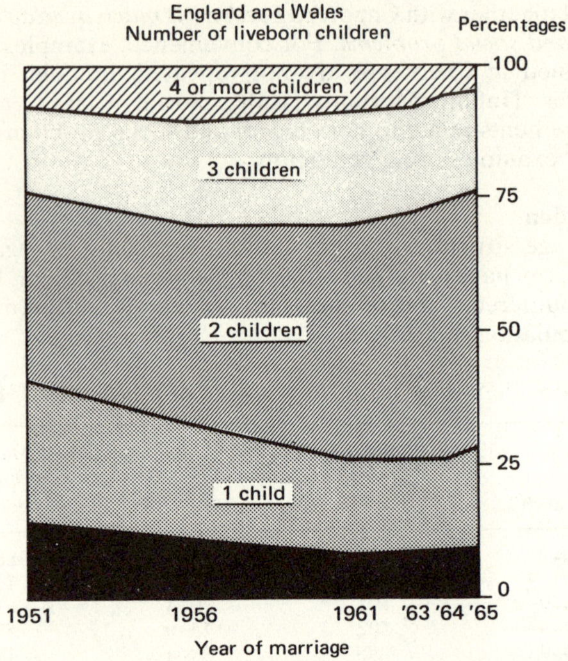

FIG. 23. Family size distribution after ten years of marriage. (From *Social Trends*, 1977, OPCS)

years, another 16% one child, another 49% two children, a further 20% three children and the remaining 5% four or more children. The changes in this pattern over this period are also interesting: there is a slight trend towards one child only and a clear reduction in four or more children. *The age of mother at the birth of a child* varies considerably with social class as seen in Table 66. Note that 21% of births in social class V occur to women under 20 years of age but this progressively falls as social class rises until it is 1% and 3% in social classes I and II. There is a corresponding higher percentage of births in ages 25–9 and 30–4 in social classes I and II.

Such statistics are significant in many ways as regards social problems. Non-accidental injury is considerably more common in the youngest mothers (who are at their most intolerant stage of

TABLE 66 Live births to married couples: by social class of husband and age of mother at birth of child, 1975, Great Britain

Social class of husband		Age of mother at birth of child: Under 20	20–4	25–9	30–4	35–9	40–4	*All births* (=100%) (thousands)
I	Professional	1	15	51	25	6	1	47
II	Intermediate occupations*	3	21	47	21	6	1	109
IIIN	Skilled occupations, non-manual	4	27	47	16	4	1	64
IIIM	Skilled occupations, manual	9	36	36	13	4	1	239
IV	Partly skilled occupations	12	38	31	12	5	1	95
V	Unskilled occupations	21	40	25	9	4	2	33
	Not classified	11	39	35	11	3	–	24
	All classes	8	32	39	15	5	1	610

* Includes most managerial and senior administrative occupations.
(from *Social Trends*, 1977 OPCS)

life). Table 66 explains one of the reasons why non-accidental injury is highest in social class V.

Projections

Estimations are made (based on current trends of mortality and birth rate, etc.) by the OPCS of the future population. These are a highly significant indication of *probable future social problems*. Table 67 gives these projections for children up to 1991. Note the quite large variations expected in the various age groups during the next 13 years. It is expected the total child population will fall from 17 090 000 in 1976 to 15 120 000 in 1991. But that statement conceals important other trends. The numbers of young children (0–4) will continue to fall until 1981 (3 201 000) but will then rise to 4 452 000 by 1991. At the same time the numbers of teenagers (15–19) will fall from a peak of 4 677 000 in 1981 to 3 685 000 in 1991. The significance for services either dealing with the very young children or with juvenile delinquency (highest in the oldest age groups) is quite obvious. The degree of change is dependent upon, of course, the future birth

TABLE 67 Children by age group, United Kingdom (thousands)

	Census enumerated		Mid-year estimates			1976 based projections		
	1951	1961	1966	1971	1976[1]	1981	1986	1991
Boys aged								
0–4	2215	2162	2451	2310	1925	1646	2010	2289
5–9	1885	1954	2181	2400	2282	1902	1622	1985
10–14	1682	2206	1956	2174	2387	2268	1886	1607
15–19	1564	1870	2158	1984	2184	2400	2281	1900
Total under 20	7346	8192	8746	8868	8777	8216	7799	7781
Girls aged								
0–4	2111	2051	2339	2192	1814	1555	1899	2163
5–9	1804	1862	2060	2278	2164	1792	1532	1875
10–14	1629	2102	1850	2057	2266	2149	1776	1516
15–19	1611	1825	2077	1876	2068	2277	2158	1785
Total under 20	7155	7840	8325	8403	8313	7773	7365	7339

[1] Provisional.
(From *Social Trends*, 1977, OPCS)

TABLE 68 Household projections of persons aged 60–65 or over, England and Wales (thousands)

			1974-based mid-year projections			
	Census 1971	1974 (base)	1976	1981	1988	1991
Married couple households (head aged 65 years and over)	1723	1824	1884	1991	2009	2055
One person households (aged 60, women; aged 65 and over, men)	1987	2420	2581	2905	3140	3284

(From *Social Trends*, 1977, OPCS)

rate but past variations are also very important. At present there is a bulge of young people corresponding with the large rise in the birth rate from 1955 to 1964 and this will be one of the most significant reasons for the expected rise in the numbers of young children from 1981 to 1991, there will be for a 10-year period a substantial increase in the numbers of women in the population at their most reproductive ages.

The elderly is another group which can produce many social problems because of the vulnerability of very old people particularly if they live alone. Table 68 gives the projections of married couple households and of one-person households for England and Wales to 1991. It will be seen that the numbers of both households are going to increase but *there is a much greater*

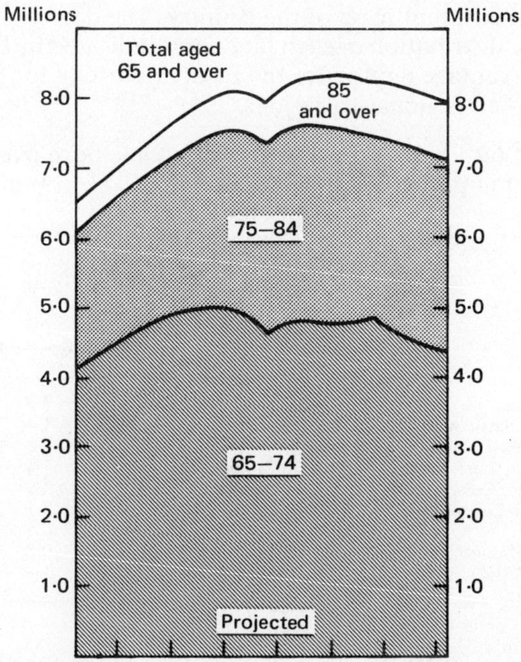

FIG. 24. Changes expected in the elderly population of Great Britain to 2000. (From *A Happier Old Age*, 1978, DHSS)

increase expected in households with only one old person. This is almost certainly going to be caused by the large increase in very old people expected in the population during the next 15–20 years.

The detailed changes expected in the population aged 65–74, 75–84 and 85 years and over are shown in Fig. 24.

The number of social and medical problems which will have to be dealt with in the next 15 years due to these population changes *are bound to increase markedly* because it is this age group 85 years and over which always produce the largest number of such problems.

Distribution in particular areas of people born overseas

The incidence of social problems connected with immigrant families is bound to be influenced by the concentration of such families in different parts of the country. The degree of unevenness in the distribution of such families is indicated in Table 69.

The percentage figures are the most interesting for they show quite marked regional variations.

TABLE 69 Selected categories of people born overseas resident in particular areas of the UK, 1971* (% of those enumerated)

	India/ Pakistan Bangladesh	*West Indies†*	*Total 'New' Common-wealth*	*Irish Republic§*	*'Old' Common-wealth‡ and foreign*
Greater London	1·8	2·3	6·4	3·3	4·7
Outer Metropolitan Area	0·9	0·4	2·0	1·4	2·8
Outer South East Area	0·5	0·2	1·5	1·0	2·6
West Midlands Conurbation	2·9	1·6	5·0	2·4	1·1
West Yorkshire Conurbation	2·2	0·6	3·2	1·1	1·7
SE Lancashire Conurbation	1·0	0·4	1·9	2·1	1·6
Scotland	0·2	—	0·6	0·6	1·3
Other Great Britain	0·4	0·2	1·0	0·8	1·4
Total Great Britain	0·9	0·6	2·1	1·3	2·1

* Final 1971 Census figures.
† Including British Honduras, Guyana and Falkland Islands.
‡ The 'Old' Commonwealth countries are Canada, Australia and New Zealand: the 'New' Commonwealth countries are the remainder.
§ Including Ireland (part not stated).
(From *Social Trends*, 1974, OPCS)

The demographic trends, particularly as regards births of various ethnic minorities are also important for they emphasize possible future social problems. In Table 70 the percentage of all live births for various ethnic minorities is given and compared with the births of the population born in the UK.

TABLE 70 Live births by country of birth of mother, England and Wales, 1971–5

	Percentage of all live births				
Country of birth of mother	*1971*	*1972*	*1973*	*1974*	*1975*
India, Pakistan and Bangladesh	2·8	2·9	3·0	3·2	3·4
West Indies	1·6	1·5	1·3	1·3	1·3
African continent	0·6	0·7	0·8	0·9	1·0
Other	0·8	0·8	0·9	0·9	1·0
Subtotal	5·8	5·9	6·1	6·3	6·7
Irish Republic	2·8	2·6	2·4	2·3	2·1
Australia, Canada, New Zealand	0·3	0·3	0·4	0·4	0·4
Foreign	2·5	2·6	2·6	2·7	2·8
Total with mother born outside UK	11·3	11·4	11·5	11·6	11·9
United Kingdom	88·1	88·2	88·3	88·2	87·9
Not stated	0·6	0·3	0·2	0·2	0·1

(From *Social Trends*, 1977, OPCS)

It will be seen that for 1971 to 1975 there was a 0·9% increase in New Commonwealth births but only a 0·2% reduction in births to UK born mothers. One of the reasons was that there was a reduction in Irish Republic births from 2·8% to 2·1% over this period. These are national figures and conceal more significant and marked regional variations in these birth rates due to the uneven distribution of people born overseas (as shown by Table 69).

Divorce

The end of any marriage in divorce can indicate a number of social problems, particularly if there are children. Likewise divorce itself can help solve social problems. The Divorce Reform Act which became operative on 1 January, 1971, has resulted in a marked increase in divorce and has made comparisons with former years difficult. In 1975, 120 500 divorces were granted in England and Wales. In Table 71, the distribution and ages of the children of such divorcing couples are given.

TABLE 71 Divorcing couples with children under 16, by number and age of children

Divorcing couples		*Ages of children of divorcing couples* (under 16 years)	
With no children under 16 years	46 000 (38%)	Under 5 years	33 400 (22·7%)
With 1 child under 16 years	28 200 (23·5%)	5–10 years	68 700 (47%)
With 2 children under 16 years	28 200 (23·5%)	11–15 years	43 000 (30·3%)
With 3 children under 16 years	11 800 (9·9%)	Total	145 100
With 4+ children under 16 years	5700 (5·1%)		
Total	120 500		

(From *Social Trends*, 1977, OPCS)

It will be seen that 38% of divorcing couples have no children under the age of 16 years, 23·5% have one or two children, 9·9% have three children and 5·1% have four or more children. Of all children of divorcing couples, 22·7% are under the age of five years, 47% aged from 5–10 and 30·3% aged 11–15 years.

The proportion of marriages ended by divorce varies with the age of those getting married.

Table 71 shows the proportion of marriages ended by divorce with the number of children under 16 years. Generally there is a *greater chance of divorce when the marriage takes place at an early age*; 14% of marriages where the wife was under 20 years of age at marriage now end in divorce compared with 6·7% and 4·6% for marriages where the wife was aged 20 to 24 and 25 to 29 years respectively at marriage.

There are marked differences in the divorce rates of various countries (Table 72). The highest rate is in USA and the lowest in France. There is an interesting difference in the rates of Scotland (1·6) and England and Wales (2·2).

TABLE 72 Divorce rates of various countries, 1974

Country	*Divorce rate* (per 1000 population)
USA	4·6
Sweden	3·2
USSR	3·0
England and Wales	2·2
Germany (Federal Republic)	1·6
Scotland	1·4
France	1·0

(From *Social Trends*, 1977, OPCS)

Housing

Many fascinating indications of possible social problems are given by statistics about housing conditions. Many of these are concerned with standards of housing. An unusual feature shown by the changing trend now apparent is the proportion of persons who own or rent accommodation compared with their age group (Table 73).

TABLE 73 Nature of household tenure compared with age, UK, 1971

	Age of head of household						
	up to 24	25–29	30–44	45–59	60–69	70 and over	All ages
Owner-occupier							
Owning outright	2	2	8	21	41	42	22
Buying	30	49	48	27	8	3	27
Rent							
L.A./New Town	21	24	29	35	32	31	31
other unfurnished	18	10	7	10	16	22	12
other furnished	23	7	2	1	1	1	3
With job/business	6	7	6	6	3	1	5
Total households	100	100	100	100	100	100	100

(From the *General Household Survey*)

It will be seen that over half of the age group 25–9 were buying or own their own houses. Since the last war, there has been a growth in owner occupation and a decline in privately rented accommodation. But the elderly still rely very much upon rented accommodation. In fact, although Table 73 does not show this, over two-thirds of both council housing and privately rented accommodation is occupied by persons over 45 years of age.

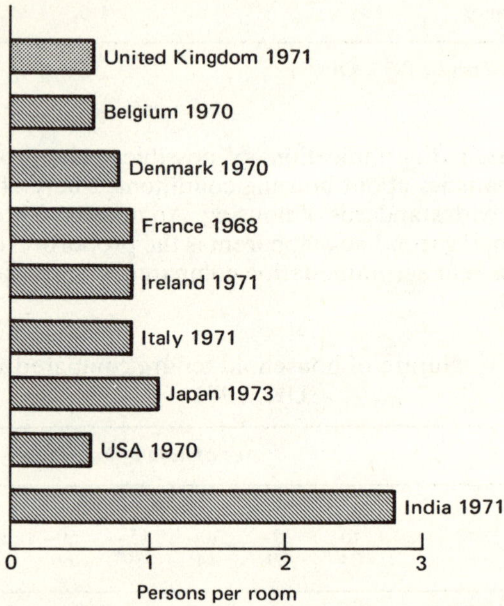

FIG. 25. International comparison of persons per room. (From *Social Trends*, 1977, OPCS)

The overcrowding in different countries of the world can be compared by an *estimate of the number of persons per room*. Fig. 25 gives the number of persons per room. In this comparison 'a room' is the UN definition and includes any space (*not* passage, bathroom or toilet) which is at least 2 m high and of a size large enough to hold a bed for an adult (4 sq m at least).

Education

The extent to which educational opportunity is available in any country is an important factor which can influence social problems. There are many ways this can be studied by comparing the opportunities for education of the under fives, the school leaving age and the academic attainment of children on leaving school, and the proportion of children going on to higher education. The increase in preschool education (the under fives) is clearly shown in Table 74 which shows that in 1976 nearly double the number of children aged 2–4 years were attending full-time or part-time education at nursery schools and classes compared with 1967. *The proportion of children aged 2–4* has more than doubled and in 1976 represented 23·7% compared with 10·1% in 1967.

TABLE 74 Education for the under-fives, United Kingdom (full-time or part time pupils in all schools as a percentage of all children)

Age	*1967*	*1976*	*no. of 1976 pupils*
Aged 2	0·4	0·5	4200
Aged 3	4·0	12·9	104 400
Aged 4	26·6	54·1	467 300
Total aged 2–4	10·1	23·7	576 000
Total (numbers)	296 100	576 000	

(From *Social Trends*, 1977, OPCS)

The academic attainment of school leavers is shown in Table 75. The changes show many interesting points. The attainment of girls is improving faster than boys. In 1975–6, 7% of girls left with three or more A levels compared with 4·8% of girls in 1965–6; in the same period the boys have improved from 8·9% to 9·9%. Also more girls than boys in 1976 (50·5% compared with 46·9%) obtained a qualification of 1–4 higher grades GCE, 5 or more O levels or A levels (i.e. 1967 boys obtaining such number 38·0% compared with girls 37·4%).

This is, of course, not a direct measure of a social problem but

TABLE 75 Academic Attainment of School leavers, England and Wales (%)

Attainment	1965–6 Boys	1965–6 Girls	1975–6 Boys	1975–6 Girls
3 or more A level passes	8·9	4·8	9·9	7·0
2 A level passes	4·0	3·8	4·1	4·5
1 A level pass	2·8	2·8	2·9	3·3
Total with at least 1 A level pass	15·7	11·4	16·9	14·8
5 or more higher grade O level or CSE passes	7·1	9·6	5·4	7·4
1–4 higher grades GCE	15·2	16·4	24·6	28·3
Total of all above	38·0	37·4	46·9	50·5
Only 1 or more other grades / No GCE or CSE qualifications	62·0	62·5	53·1	49·5

(From *Social Trends*, 1977, OPCS)

is an indication of inequality of educational achievement within the same family (between generations and sexes) and may indicate particular stresses. Perhaps the *greatest value of such an example is the ever changing or dynamic nature of what is being measured.*

General

The examples of objective social indicators given here and in Chapter 3 are not in any way intended to be comprehensive, for such a study would be far beyond the scope of this book. They are, however, meant to illustrate the way in which social conditions and problems can be measured. Unless the social services provided in an area are being constantly checked against needs, it is very easy for them to become unbalanced. It is, therefore, important that all field work staff become used to using and referring to such data, but they must always realize that *no single social indicator can ever give a complete picture.* All social problems have complex causes and an appreciation of these will only be obtained by consideration of many factors.

SUBJECTIVE SOCIAL INDICATORS

Whereas objective social indicators measure conditions such as housing, education, employment, etc. there is another aspect which is also important to assess—that is the degree of satisfaction or dissatisfaction felt by people with various aspects of their lives. Recently, in the USA and this country, a number of attempts have been made to measure the *subjective* factors—to assess each individual's reactions and perceptions and to weigh these against his expectations, experiences, attitude and present circumstances. Such measurements are spoken of as *subjective social indicators*.

These studies were developed because many people pointed out that objective social indicators are crude measurements and, although useful to give a general background picture, have many limitations. For instance, the quality of life in a community depends very much on the life which people lead—their participation in community events, their concern for the community they live in, racial equality, etc. Small communities, villages and small towns are well known to be pleasanter places to live in than cities, and often this is principally because the person is more integrated into that community and is therefore more useful and feels needed.

Two small surveys were carried out in the UK by the Social Science Research Council Survey Unit and by the Social and Community Planning Research in 1971. The results are fully reported in *Social Trends* No. 4, pp. 35–49.

The method of carrying out these surveys is interesting for an 11 point scale was used to indicate 'satisfaction ratings'. The levels 0 and 1 represent very low satisfaction, 9 and 10 very high satisfaction. Each person interviewed was asked to classify his satisfaction rating at the time, 4 to 5 years ago and what he thought it would be in 4 to 5 years under the following headings (or domains):

Marriage, family life, health, standard of living, house, job, spare time, district, religion, democracy.

First of all, each person was asked to say which of these items was most important in determining his satisfaction or dissatisfaction with life in general.

The results, in order, were:

Marriage, family life, health, standard of living, housing, job, spare time, district, religion, democracy, education.

Next persons were asked to put in order their *satisfaction levels* in these features and the order was:

Marriage, family life, job, district, health, spare time, housing, standard of living, education received, religion, and democratic standards.

The majority said that marriage, family life and health, were very important and also that their levels of satisfaction in these aspects were high. But in two of the features, standard of living and housing, there was a marked disparity between the levels of importance (both were considered important) and the levels of satisfaction (both were scored low).

Studies of this type introduce a completely new dimension into the ways of measuring social problems. Although such researches are subjective (they depend on the assessment by the people tested) they are measuring features which everyone recognizes as most important. Social problems follow dissatisfaction and it is well known that satisfaction is not the inevitable sequence of a high standard of living and an excellent house to live in. By measuring only objective conditions such as salary levels or housing standards, only very crude indications can be reached into how many social problems are produced. By also studying subjective social indicators, a much deeper impression is gained of what people themselves consider important and how far their hopes and expectations are met.

In the next survey being undertaken in the UK, it has been decided to concentrate upon the four factors considered most important, *marriage, health, standard of living and housing*, and these will be studied as priorities and examined in much greater detail. These results should be most interesting and make a useful addition to the measurement of social problems.

23 Care of Children in Need

DAY CARE

Day Nurseries

Day nurseries are provided by local authorities to help care for young children who, due to social circumstances, cannot remain at home during the daytime. In this way, young children need not be admitted to a residential home. Day nurseries are of great help (*a*) to the unmarried mother who has to go out to work; (*b*) to a widow or widower with a young family to support; (*c*) where the mother of the family is suddenly taken ill, resulting in her admission to hospital; (*d*) to a family with a mild or moderately handicapped child.

Day nurseries are open five days a week from about 7.30 a.m. to 5.30 p.m. Children from a few weeks old to five years of age are admitted and the parent usually brings the child on the way to work. The child normally has all his meals at the day nursery and will be completely looked after there during the day. A small charge is usually made for this service. Most day nurseries care for about 50 children who are usually looked after in 'family groups' consisting of eight to ten children aged from six to eight months to five years as it is thought that this gives a more normal homelike life and enables the children to keep a close relationship with the two nurses who care for them. It also enables children from the same family to be kept together. The older children from all family groups have periods of play together while the babies under the age of six months are usually kept together.

A qualified matron and a deputy matron are in charge of the nursery and, to assist them, there are a number of *trained nursery nurses*. The health of the children must be carefully supervised; usually a doctor from the child health service makes regular visits and examinations. It is important to ensure: (*a*) that every child is fit before being admitted; (*b*) that every child is fully immunized; (*c*) that any case of infectious disease is carefully investigated. It is essential that dysentery or gastroenteritis is never allowed to develop in a day nursery. Any child with diarrhoea should be immediately excluded until a bacteriological stool examination is normal.

There are four other types of day care provision for young children: (1) playgroups, (2) preschool playgroups, (3) private day nurseries and child minders, (4) nursery schools and nursery classes.

The first three must be registered with the social services department which has the responsibility for inspecting periodically. Nursery schools and classes are the responsibility of the local education authority.

Playgroups

Many playgroups are provided by voluntary bodies and often by groups of mothers. They provide sessional care for children between two and a half years and five years of age. Local arrangements vary and playgroups may meet two to five times per week. Usually playgroups are used to help mothers, especially in the more deprived areas, as well as helping generally in the day care of children.

Preschool playgroups

Many of these playgroups have been formed during the last 14 years with help from the national Preschool Playgroups Association. Their functions are very similar to playgroups and before the reform of social services had a very close link with education. Many preschool playgroups concentrated upon helping mothers and used the involvement by individual mothers in the playgroups as a means to teach parents more about their children, and in this way help parents to provide a better home environment for their children. Many preschool playgroups have become closely linked with various community groups and help to develop closer links within local populations especially in new housing areas. Preschool playgroups have, in this way, reduced the isolation felt by many mothers especially when they have recently been rehoused in a new housing area where they know very few people.

Private day nurseries and child minders

There are not many private day nurseries although a number are run by local industry for their workers. The 'child minder' is the term used for *those caring for more than one child in their own home, whether for profit or not.* Anyone acting as a child minder must register with the social services department of the local authority.

In private day nurseries the social services department stipulates the numbers of children to be looked after and the general requirements as to staff, diet, equipment and fire precautions. In the case of child minders inspections also take place to ensure that the premises used are suitable.

Nursery schools and nursery classes

These provide part-time education for three and four year olds. Many variations of service exist, but increasingly nursery classes are being developed in conjunction with primary schools. During 1973, the Secretary of State for Education announced a large expansion development in this field and there has been a marked increase in the percentage of children attending. By 1976, 23·7% of all children aged 2–4 years attended a nursery class or school.

Although day care provision for young children is provided in both the social service and education fields, it is important that *every local authority plans its day care provision in such a way that maximum coordination is achieved between both services and the voluntary field.* In the training of nursery nurses, a period of teaching is always arranged in both day nurseries run by social services departments and in nursery schools run by education departments.

In some local authorities experimental units have been introduced containing both a day nursery and nursery school.

CHILD CARE SERVICES

Under the various Children Acts, 1948, 1958 and 1975, and the Children and Young Persons Acts, 1963 and 1969, County Councils, Metropolitan District Councils and London Boroughs have many special responsibilities especially in supervising or caring for children and young persons under the age of 18 years.

In particular these responsibilities cover four main groups of children:

1. Those who have to be cared for by the local authority because their parents are temporarily absent (i.e. illness) or because they have no parents or guardians or because their parents or guardians are unable to look after them properly or have abandoned them. The reason may be temporary or permanent, and local authorities can either receive the children into voluntary care (see p. 417) or, through a court, have a statutory care order made transferring the parental rights.
2. Children and young persons who have been brought before a court for criminal proceedings.
3. Children placed by a court in the care of the Social Services Committee of the local authority in connection with matrimonial proceedings.
4. Children who have been placed in foster homes or who have been placed privately for adoption (see p. 430).

Most of these responsibilities are now undertaken by the Social Services Committee and the social services department under the control of the Director of Social Services. In 1971, the responsible central government department became the Department of Health and Social Security and the Secretary of State for Social Services (formerly it was the Home Office).

Under these child care services the local authority through its Social Services Committee and department can help in many ways and has certain duties imposed upon it. Every social services department will aim at ensuring that children in its care are brought up in good conditions and, *if possible, in conditions which are similar to those of any normal family.* It is most important that every child is cared for in an atmosphere of security and affection.

Any local authority may pass a resolution assuming parental rights over a child if there are no parents or guardians or if the local authority considers the parent or guardian unfit to care for that child. If the parents object, *the matter must be referred to a juvenile court.* In practice, in those cases where a local authority claims statutory care (Section II of Children's Act, 1948) the case is dealt with by a juvenile court.

In many instances, the social services department cares for the child by agreement—*voluntary care*, under Section I of the Children Act, 1948.

Voluntary care

Under Section I of the Children's Act, 1948, the local authority has a duty to investigate when it comes to their knowledge that a child is in need of care and protection due to neglect, abandonment or inability of the parents to cope. Moral danger may be another reason. Social workers undertake an inquiry; in many cases, the child is taken into care with the consent of the parents and, in this instance, the parents can later claim the child when the problem is over. But in more serious cases court action is started which may result in the child being committed to the care of the local authority (see below—statutory care). Voluntary care may last less than six months, i.e. 'short-term care', or it may last longer than six months when it is called 'long-term care'. Obviously the length of stay of each child in the care of the local authority depends upon the circumstances of each case.

Short-term care is particularly used for a sudden family crisis, such as the illness or confinement of the mother. The local authority provide a short-term care service in which they look after the children temporarily. Short-term care never lasts longer than six months and often for a few days or weeks. In all cases it is usual for very little deprivation to occur to the children and once the family crisis is over the children are returned to their natural parents.

Under the Children Act 1975, any local authority, through its social services committee will eventually be able to:

a. require up to 28 days notice from any parent who wishes to remove a child who has been in their care for 12 months or more

b. assume parental rights over a child who has been in their care or that of a voluntary organization for three years.

Any doctor who comes across a child in his practice who is in need of care and protection should immediately report the case to the Director of Social Services who will then arrange an investigation and will safeguard the child.

Statutory care

Under Section II of the Children Act, 1948, a court may commit a child, whom it considers is in need of care and protection, to the care of a local authority and in such cases the parental rights are transferred to the local authority. Once a child has been committed to the care of a local authority, the only way that the natural parents can reclaim that child is by petitioning the same court who originally made the order for its revocation. The court then will decide whether the parents are now responsible enough to justify again committing the child to their care. Under the Children and Young Persons Act, 1969, statutory care covers both deprived and delinquent children.

In urgent cases, an *interim care order* is obtained which has the effect of placing the child in care temporarily until a full court hearing can be arranged.

Statutory care orders will remain in force until the child reaches 18 years of age or the local authority agrees to the child returning home.

Financial provisions

Parents of children who are in the care of the local authority are liable to make contributions to the cost of maintenance until the child reaches 16 years of age.

When a child comes into *voluntary care*, the parent is allowed to keep child benefit payments for the first eight weeks. For any child in *statutory care*, child benefit payments cease immediately.

Transfer of voluntary care of children to statutory care

In some cases, the child is first placed in voluntary care, but the circumstances deteriorate and the local authority may then consider that the child requires the added protection of statutory care. The local authority in such cases has power to assume the parental rights under Section II of the Children Act, 1948, on grounds which must meet the specifications laid down in the Children and Young Persons Acts of 1933, 1963 and 1969. Whenever parental rights are assumed in this way, the natural parents must always be notified and can challenge the decision of the local authority in the courts.

Children who are victims of divorce

There are special provisions to care for children who are the victims of divorce. These are a relatively small percentage of cases, but under the Matrimonial Cause Acts, the High Court can make the local authority the guardian of the child acting under the directions of the Court. The social services department then looks after the child in the usual way.

Cessation of parental rights

In all cases where parental rights have been transferred to the local authority, these cease when the young person reaches the age of 18 years.

Definition

The Children and Young Persons Act, 1933, defines a child as a person under 14 years of age and a young person as one between the ages of 14 and 18 years.

In 1976, 61 100 children came into the care of the local authority. The majority are admitted for some 'home problem' or crisis and a smaller proportion for the juvenile delinquency of the child.

In the same period (1976) 48 294 children went out of the care of local authorities. The vast majority of these (33 430), either became self-supporting or their care was taken over by a parent, guardian, relative or friend.

Approximately 100 000 children are in the care of local authorities in the UK. It is most important that the needs of every child should be carefully assessed on admission into care, and as far as possible the wishes of the child should be taken into consideration. This process is often spoken of as *observation and assessment* and in certain cases (i.e. delinquent children) should be carried out in special units with expert facilities including psychiatric help. Under the Children and Young Persons Act,

1969, *assessment is a duty* imposed upon the social services department who *must review each case every six months*. The aim is to place every child on the basis of its assessed needs. In practice, placements include:

1. *Boarding out of the child with foster parents* is ideal and is used wherever possible. Each foster parent looks after either one or a number of children in conditions very similar to a normal family. Each foster parent is paid an allowance by the local authority to meet the costs of looking after the child. Approximately 33% of children in care are fostered out.
2. *Placement in a community home* (formerly called children's home) provided or controlled by the local authority: There

   a. Small community home containing from 12 to 18 children.

   b. Family group home containing from 4 to 6 children. Such homes are usually one or two ordinary council houses in a normal residential area. They are particularly useful to keep together brothers and sisters under natural conditions as in a large family and where fostering has proved impracticable.

   Approximately 22% of children live in either small or family group homes.

   c. Community homes with education on the premises (CHEs) which are used for longer-term boarding school placements or for observation and assessment. Approximately 12% of children are accommodated in other observation and assessment units or in community homes with education on the premises (see p. 423).

   d. For very young infants and children, initial care may be undertaken in a residential nursery; 2% of children in care are looked after in such units.
3. *Placement of the child in its own home under supervision* of his parent, guardian, relative or friend; 18% of children 'in care' are looked after in this way.
4. *The child may be placed in a children's home run by a voluntary body* (such as the National Children's Homes, Barnardos, etc).

5. *Placement in a hostel or lodgings*, for older children (2·5%).
6. *Certain handicapped children in care* may be placed in special accommodation (3%).
7. *The remainder* are placed in various other types of accommodation.

When a child is admitted into a children's home an attempt will always be made to rehabilitate him later into a foster home or back to his natural home so that the child can have the advantage of a normal family atmosphere. In this way, the social services department tries gradually to make the child more independent and secure so that before the child reaches 18 years he has returned to normal living conditions.

Supervision over fostering

When a child is placed with foster parents, it is the duty of the social services department to arrange regular visiting. Under the Boarding-out Regulations this must be at not more than six week intervals.

Whenever there is a private agreement or contract between one private individual and another for the placement of a child or children, the social services department *must* be notified and has a duty to satisfy itself about this placement and to ensure the child is well looked after.

Custodianship

Under the Children Act 1975, a new legal status called '*custodianship*' will eventually be introduced (by early 1979, it had not yet been implemented). This is a half-way stage between adoption and fostering under which legal custody is transferred but the child keeps his name, and his family contacts are not cut off.

Custodianship can be granted by the Court on application of a relative, step-parent or any other person who is not the mother or father of the child but who has the child in his care. In the case of a relative or step-parent the child must have had his home with the applicant for at least three months; if the applicant is not a relative or step-parent the child must have been living there for at least 12 months. The application can be made without the consent of the parent or guardian if he has had his home with the applicant for at least three years.

It is hoped that this part of the Bill will give greater security to children who are in the long term care of local authorities, voluntary organizations and others, and to prevent some of the difficulties which lead to 'tug of love' situations.

Special Residential Units

In addition to providing ordinary community homes (children's homes), it is usual for the larger local authorities to provide a number of special residential units—an admission unit, a residential nursery, observation and assessment units (reception centres) and community homes with education on the premises (CHEs).

Admission unit

This is the place into which all urgent cases are admitted. Size varies but most look after 40 to 50 children and enable skilled assessment to be undertaken. The child who is looked after for a short time (as in short-term care) will probably stay in the admission unit until discharged, but others move on from the admission unit to other forms of care—residential nursery, reception centre, boarding out or a children's home.

Residential nursery

This caters for young babies and children under the age of five years and may care for from 20 to 40 infants. It is usual to segregate the very young infants, but the others are usually accommodated in groups.

Observation and Assessment Unit (Reception Centre)

This allows for the longer assessment of children, particularly those who have some difficulty in settling down, or those who are maladjusted. Children are admitted to an observation and assessment unit from other forms of care—from admission units and from children's homes. The main function of this centre is to allow a longer expert assessment of the child to be carried out.

In both admission units and an observation and assessment

unit, it is usual to have one or two classes which children can attend, the teaching staff being provided by the Local Education Authority. In other forms of care—boarding out, family group homes and community homes—the children attend normal schools in the community.

Community homes with education on the premises (CHEs)

This is the name now given to all the various types of residential accommodation for children including children's homes, reception centres, nurseries and those special units which were formerly called remand homes and approved schools.

'Group A' community homes are the former approved schools.

'Group B' community homes are equivalent to boys' remand homes and hold boys on interim or remand orders, but now also act as assessment centres for boys already dealt with by the courts and placed in the care of the social services department.

'Group C' community homes are equivalent to the former girls remand homes and hold girls on interim or remand orders, but now also act as assessment centres for girls already dealt with by the courts and placed in the care of the social services department.

Provision of education in community homes with education on the premises (CHEs)

There are two arrangements for providing education in CHEs. In most such homes the social services department provides the education directly and employs the teachers; in other the teachers in such homes are seconded from the local education authority. The Warnock Committee on special educational needs, which reported in 1978, was concerned about the standard of education in CHEs and made the recommendation that 'as a first and major step in improving the quality of educational provision in CHEs and observation and assessment centres, teachers in those establishments should be in the service of local education authorities.

Most of the larger local authorities provide these community homes with education on the premises, but many large voluntary bodies also provide such units. Under the Regional Plan (see below) CHEs run by voluntary bodies are of two types:

Assisted community homes

These are provided by the largest voluntary bodies (usually national organizations) which are backed by a full child care social service. Each has to be approved in the Regional Plan by the Secretary of State and must nominate a neighbouring local authority which provides a minority of members on their governing local body as managers of the community home. Advice and support is provided by the social services department of the nominated local authority.

Controlled community homes

These are provided by voluntary bodies which do not provide a full child care service. Each has to nominate a neighbouring local authority which must provide a majority of managers on the local governing body and who must also provide the supporting child care services. Under the Regional Plan, all these arrangements must be approved by the Secretary of State.

Juvenile Proceedings

Care order proceedings

Care proceedings (to take a child into the care of a local authority) are at present taken in a juvenile court (eventually under the 1975 Children Act it is likely that this work will be transferred to Magistrates Domestic Courts).

A care order granted under Section II of the Children's Act, 1948 (which has the effect of transferring the parental rights from the natural parent to the local authority) may be granted by a juvenile court on the following grounds:

1. that the child is being ill-treated and neglected
2. that he is exposed to moral dangers
3. that he is beyond the control of his parent or guardian
4. that he is of compulsory school age and is not receiving efficient full-time education
5. that he is guilty of any offence *excluding homicide*

Representation of children and parents in care proceedings

The Children Act 1975 extended the provisions relating to the representation of children and parents, in all care proceedings, where there is a potential conflict between the parents and the child. In such cases, the court has discretion to direct that:

1. the parent shall not act for the child
2. the parents may be granted legal aid so that they may be separately represented. This is in addition to any legal aid in respect of the child
3. an independent experienced social worker shall be appointed to act for the child and shall be free to retain the services of a solicitor if he thinks it necessary, *or*
4. a solicitor alone shall be appointed to act for the child

Where the parents apply for discharge of a Care of Supervision Order and this application is unopposed, *separate representation of the child is mandatory*.

Criminal proceedings against a child

The criminal law relating to children is now primarily dealt with by the Children and Young Persons Act, 1969, which enables the minimum age for prosecution to be raised to 14. However, this provision has not yet been brought into force.

The Act has, however, abolished approved school orders and fit-person orders. If a juvenile court (which deals with all criminal proceedings in persons under the age of 16 years except homicide) wishes to send a child offender to a Group A CHE (formerly an approved school), the court can now only make a care order committing the child to the care of a local authority (to the social services department) who *then assesses the child professionally and decides which form of further treatment is appropriate to his case.* This assessment process usually takes six to eight weeks and may involve psychiatric and psychological examinations. After assessment, the social services department may decide to:

1. send the child to a Group A CHE (former approved school)
2. send the child home under supervision
3. order intermediate treatment

There has been considerable disquiet voiced by juvenile magistrates, to Parliament about the way the Children and Young Persons Act, 1969 is working. In 1978, a report of a joint working party of the Magistrates Association and local authority associations was published. In an attempt to improve the workings of the Act particularly as regards children who had committed offences and who were then put in the care of the local authority by the Court, an *agreed code of guidance was published.* This indicated that wherever such a care order is made by a juvenile court, there is a presumption that the *child or young person will be removed from his home to be cared for in a residential home or foster home* for an intensive period of observation and assessment. It is not acceptable for the local social services authority to return to his own home any such child merely because the local authority does not have adequate facilities for him. Suitable alternative accommodation must be sought in co-operation with the regional planning committee or in other regions. (If no place can be found, the DHSS must then be consulted.)

Supervision orders

Probation orders for young persons under 17 years have been replaced by *supervision orders* which may be made in both criminal and care proceedings. These supervision orders are now administered mainly by the social services department.

Intermediate treatment

Since 1973, schemes of intermediate treatment have to be provided by children's Regional Planning Committees. Such schemes set out the facilities which the supervisor may use (on the conditions laid down by the Court as to residence, attendance and the facilities to be provided). The object of intermediate treatment is to provide a new dimension in the treatment of children and particularly to introduce the child into new constructive activities. Examples of intermediate treatment schemes are carrying out community work such as helping old people by decorating their homes or assisting in the running of club activities, and adventure training along the 'Outward Bound' principles.

The Juvenile Court may make an *attendance order* to enable intermediate treatment to be carried out or it can specify in a supervision order a condition that intermediate treatment be insisted upon for the child.

Other Residential Establishments Dealing with Children

The following are units set up specially to deal with difficult and disturbed children.

Youth treatment centres

These are provided for in the Children and Young Persons Act, 1969, to meet the needs of boys and girls who cannot be dealt with in the normal community home system. It is eventually planned to provide three such units nationally which will combine the facilities of a home, school and hospital. Two are now operating: at St Charles, Brentwood, Middlesex, and at Glenthorne, Birmingham. Both are run by the DHSS and both look after very serious long-term cases such as psychopathic children sentenced 'to be looked after at Her Majesty's pleasure'.

Detention centres (under the Home Office)

These are available to deal with young offenders aged 14 to 21 years who do not need a long period of residential training away from school, but *who cannot be taught respect for the law by fines or probation.* Usually young offenders are committed to detention centres for periods of three to six months. The regime is under conditions of security and is strict and vigorous, but emphasis is on education and physical training.

Borstals (under the Home Office)

The Borstal system of training was introduced in 1908. The aim is *to provide training for offenders from 15 to 21 years of age* and the sentence is in two parts: (1) a period of training in a borstal establishment (minimum six months, maximum two years); (2) a period of supervision up to a further two years.

Summary of the ways in which a juvenile court may deal with young persons under the age of 17 years (they cannot deal with homicide)

1. grant an absolute or conditional discharge
2. bind over the offender
3. bind over the parent or guardian
4. fine or compensation

5. make a hospital or guardianship order under the Mental Health Act (see p. 487)
6. make a supervision order (see p. 426)
7. make an attendance centre order to enable intermediate treatment to be carried out (see p. 426)
8. make a care order committing the child to the care of the local authority
9. make a detention centre order (if 14 or over)
10. commit the child to borstal (if 15 or over)

CHILDREN'S REGIONAL PLANNING COMMITTEES

There are 10 Children's Regional Planning Committees for England and they were set up by the Children and Young Persons Act, 1969 covering the 10 regions shown in Fig. 20, p. 387. They consist of representatives from the Social Services Committee of the local authorities making up each Region, and their function is to rationalize the provision of all types of residential accommodation for children (community homes) provided by local authorities and by voluntary bodies so that the requirements of the region are met.

A Regional Plan has been published for each Region classifying all the accommodation available and the voluntary community homes designated either as 'assisted' or 'controlled'. It is the intention to update the Regional Plan from time to time.

Each local authority wishing to add to its accommodation must notify the Regional Planning Committee which must approve the development as being suitable and appropriate to the needs of the Region.

Each local authority is responsible for the costs of its own units, but centre establishments, Groups A, B and C Community Homes (CHEs) (the former approved schools and remand homes) are classified as 'high cost premises' and the costs of these units are pooled—their costs are distributed over the whole number of local authorities making up the Region.

PROBLEM FAMILIES

The causes of various social problems in families are multiple and complex and it is essential that a close degree of coordination is maintained between the various officials and voluntary workers helping them. These include the Director of Social Services and his staff of social workers, the District Nursing Officer and her staff (especially health visitors), education staff and staff of the Area Medical Officer. *Case conferences* are arranged to discuss these difficult cases and to the meetings are invited social workers of the local authority who may be concerned and appropriate officers of the AHA as well as representatives of various local voluntary bodies including the National Society for Prevention of Cruelty to Children (NSPCC). When a general practitioner has to deal with illness in a problem family and is worried about the ability of the family to cope he should report the case to the Director of Social Services, the health visitor or social worker. *When non-accidental injury in a child is suspected, action should always be taken as outlined on p. 433.*

The powers of prosecution in cases of neglect and cruelty to children lie with the local authority and the NSPCC in addition to the normal powers of the police.

Under the Children and Young Persons Act, 1969, there is now no distinction made between deprived and delinquent children.

PREVENTIVE SOCIAL AND REHABILITATION WORK

The local authority is *always required to develop and promote methods of preventing children coming into care or appearing before a Court.* The Children and Young Persons Acts, 1963 and 1969 emphasized the importance of this preventive work and of avoiding family breakdown. In certain circumstances the social services department is empowered to *make financial payments (to pay rent arrears, etc.) under the 1963 Act, to prevent the child coming into care.* The local authority must also do all in its power to endeavour to rehabilitate each child in its care so that he may eventually return to his family.

ADOPTION OF CHILDREN

Doctors very often are asked about the law relating to adoption of children. Locally the most reliable source of information is the Director of Social Services who undertakes many responsibilities in this respect. The Children Act 1975 introduced many changes in relation to adoption procedures. These are being introduced in stages and those already in operation by mid-1978 are included in the correct legal requirements for adoption listed below. The further future changes which the Act makes possible are then described separately. The detailed legal requirements for adoption are beyond the scope of this book but some of the more important points are as follows.

1. A legal adoption is by an *adoption order* granted by a Court of Law.
2. Persons who may adopt include the mother or father of the child and either can only *singly* adopt if (*a*) the other parent is dead or cannot be found or (*b*) there is some other reason justifying the exclusion of the other natural parent.
3. A married couple may adopt where each has attained the age of 21 years (this is the only exception to the general rule that an adoption order shall only be made to one person).
4. An adoption order may be made on the application of one person where he or she is 21 years of age and is:
   a. not married, *or*
   b. is married and the Court is satisfied that:
      i. the spouse cannot be found, *or*
      ii. the spouses have separated and are living apart and the separation is likely to be permanent, *or*
      iii. the spouse is by reason of ill-health (physical or mental) incapable of making an application to adopt
5. Normally a male person cannot adopt a female child.
6. A child who is or has been married cannot be adopted.
7. An adoption order may contain such terms and conditions as the Court thinks fit.
8. The *Court hearings must be in private.*
9. The child must have been in the care of the applicant for at least three consecutive months.
10. The applicant must notify the local authority.
11. The persons whose consent is necessary (parent or guardian) must fully understand the nature of consent—full parental rights pass with adoption. Parental consent to adoption may be dispensed with where a parent cannot be

found or is incapable of giving agreement or where a child has been seriously ill-treated.

12. That adoption is in the best interests of the child.
13. That the adoption has not been arranged for reward.
14. Social workers must visit prospective applicants during the three-month period.
15. The local authority can make arrangements for adoption and/or register locally 'adoption societies'.
16. The Court appoints a 'Guardian *ad litem*' which is an officer who is appointed to safeguard the interests of the child on behalf of the Court. The Director of Social Services usually has officers on his staff who can act as 'Guardian *ad litem*'. Very considerable safeguards are specified and most of those depend on independent visiting and reports from staff of the Director of Social Services.

The doctor should realize that there are important medical considerations relating both to a child to be adopted and to the adopting parents. It is important that the general health of the child and any defects of sight, hearing, speech or mental subnormality are known to adopting parents. Serological tests for syphilis should be carried out. In the same way, the adopting parents should be in good general health, be suitable temperamentally and psychologically to care for a child and have a good family history. The circumstances which should be considered include mental illness, mental subnormality, epilepsy, tuberculosis and any serious chronic illness.

If any problems arise, the general practitioner is advised to contact the local Director of Social Services.

Further future changes in adoption procedures likely to be introduced by full implementation of the Children Act, 1975

The further changes which the Children Act, 1975, provides for (these clauses have yet to be implemented) include:

1. All local authorities will eventually have to establish and maintain an adoption service as part of their general social services either by providing the service themselves or by doing so in conjunction with approved adoption agencies (the majority of local authorities do this now).

2. All responsibility for approval and registration of adoption societies in England will be transferred from local authorities to the Secretary of State for Social Services. It is hoped that this will ensure uniformly good standards of practice throughout the country.
3. Parental consent to adoption will in future be given by the parent *before* an adoption order is made. Under existing law this is not possible and the natural parent can withdraw consent at any time up to the making of the adoption order. At present, it is not even possible for parental consent to become final before then. This results in a period of great uncertainty for all adopters, and also for the mother, who is asked to re-affirm her consent a number of times. The Children Act, 1975, includes clauses which were described by the Houghton Committee as *relinquishment* or *freeing of children for adoption* which will enable any child to be freed for adoption and the natural parent to give early consent to adoption *before* an adoption order is made. This will mean that adoption arrangements can be proceeded within the certain knowledge that they cannot be upset by a sudden change of mind on the part of the natural parent. Such agreement by the mother must be given *after* at least a period of six weeks from the birth of the child.
4. In future it will be possible for an Adoption Agency to apply to the Court for an order freeing for adoption any child who has been in the care of a local authority or adoption agency for a long time but whose parents will not consent to adoption and are also unwilling to make plans for the child's future. In all such cases, the natural parent must be given three months' notice of a Court Hearing of such an application and would be eligible for legal aid to contest it;
5. Foster parents and others who have looked after the child continuously for five years will, in future, be able to apply to adopt the child without any fear that the child can be removed before the Court hearing without leave of the Court. This will ensure that foster parents who have satisfactorily cared for a child for five years can apply for adoption without being worried that the local authority or natural parent can immediately remove that child from their care;

6. Adoptions may only be arranged through an approved adoption society unless the person wishing to adopt the child is a close relative of that child.

NON-ACCIDENTAL INJURY TO CHILDREN (CHILD ABUSE)

During the past six years, much emphasis has been laid upon the problem of non-accidental injury to children. This was first called the 'battered baby syndrome', but since it is now known to involve older children as well it is now called child abuse.

Non-accidental injury is the deliberate injury of children, usually by parents, and is caused by many different factors. In some cases, criminal neglect by parents may be associated with other forms of anti-social behaviour—assaults or drunkenness, but in many instances, frustration, bad living conditions, unsympathetic neighbours or landladies complaining of babies who cry continuously, or psychiatric illness in a parent are the main factors. The problem can present itself in many forms but usually starts by one or both parents slapping, hitting, punching or severely shaking the child causing bruises and occasionally more serious injuries. Ill-treatment usually starts gradually but if it is unnoticed, it is quite possible for the child to be seriously injured and it is now estimated that approximately 300–400 deaths per year in children may be caused in this way.

Diagnosis and Early Recognition

The following may be the first signs of non-accidental injury:

1. Minor bruises which show that the child has been gripped tightly or shaken.

2. Minor injuries (such as facial bruises) probably caused by slapping or hitting the child. The type of injury is usually similar, 70% being soft tissue injuries to the head and face. There may be 'finger bruising' in which the outlines of the fingers which slapped the child are clearly seen within the bruised area. Such bruising tends to pick out the bony prominences. In many cases, the lips are thick and bruised and there is a torn upper lip frenum. Ribs are frequently bruised or broken and X-rays often indicate that

these injuries have been caused at different times. Occasionally small burns or scalds may be present.

Surveys have shown that 1–2% of such injuries prove fatal, about 30–40% of cases have serious injuries, the remainder being moderate or mild.

3. An unexplained failure of the child to thrive.

4. Unusual behaviour by the parents. This may take many different forms—over-anxiety and frequent attendance with the child at clinics or surgeries, plausible explanation of an injury which does not fit the case, or unnatural lack of concern for the child's condition.

In many instances, the circumstances of parents involved in cases of non-accidental injury show many similar characteristics; stress of various kinds is common including poverty (in one survey 80% were in receipt of social security), unemployment (many fathers batter their children when engaged on maternal tasks), overcrowding and unsatisfactory housing conditions and many have unstable marriages. Another interesting finding is that the parents are often very young (about four years below the national average). Studies have shown that teenage parents are less tolerant and have a low tolerance towards the baby's crying. A high proportion of the women involved are pregnant at the time. Any additional stress will tend to precipitate problems.

A proportion of parents shown to be responsible for non-accidental injury are mentally disturbed or inadequate emotionally. It is interesting that the 'innocent' parent (usually the mother) does not do more to protect her child. The most likely explanation is that she has never learnt how to stick up for herself and for their children. Certainly many of the parents involved have never received any affection in their homes and consequently find it very difficult to relate as a normal parent does towards their child. In practice, approximately 70% of injuries are caused by men and 30% by their mother.

Where any allegation of non-accidental injury has been made and the child and parents cannot be found within 48 hours an immediate case conference must be held.

Early diagnosis of non-accidental injury to children depends upon the alertness of many professional staff including general practitioners, paediatricians, health visitors, district nurses, midwives, social workers, teachers, police and staff of many voluntary organizations including the NSPCC. Because injury to the child is always a dominant feature, all those working in casualty or accident departments of hospitals should be especially vigilant.

Management and Treatment

Once there is a reasonable degree of suspicion of non-accidental injury, the child should at once be admitted to a hospital (or very occasionally a children's home) for diagnosis and for his own safety. In many instances, a *place of safety order* will be obtained from a court (this can most easily be arranged by the social services department) but the child may be admitted voluntarily.

In all cases an immediate *case conference* should be arranged which should include those concerned with the case, the paediatrician, general practitioner, health visitor and social worker, as well as the NSPCC and a senior police officer. As the social services department has the statutory duty to protect and care for all children, it is best if each case conference is arranged by the social services department within 24 hours.

In those instances in which the professional worker does not feel that the suspicions are firm enough to arrange immediate admission to a hospital, it is still advisable to hold a case conference to decide on the next action. If suspicion is very slight, in every instance at least the doctor, health visitor or social worker should:

1. consult the family doctor
2. discuss the details of the case with a senior colleague
3. make a record of such consultations and discussions

Area Review Committee

An Area Review Committee has been set up in each Area Health Authority or local social services area, to act as a policy forming body to ensure that the arrangements in that area for dealing with the problem of non-accidental injury are satisfactory. Each Area Review Committee should include representatives of the appropriate local authority, from the social services department who usually provide a convenor; education department; the health services (especially paediatric and other consultants; the Area Medical Officer; the Area Nursing Officer; plus the Area Specialists in Community Medicine for Social Services and Child Health) and a senior police officer; senior inspector of the NSPCC; and the Chief Probation Officer.

Area Review Committees should meet regularly (three or four times per year) and should:

1. review local practice and procedure for dealing with such cases
2. ensure that immediate hospital admission for children at risk is accepted
3. Approve written instructions defining the exact duties and responsibilities of professional staff in connection with non-accidental injury
4. provide education and training programmes for staff in the health and social services
5. review the work of case conferences
6. inquire into the circumstances of cases which appear to have gone wrong and from which lessons could be learned
7. ensure that procedures are in operation to safeguard continuity of care between neighbouring areas and in those instances when families move to another area
8. agree arrangements for the operation of a total register of cases which have been dealt with by case conferences or other action

Specialist Social Worker for Non-accidental Injury

A number of large urban authorities have appointed a full-time specialist social worker for non-accidental injury. The officer is responsible for coordinating all this work in the social services department, for arranging case conferences, for advising on difficult cases and for liaison with the health, education and voluntary services, as well as maintaining the register. In 1978, a joint working party of the British Paediatric Association and the British Association of Social Workers studying non-accidental injury registers *strongly recommended that every social services department should appoint such a specialist.*

Registers

A register of information is essential in each area to ensure there is good communication between the many services involved. The name of the child and the names of both parents, if known, in cases of non-accidental injury should be kept in such registers *until that child or his brothers and sisters are at least 10 years old. Absolute confidentiality is most important* and there should also be arrangements to share information between neighbouring authorities. Registers may be set up by voluntary bodies working in this field (e.g. the NSPCC) or by social services departments or by AHAs. The most *important feature of registers is that they should be readily accessible (at all times—on a 24 hour basis)* to doctors, nurses and social workers, and that they should include accurate up-to-date information. The ability of a doctor in a casualty department or a health visitor or social worker in the community to seek information from such a register could be vital to early and effective diagnosis of non-accidental injury. Notes of all referrals to the register are kept and where two separate enquiries are made within 18 months, the two officers are informed.

Treatment and Rehabilitation of Known Cases of Non-Accidental Injury

Most cases will initially be in the care of the paediatrician who will be responsible for the assessment and treatment of the case in hospital. Assessment should include both physical and psychiatric investigations. A case conference will be held and should indicate the most likely methods of treatment. These will vary considerably in different cases and will include:

1. Receiving the child into *statutory care* by the local authority (by Court Order). In the very worst cases there will also be prosecution of the parents.
2. Accepting the child into *voluntary care.* (This may be risky in some cases because parents may suddenly remove the child from hospital or children's home. Therefore, in all cases received into voluntary care, the Social Services

Department must always be prepared to seek an urgent *Place of Safety Order* if that need arises.)

3. Arranging for the child to remain under supervision in the home by a Court Order.
4. Returning the child home with planned help to the parents.

In all instances the aim is to ensure that the short and long term interests of the child are met as far as possible. It is important to realize that, although there are a number of serious cases of intentional injury and neglect that can only be properly treated by permanent removal of the child from the parents, *the majority of cases are quite different.* In these the non-accidental injury has been caused by many other factors—bad living conditions, unemployment, poverty, threat of eviction especially if babies cry repeatedly and by minor psychiatric illnesses. *These parents urgently require help* and if this can be satisfactorily given they may be assisted to develop into perfectly satisfactory parents and families. However, the causative factors *must* be discovered. In many instances, the temporary provision of residential care (in a residential nursery or children's home) may be required to enable the parent to be treated.

Day Care

Many mothers who have been found to ill-treat their children are very young and often very isolated and lonely. It is usual to find that the mother herself had an unhappy childhood or was brought up in a broken home.

A very useful method of helping is *to admit the child to a day nursery or play group* and then to arrange for the mother to help in the group. In this way, the mother is assisted to make new friends and to obtain the support she needs. Indirectly she will be taught to improve her relationship with her own child from the example of care she will see in the nursery or play group.

More and more social services departments are now developing day care which can be extended to older children in the same family who come along to the unit after school.

Many girls' schools now arrange for senior girls to help periodically in play groups and day nurseries, and thus to learn more about the methods of care of young children. This is particularly important because more girls now marry before twenty and the incidence of non-accidental injury is highest in teenage mothers.

Some local authorities have arranged to deal with many cases in nurseries close to a paediatric department which makes the development of special working arrangements between the health and social services easier.

Periodic Review of Long Term Cases

Some of the most difficult problems are found in long term cases. It is absolutely essential that *periodic reviews* of such cases are undertaken. These must involve the many professional workers who would normally be concerned with the care of that child and especially general practitioners, teachers, school nurses, health visitors, education welfare officers, social workers (including those working in child guidance) as well as those working with voluntary agencies in that area. In all older children (and some of the worst cases of non-accidental injury occur in older children) it is most important that the *levels of communication between teaching staff* and others concerned with the child in school and health visitors and social workers are always good.

The statutory duty to protect and care for all children who are in need is that of the Director of Social Services and his staff. But unless there is an effective network of information between all staff working in education, health and social services, action by the social services department may be delayed until it is too late to prevent further injury. For this reason, long term cases should never be written off if there is a younger child in the family and until a case conference agrees that no risk remains. Unless this multidisciplinary team approach is always used, mistakes of the past will be repeated.

In any serious case of doubt, a doctor should always arrange immediate hospital admission for the child to enable more detailed investigations to be undertaken. It is obviously better to admit unnecessarily a few children in this way than to miss one serious case of non-accidental injury. In cases of difficulty, the problem should always be reported by telephone to the Director of Social Services.

24 Care and Rehabilitation of the Disabled

The prevention of serious after-effects of chronic illness or disabilities is an important part of the social services. The provision of services for a varied group of physically handicapped involves many different bodies including voluntary and statutory authorities, but in all cases a close link must be maintained with the consultant hospital services which undertake the acute or sub-acute treatment. Training and resettlement will usually involve hospital staffs and general practitioners as well as Manpower Services Commission officials, the Director of Social Services and his social work staff, together with many voluntary bodies. The groups for which special facilities are available include those suffering from : (*a*) blindness; (*b*) deafness without speech (deaf and dumb); (*c*) deafness with speech (hard of hearing); (*d*) all types of physically handicapped persons; (*e*) cerebral palsy; (*f*) epilepsy. In many instances, disabled persons suffer from multiple handicaps.

Legislation

The three main Acts dealing with the handicapped are the Disabled Persons (Employment) Acts, 1944 and 1958, the National Assistance Act, 1948, and the Chronically Sick and Disabled Persons Act, 1970.

The Disabled Persons (Employment) Acts, 1944 and 1958, mainly deal with employment problems of the handicapped and under them the Employment Service Division maintains a register of disabled persons. A 'disabled person' for employment purposes is one 'who on account of injury, disease or congenital deformity, is substantially handicapped from obtaining and keeping employment'. Every employer who has twenty or more persons on his staff must always employ a minimum of 3% of disabled persons, and in this way encouragement is given to the employment of handicapped people.

Chronically Sick and Disabled Persons Act, 1970

The Chronically Sick and Disabled Persons Act, 1970 gives many special responsibilities to local authorities in respect of those who are substantially and permanently handicapped (including mentally handicapped). The main duties of Local Authorities are:

Information

Local authorities must ensure (*a*) that they are adequately informed of the numbers and needs of the handicapped so that they can properly plan and develop their services, and (*b*) that the handicapped and their families know what help is available to them by general publicity and personal explanations.

Provision of services

Local authorities, when satisfied that the following services are necessary to the handicapped person, can provide the following:

a. practical assistance in the home (such as the provision of social workers, home helps, occupational therapists)
b. wireless, television, library or similar recreational facilities in the home
c. recreational facilities outside the home (access to parks, sports centres and gymnasia and all club activities), and assistance in taking advantage of educational facilities
d. travelling facilities for handicapped persons (group transport)
e. assistance in carrying out adaptations to the home
f. facilitating the taking of holidays
g. meals at home or elsewhere
h. a telephone and any special equipment necessary for its use (usually installation and rental)

Housing

Every local housing authority must have regard to the special needs of the disabled and any new houses planned must show that special provision is made for the disabled. *This clearly gives housing authorities a duty to plan and provide special housing accommodation for the handicapped.*

Premises open to the public

There is a series of requirements for public buildings. These deal specially with:

1. Providing means of access to and within the building and in the parking facilities and sanitary conveniences for the disabled. Such provision must be considered before planning permission is given.
2. Need for a local authority to provide public sanitary conveniences for the disabled.
3. Need for anyone providing sanitary conveniences in premises open to the public for accommodation, refreshment or entertainment, to make provision, as far as is practicable, for the disabled.
4. Adequate sign-posting for the above provisions from outside.
5. Need to provide facilities for access, parking, sanitary conveniences suitable for the disabled as far as is practicable at school, university and other educational buildings.

In addition, there are special clauses about Advisory Committees for the handicapped either nationally or locally and these insist that members of such committees must include persons with experience of work for the disabled and persons who are themselves disabled.

Employment and Training for the Disabled

The employment and training of disabled persons of all ages is very complex. Careers guidance and assessment at school is mainly the responsibility of the specialist careers officers of the education authority (see p. 142). The main government department is the *Manpower Services Commission* and its two executive arms, the *Training Services Division (TSD)* and the *Employment Service Division (ESD)*.

The TSD is responsible for training and promotes all forms of training through the *Industrial Training Boards* on which employers are widely represented. The TSD runs the Training Opportunities Schemes (TOPS) which are designed to help those who for any reason (including disability) need training for new employment. Disabled young people leaving school can benefit from a TOPS course (young persons who are not disabled cannot enter TOPS courses) which can be provided at skill centres, establishments of further education or private colleges and arrangements are also made for residential courses. These vocational training courses give training in various industrial skills to disabled persons; training is also carried out for those who later will be self-employed.

The ESD is responsible for helping place disabled persons in employment. It maintains 26 *Employment Rehabilitation Centres* which offer special courses for people who following injury or illness or prolonged unemployment find it difficult to obtain a job. In 1976, over 15 500 persons were trained at Employment Rehabilitation Centres (including 2250 young handicapped persons aged 16–18 years). These industrial rehabilitation courses have three main functions (*a*) assessment for employment; (*b*) selection of the most suitable employment; and (*c*) completion of the rehabilitation regime.

The key local officer of the ESD is the *Disablement Resettlement Officer (DRO)* whose main function is in assisting and placing handicapped persons into occupations.

There are two main ways in which the handicapped can be employed full-time: (1) in open industry, (2) in sheltered employment.

1. *Open industry* refers to ordinary occupations in which the handicapped person works with and under the same conditions as normal people and full wages are paid. It is the best solution but is only possible in a proportion of the employable handicapped, but every effort should be made to encourage open industry. It is usually possible to place a few intelligent well-trained handicapped persons in most industries. In some cases, as with the blind, specially trained officers are employed to assist in the placement of the handicapped in open industry.

2. *Sheltered employment* is subsidized full-time employment of the handicapped in either a special workshop or in a 'home workers' scheme. Widespread use of sheltered employment occurs with the blind (see p. 455). For others, the Employment Service Division runs special Remploy factories and various voluntary bodies run sheltered workshops usually with financial help from local authorities.

SOCIAL SERVICES

The DHSS is centrally responsible for all social services for the handicapped. Each relevant local authority has its Social Services Committee reponsible locally, and the chief officer in charge of these services is the Director of Social Services (see page 389). Many local and national voluntary bodies assist in carrying out this work—examples include the Royal National Institute for the Blind, Spastics Society, various deaf and dumb associations, The Royal Association for Disability and Rehabilitation, Disabled Living Foundation, British Epilepsy Association and many voluntary homes or hostels. Occasionally a local authority will arrange for a local voluntary body to provide services on an agency basis and there are increasing numbers of local voluntary Associations for the Disabled.

General principles of social services for the handicapped

In the rehabilitation and training of handicapped people there are four basic principles which are essential: (1) the problems of every handicapped person are *highly individual and personal.* (2) The best solution for any handicapped person is the one which is as *near normal as possible.* (3) *Much improvisation* will be necessary. (4) Great determination and *singleness of purpose* are essential for success.

1. The problems and difficulties of any handicapped person are highly individual and depend on: (i) the nature and extent of the handicap, and (ii) the response and reaction of the handicapped person to the difficulties he faces.

An example is shown by the fact that many blind people are able to hold down an important job while others, who are also blind, may be quite unable to carry out successfully even a simple occupation. In both the handicap—complete blindness—is the same, but residual problems vary greatly. The reaction of the handicapped person to his difficulties depends very much on *the attitude of those who have tried to help him in the early and crucial stages of his handicap* and a correct approach and attitude of mind at this time is important. Very often the best approach is a fairly tough one which promises the handicapped person little but many hard struggles and disappointments. At all costs, self-pity in the individual must be avoided.

For these reasons, *individual visiting and assessment* are always an important first step in training or rehabilitation because the social background of the handicapped person—his home and his family—will always play a significant part in his efforts to overcome his handicap.

2. There is a very simple rule to follow in determining what should be attempted by any handicapped person. The best solution is always the one which is *as near normal as possible* and this basic rule is true for educational or employment problems. For example, a normal person works in industry or office and is in no way protected and this is equally the best solution for any handicapped person. This means that 'open industry' is better than 'sheltered workshops' which in turn are preferable to home workers schemes. When it is difficult to suggest the next stage in the rehabilitation of any individual, this 'as near normal' rule is a valuable guide.

3. Just as the problems and difficulties of any handicapped person differ, so will the solutions. Hence, an *ability to improvise* in overcoming inevitable or unexpected difficulties is most important and no social worker with the handicapped can ever afford to be narrow minded or too set in his ways. All the most successful social workers with the handicapped are resilient and are often unconventional people to whom improvisation comes naturally.

4. It is usually easy to find an excuse for failure when working with the handicapped. Therefore, to succeed, it is important to concentrate solely upon success however remote this might seem to be. If possible, the handicapped person and those immediately around him should be fired with an enthusiasm to succeed irrespective of the difficulties and inevitable disappointments. A

complete *singleness of purpose* should be encouraged and this often helps to overcome difficulties.

Registration of the disabled

Social services departments arrange for the *registration of disabled persons.* Table 76 shows the numbers on the register in England in 1976. Note the concentration of disabled persons of all other types (except totally deaf in the 65 years and over age group).

TABLE 76 Persons registered as substantially and permanently handicapped, England, 1976

Blind	
All ages	101 100
Aged 50–64	14 300
Aged 65+	74 000
Partially sighted	
All ages	42 900
Aged 65+	28 400
Deaf	
All ages	27 500
Aged 65+	6900
Hard of hearing	
All ages	25 600
Aged 65+	18 600
All other disabled (physically)	
All ages	657 200
Aged 65+	400 800

(From *Health and Personal Social Services Statistics*, DHSS, 1977)

Domiciliary services for the disabled

Among the domiciliary workers visiting the handicapped at home are social workers, specially trained workers for the blind and deaf and dumb, occupational therapists and health visitors. Much domiciliary visiting by social workers is concerned with assessment of individual problems. Occupational therapists particularly concentrate on *teaching clients to live with their handicaps* rather than on instruction in craft-work. Those working in special centres for the handicapped include occupational therapists, social workers, handicraft instructors and voluntary workers. Health visitors are especially useful in maintaining a close link with hospital services or with general practitioners. Social workers usually play an active part in the administration of these services and in arranging residential accommodation for the handicapped. *Home helps* (see p. 508) and *meals on wheels* (see p. 511) are also provided for some seriously disabled persons living at home.

Day centres

Occupational therapy and rehabilitation centres

Many social services departments run *occupational therapy and rehabilitation centres for the handicapped* where training is given with the assistance of various aids and machines, including knitting machines, fretsaw machines, various looms, etc. Many crafts—rug making, simple carpentry or basketry—are also taught. There is also a *training kitchen* which helps the handicapped housewife to become more independent. Usually special transport collects the handicapped from their homes and this makes it possible to extend the range of those who can be helped.

The rehabilitation centre is open for people to attend either for half a day or a full day and one of the valuable features of these units is the social one, whereby various handicapped people meet other persons. In many long and chronic illnesses there is a tendency for the person to become more and more withdrawn as he stays permanently at home meeting only his family or close friends. Attendance at an occupational therapy rehabilitation centre and travelling to it increases greatly his self-confidence and does much to prevent permanent invalidism.

Community or domiciliary occupational therapy may also be run by AHAs. Thus community occupational therapy services in England at present are run in some cases by AHAs and in others by the local social services department.

Handicraft centres

Handicraft centres for the disabled and handicapped (including the elderly) are also provided by local authorities and staffed by handicraft instructors. The aim of such centres is to help those handicapped to maintain interest and to enjoy recreational facilities even when rehabilitation is not practicable.

Social centre and clubs

Most local authorities run clubs for the handicapped or give financial support to such centres provided by voluntary bodies.

Housing for the handicapped

The design of the home is important for many severely handicapped people. Doors may have to be widened to allow wheelchairs free access and bathrooms may have to be provided at ground level. The Chronically Sick and Disabled Persons Act, 1970, encourages help with housing for the handicapped and many local authorities now build special houses or bungalows as it is more satisfactory to do this than adapt existing premises, especially if many alterations are needed. Many *Housing Associations* also build special flats and bungalows for the disabled.

Adaptations

An important function of social services departments is to arrange and assist with the adaptations of any disabled persons home. Such adaptations include minor additions such as handrails or ramps, but may involve much more radical alterations to the home such as the building of a downstairs bathroom and lavatory, the widening of doorways or passages. In most instances, the local authority will either pay all the cost of the adaptations or a substantial portion of them *provided that permission to carry out such adaptations is first obtained from the social services department.*

Aids and gadgets

Under the Chronically Sick and Disabled Persons Act, 1970, local authorities are given power to provide a wide range of aids for the handicapped. These include the following:

1. *Hoists* in bedrooms and bathrooms for those paralysed in the legs so that they can become more independent and mobile.
2. *Lifts and stair lifts* can be provided.
3. *Modifications to table implements*, knives, forks and spoons, to make them more easily used by those whose grip is weak or whose hands are deformed.
3. *Various kitchen fitments* for the handicapped. These include many gadgets for one-handed people or those who have power only in one hand. Other aids are provided for

those whose balance is poor (slings are fitted to sinks to support the housewife while standing).

5. *Kitchen management and planning* are important, including the heights of various working surfaces and the design of kitchen furniture.
6. Various *personal aids in dressing* encourage independence in the client. The occupational therapist also attempts to increase the mobility of crippled persons. Special walking aids are provided and the handicapped person is trained in their use. Whenever rehabilitation has reached a certain stage, the individual should be encouraged to attend a rehabilitation centre.
7. An extensive range of special clothing is now available for the disabled. Many of the garments have special arrangements for fastening to enable a disabled person with a poor grip to dress himself and to be completely independent.

Aids centres

Permanent aids centres containing a wide range of equipment suitable for the disabled have been established in London by the Disabled Living Foundation and recently in Liverpool, Newcastle, Birmingham, Wakefield and Leicester. These aids centres set out to enable the severely disabled to see for themselves the range of equipment and to compare the various facilities available. It is usual to staff such units with experienced *occupational therapists* and to run the centre on an appointment system as it usually takes 1½ to 2 hours to demonstrate all the appropriate equipment.

Disabled or their families wishing to visit such centres should contact either the Disabled Living Foundation, 346 Kensington High Street, London, W.8, or the Directors of Social Services for Liverpool, Newcastle, Birmingham, Wakefield or Leicestershire.

Holidays and outings

Outings in summertime and special holidays for the handicapped may be arranged and many of these are in seaside hotels or holiday camps at the start or end of the season. It is usual to send special staff with such holiday groups to assist with wheelchairs and help those who are severely disabled. In this way, many handicapped people are able to enjoy a holiday who otherwise could not do so. There has been a wide extension in the range of holidays during the past five years, and more and more of the handicapped can now enjoy what has become normal to many ordinary persons—an annual holiday abroad.

Mobility and Transport for the handicapped

Individual transport (motorized or non-motorized) can either be provided by the DHSS if the handicap is permanent and serious or a mobility allowance paid. The procedure is for the appropriate hospital consultant (usually the orthopaedic specialist) or the patient's general practitioner to complete the form and send it to the local appliance centre of the DHSS. If the application is accepted, there is usually a long delay before the vehicle is delivered. There are many different types of wheelchair provided and four types of motorized transport—motor car, motor tricycle, electrically propelled tricycle and electrically propelled indoor chair. The type of transport ordered is always the one which is best suited for the handicap. Motor cars can only be provided to those who have considerable power in their arms—say paraplegics below T 10.

Local authorities provide wheelchairs on a *temporary* basis, but this aid should not normally last longer than six months.

Group transport for the disabled

Personnel carriers of various types and small buses may be provided to take the disabled to day centres, clubs, etc. Most of these vehicles have hydraulic lifts attached so that a wheelchair and occupant can easily be loaded.

Mobility allowance

The *mobility allowance* is a cash benefit which is payable to severely handicapped persons to help them to be more mobile. It is additional to any other social security benefit, is taxable and, at the end of 1978, was £10 per week.

In order to qualify, the disabled person must fall within the age groups 5–60 for women and 5–65 for men (by late 1978) and be unable, or virtually unable to walk because of a disability which is likely to persist for at least 12 months. He must be able to make use of the allowance—a person who for medical reasons cannot be moved or who is in a coma, would not qualify. He must also be living within the UK (Isle of Man qualifies and there is in Northern Ireland a parallel scheme), and must have been living there for at least 12 months in the 18 months preceding the date from which he is claiming.

The allowance is intended to be spent on outdoor mobility but may be spent in any way—towards a vehicle, to pay for taxis, to hire a car or other vehicle, to pay for holiday transport. *The way it is used is entirely left to the discretion of the severely handicapped person* or parent (in the case of a child). The mobility allowance is paid to more than one person who qualifies living in the same household.

Disabled persons who at present have a car or invalid tricycle provided, or had at any time before November 1976, are able, if they wish and are still medically eligible, to switch to the Mobility Allowance *without further medical examination and without age limit.*

A claim for the mobility allowance can be made by completing the form attached to the mobility allowance leaflet N.1 211 and then sending it to the Department of Health and Social Security Mobility Allowance Unit at Norcross, Blackpool, Lancs. A medical examination will usually be arranged for applicants.

Recipients of the mobility allowance (or persons nominated to receive the allowance on their behalf) will, from 1st December, 1978, no longer have to pay vehicle excise duty on a vehicle used by or for the purpose of a disabled person. This vehicle excise duty exemption can also be claimed for those outside the mobility allowance age groups if (*a*) they are unable to walk; (*b*) have a car registered in their name: (*c*) they need to be driven; (*d*) they need to be cared for by a full-time attendant.

Telephones

Telephones have been provided in most areas for very severely disabled persons living alone or left on their own for long periods of the day. Criteria vary slightly in different areas, but usually include a minority of *medical reasons* (a medical condition which might require urgent medical help) and many *social reasons* usually including such a degree of disability that the person cannot go out of his home in normal weather conditions (in addition to living alone).

Special homes or hostels for the handicapped

Many voluntary bodies and a number of local authorities have built hostels for handicapped persons. Examples of the former are the Cheshire Foundation Homes for seriously crippled persons. It is usual for local authorities to pay the *per capita* charge for any of their residents living in such homes. In addition, a number of *sheltered housing units* for the disabled are being developed to encourage independence in the disabled.

Financial assistance

Attendance allowance

This is a tax-free allowance for a person who, because of his severe physical or mental disabilities has needed, for six months or more, frequent attendance throughout the day and/or night. The requirements which have to be met are:

By day: frequent attention throughout the day in connection with his bodily functions *or* continual supervision throughout the day in order to avoid substantial danger to himself or others.

By night: prolonged or repeated attention during the night in connection with his bodily functions *or* continual supervision throughout the night in order to avoid substantial danger to himself or others.

From the end of 1978, a higher rate of £14 a week is paid if one of the day requirements and one of the night requirements are satisfied for a period of at least six months. A lower rate of £9.30 is paid if one of the day or night requirements is satisfied for a period of six months.

Claims are made by completing the form attached to the attendance allowance leaflet. A medical examination will be made and all claims are decided by an Attendance Allowance Board based in Blackpool.

LINKS BETWEEN THE HEALTH, EDUCATION, EMPLOYMENT AND SOCIAL SERVICES

With disabled persons of all ages, it is essential that there are effective links between the health, education, employment and social services. For congenitally disabled children, the *health visitor usually plays an important role* and is assumed to be the person to act as 'the named person' (see p. 138). The satisfactory education of such a child depends largely on the cooperation of the health and education and social services. In particular, these links become even more important during that difficult period of transition from school to adult life. The Warnock Committee in its report emphasized how vulnerable many disabled children and their families were at this critical period. The specialist careers officer of the local education authority should play a crucial role in advising the disabled young person about what further training and careers are most suitable. Some of the facilities for preparation for work made available by the TSD have already been briefly discussed (see p. 443).

Any individual disabled person who is having difficulty in obtaining or retaining a job, can often be helped by a brief case conference between the DRO, the social worker, the occupational therapist and doctor to ensure that all the difficulties and potentials are fully understood. It is very easy to assume that many seriously disabled persons are unemployable but this is rarely so. However, if such individuals are allowed to remain at home just idling away time, they can soon become disillusioned and may never reach their true potential. For this reason, *day centres, education and training of all kinds are so important in rehabilitation* because the individual handicapped person is given some clear sense of purpose as regards his future life.

DETAILED SOCIAL SERVICES FOR DIFFERENT GROUPS OF HANDICAPPED PERSONS

The Blind

Registration

Each person suspected of being blind must be examined by a consultant ophthalmologist who carries out a complete examination of the eye and indicates, in his report, the degree of sight and prognosis. A person is considered blind if *'unable to perform any work for which sight is essential'*. In practice, this means that any person with vision less than 3/60 (Snellen), with a full visual field, is blind; if the field is considerably contracted then visual acuity up to 6/60 may come in this category. Those whose vision is better than these standards but still defective are *partially sighted.*

In 1976, there were 10 100 (39 000 men and 62 100 women) registered blind persons in England; 88·3% of blindness occurs among persons aged 50 years and over. This means that many of the problems accompanying blindness are those of old age.

Individual assessment

The age of onset of blindness is an important factor in relation to the social problems created. A child born blind must be educated and employed as a blind person as well as facing the problems of old age with the same handicap. But a very old person going blind has only a few years of blindness to face. As well as age, personality, past training, intelligence and home conditions have a marked effect on either reducing or increasing difficulties.

Each blind person must therefore, be carefully and individually assessed by expert social workers (home teachers for the blind). With newly blinded people aged 20 to 50 years, assessment is never easy for the sudden onset of blindness often leaves the person uncertain and full of bitterness and self-pity. The Royal National Institute for the Blind runs an excellent *special assessment centre at America Lodge, Torquay*, for such patients where, under expert guidance, the newly blinded person spends four to six weeks. After a visit to this centre, most lose any self-pity and return home to approach the difficult period of industrial retraining with a new and essential spirit of hope.

Periodic visiting should be carried out by social workers to continue in an unobtrusive way observation of current problems.

Employment

Under the Disabled Persons (Employment) Acts 1944 and 1958, the social services department of the local authority and the Employment Service Division have a joint responsibility for the vocational training and employment of the blind.

Approximately 15% of blind people are aged 16 and 60 years and it is in this group that the problem of employment occurs. Full-time employment is undertaken either in 'open industry' or in sheltered employment in workshops or home workers' schemes.

Employment in 'open industry'

There are many different types of occupation in which the intelligent, highly trained blind person can succeed and these include a number of industrial processes such as capstan lathe operatives, telephone operators, piano tuners, etc. Two essentials are needed for the successful placing of blind people in industry: (*a*) a helpful and sympathetic employer who is prepared to try one or two blind people in his factory, and (*b*) proper training of the blind person before and during early employment.

In both respects, the Blind Persons Resettlement Officer of the ESD is invaluable. He is usually *a highly trained blind person* who acts as liaison officer with industry, finding suitable vacancies for blind people. He then assesses the potential of the blind person, trains those whom he selects and then introduces him to his new post and stays to help and train him in his new job. Later follow-up visits are made to ensure there are no problems.

In general, the aim should always be to place as many blind people as possible in open industry. In many areas, up to 70% of the employable are working in open industry. No special arrangements are made as regards remuneration.

Occupation in sheltered employment

Sheltered employment is specially subsidized full-time occupation and there are two main types:

Workshops: A blind worker needing sheltered employment should, if possible, be sent to a special workshop for the blind where, after training, he is employed in one of the traditional trades including basket making, chair caning, rug making, brush making or machine knitting. Sighted foremen help with the finishing off of the articles and also arrange for the marketing of the products.

Each blind worker receives the usual wage for the occupation although, because of his handicap, it is unlikely he could earn this on 'piece rates'. The difference between what he actually earns and what he is paid is called '*augmentation*' and is provided by the local authority, which receives a large grant (in 1978 up to a maximum of £1187 annually per blind worker employed) from the ESD.

An example of augmentation in a workshop is as follows: A blind person employed as a basket maker in a workshop earns weekly £55.00. This is made up of approximately £10.50 actual earnings and £44.50 augmentation (1978 figures).

Home workers' schemes: In rural areas or small towns, it is never possible to collect together enough blind people to run a workshop. *Home workers' schemes* are then used. The blind worker is trained in an occupation, supplied with materials at home and makes a certain quota of goods which are later collected and marketed. Provided the blind person averages a certain agreed minimum output, he receives *augmentation* as in the workshop scheme. Although home workers' schemes are valuable, they are not as satisfactory as sheltered workshops. Difficulties include inadequate supervision and consequently the quality and quantity of work are usually lower.

Part-time employment

Arrangements are made to help elderly blind people wishing to do some part-time employment and the home teacher for the blind assists with the provision of materials and with the marketing of finished products. No augmentation is paid for part-time employment.

Other services for the blind

Learning to read

Braille is the best method of reading used by the blind. It is taught to all children and younger blind adults and others who have the ability and desire to learn. Home teachers instruct with the aid of a widespread library maintained by the Royal National Institute for the Blind. It usually takes an intelligent person at least six months' hard concentrated study to learn Braille and is, therefore, beyond the scope of many elderly persons. A useful indicator of the likelihood of an elderly person learning Braille is given by inquiring about his reading habits before he lost his sight. Avid readers should always be taught Braille but others find reading substitutes more useful.

Substitutes for reading

A large lending library of *tape-recorded books* is maintained by the Royal National Institute for the Blind and a tape recorder is lent to each blind person wishing to take advantage of this service. By borrowing these, the blind person can have a continuous and changing supply of books read aloud to him. Each local authority makes a financial contribution to the Royal National Institute for the Blind in respect of each blind person making use of this service.

Wireless for the blind

The radio is most useful and is greatly enjoyed by all blind people. There is a special voluntary society (Wireless for the Blind Fund) financed by the traditional radio appeal each Christmas Day, whose object is to ensure that every blind person has a wireless. Maintenance of the radio is arranged by most social service departments.

Special aids

There are many special aids in the home available for the blind. An example is the special Braille form of 'regulo' which can be fitted to gas stoves.

Provision of guide-dogs for the blind

A society exists which provides and trains special guide-dogs for use by the blind. The selection and training of the dogs and blind person is lengthy and limits the number who can be helped in this way. *Guide-dogs are especially useful to those blinded in early adult life* and those living on their own. Local authorities assist with the cost of training which is usually about £1000 (1978 figure).

Holidays and hostels

There are a number of special holiday homes for the blind, adapted to make it safe for them to go on holiday alone, and many of these are run by voluntary bodies but local authorities assist with the running costs on a *per capita* basis.

For the elderly blind, it is better to look after them in an ordinary elderly persons home (perhaps 2–3 per home) than to provide special homes.

Financial help

Special pension facilities are available for blind people: (*a*) all blind persons are eligible for retirement pension at 40 years of age; (*b*) supplementary pensions may, in certain circumstances, be paid by Social Security.

Voting

A blind person has the right to vote by post in parliamentary and local elections or to have his ballot paper marked with the help of a sighted person.

Free postage is allowed for a number of 'articles for the blind' including embossed literature, paper for embossing and recordings acting as an alternative to an embossed book.

There is a reduction of £1.25 in the cost of a black and white television licence and the blind person does not need a dog licence for a guide dog.

There is a special £180 (single person) or £360 (married couple) income tax allowance for blind persons—less any tax-free disability payments.

The Deaf and Dumb

Because normal speech is learnt by imitation, in the past the congenitally deaf have been unable to speak. Today, with special instruction methods, it is usually possible to teach some speech to most congenitally deaf children. The deaf and dumb often suffer from isolation and communicate by a mixture of lip reading, sign and finger language. They benefit from club and recreational facilities where they can meet others with similar problems.

There are few employment problems provided interpreter services are available to help with interviews. Skilled trained social workers who freely speak sign and finger language are employed usually by a voluntary society financed by local authorities. Many of these societies are connected with church bodies—a legacy from the past when the main object of welfare services was to provide special church services for the deaf and dumb.

The Hard of Hearing

People who become deaf, having in the past enjoyed good hearing, are usually referred to as '*hard of hearing*'. Such persons have normal speech and this is the usual method of communication although a hearing aid and lip reading may be used. Most of the hard of hearing are elderly persons as deafness, like blindness, often accompanies old age.

The difficulty of communication, leading to loneliness and isolation, is the biggest problem. It is essential that the fullest use is made of any residual hearing which should be correctly assessed by *pure tone audiometry* and the fitting and maintenance of a hearing aid. In many instances, medical social workers of departments of audiology in large general hospitals organize clubs and recreational facilities. This arrangement helps surveillance, as does periodic home visits by social workers or health visitors to check that the deaf person is managing his hearing aid. As most hard-of-hearing persons are elderly, employment problems are not great and sheltered workshops not required.

The Physically Handicapped

This large and diverse group contains many conditions which are chronic and sometimes progressive, such as hemiplegia, paraplegia, multiple sclerosis, rheumatoid arthritis, osteoarthritis, poliomyelitis and muscular dystrophies. With the exception of paraplegics, there is generally a shortage of welfare facilities.

The rehabilitation of paraplegics was greatly advanced by the establishment in the 1939–45 war of special regional hospital spinal centres, the largest being at Stoke Mandeville. Insistence on the importance of independence for paraplegics whenever possible has completely changed the outlook of this group and now 85% of such patients are gainfully employed.

By careful training, it is usually possible for bladder functioning to be either controlled by abdominal muscles or, in higher lesions, to become automatic. With development of arm and shoulder muscles, many functions can be carried out by paraplegics including raising the weight of the body when climbing into chairs. Various motor vehicles are used making the patient even more independent. Recreational and sporting facilities have been developed extensively for paraplegics and include archery, basket ball and swimming and many clubs have been formed to encourage these activities. Local authorities help in this work by providing gymnasia and swimming baths. Reference has already been made to the types of wheelchairs and special motorized transport that are available (see p. 450).

For the very severely crippled persons many additional facilities are available. The full range of home nursing services is used together with specialized lifting equipment—hoists, and special beds which are lent by the local authority to the patient. It is essential to encourage such patients to be as active as possible even if they are bedridden or the eventual prognosis is poor, and they should be visited by the occupational therapist at home and taught various crafts and handicrafts, a most valuable local authority service.

In many serious cases where the patient is almost completely paralysed, a new electronic machine operated by sucking or by blowing into a mouthpiece or by similar light pressure has been developed. It is called *Patient Operated Selector Mechanism* (POSSUM) and enables a tetraplegic or completely paralysed patient to make a telephone call, turn on and off a radio or television, switch off lights and use a typewriter etc. This machine adds much to the independence of a grossly paralysed person. It is now available on the National Health Service but the local authority is expected to undertake the electrical fitments needed and to provide a stand. Inquiries should be made to the AHA who will send out a consultant to assess each client individually.

For patients crippled with *rheumatoid arthritis or osteoarthritis* there is a large range of gadgets now available to assist with everyday tasks of cooking, dressing and life at home. Such patients should attend the occupational therapy or rehabilitation centres (see p. 447) where their needs can be expertly assessed.

Cerebral Palsy

The incidence of cerebral palsy in the United Kingdom is about two per 1000 schoolchildren. This means there are approximately 28 000 persons with some form of cerebral palsy under the age of 20 years. About 88% are caused by prenatal or intranatal conditions, while the remainder are of postnatal origin (anoxia, meningitis). In the prenatal group 20% have a history of prematurity. Lack of oxygenation of the brain is an important cause. There is a marked increase of mental handicap in cerebral palsy (in one survey, 48% of such patients had IQs below 69 compared with 3% of the normal population). But there is much variation and the mildest cases usually have a normal IQ although there are few instances of very severely crippled cases with a normal IQ. *Accurate and early diagnosis is important, so that full benefit can be obtained from special education.*

In early adult life, assistance may be required to find suitable employment. It is of value to designate a social worker to help with coordination with the Disablement Resettlement Officer and with the specialist careers officer (see p. 142). In those with mental handicap, many of the services available to that group (Chapter 25) are important. The value of a good home is important and, if this is lacking, young adults should, if possible, be placed in a hostel and given special industrial training.

A special fund for the families of handicapped children—the Joseph Rowntree Memorial Trust—was fully set up in 1973 to help the parents of *severely congenitally handicapped children under the age of 16 in the United Kingdom.* It aims to help in relieving stress in families by complementing the provision of services and cash benefits from both statutory and voluntary sources. Application forms can be obtained from the Trust at its offices at Beverley House, Skipton, Yorks.

Epilepsy

Persons with epilepsy present many problems not found in other handicapped people. This is not due to the difficulties of treating epilepsy, but to *ill-informed public opinion which, quite wrongly, considers that epileptics are usually dangerous.* The truth is that the majority are well controlled and can quite satisfactorily be educated and employed normally. Adverse public reaction results in many patients concealing the fact that they have had occasional epileptic seizures, because they fear if it becomes known they may lose their jobs or find it difficult to obtain employment. This in turn leads to considerable strains which produce other difficulties including minor anxiety states.

In order to help the person with epilepsy, it is important to realize these environmental pressures and *to arrange for his employer or prospective employer to be told the full facts* and particularly that his epilepsy, if properly controlled, is no problem. Many have some warning of an impending attack and, apart from avoiding a few very dangerous occupations in which those with epilepsy will rarely want to work, there are few jobs which are not suitable. But a watch should be maintained to ensure that the disease is being controlled. This follow-up can be carried out by a specially trained health visitor who maintains a close liaison with the patient's doctor. The social aspects, which are so important to successful treatment, should always be carefully considered—including conditions in the patient's home and his occupation, so that problems can be avoided or corrected before they have a serious effect.

Occasionally, it is necessary to admit the patient to an *epileptic colony* which mainly deals with those rare cases whose illness cannot easily be controlled by treatment and with those with antisocial behavioural problems. Those in such a colony may remain there permanently and, if possible, do some productive work on a farm or in a small workshop. Most colonies are run by voluntary bodies with local authorities meeting the *per capita* cost.

Ischaemic Heart Disease

This disease is becoming an increasing problem (see p. 249) and it is important to consider how the rehabilitation of the patient can be assisted. *There is a danger of too much overprotection of the convalescent patient* and many families show too much anxiety. In rehabilitation it is important to encourage the patient early and to concentrate on normality. Extra rest may be needed but moderate exercise, walking, golf, swimming, horse riding or cycling are valuable. It is best to avoid competitive sports because of the emotional stress involved. Rehabilitation will vary with the age of onset. In the younger coronary thrombosis, return to work is desirable as soon as the convalescence is over. Most can return to their former occupations with the exception of those in heavy unskilled occupations. *Smoking should always be given up* and *overweight corrected* but it is a mistake to stress particular diets for they tend to make the patient introspective and afraid to take meals out.

Even for those who have symptoms, a light job should be found. Many seriously incapacitated young patients can work in sheltered workshops. *Occupational therapy* should always be encouraged for any unable to find work.

25 Care of the Mentally Disordered

The term 'mentally disordered' includes two main categories of persons:

1. Those suffering from all types of *mental illnesses*. These include the various psychoses (schizophrenia, affective psychoses, dementia and other types of psychoses), neuroses (anxiety states), various personality disorders, drug addiction and alcoholism.

2. Those suffering from *mental handicap* (or mental subnormality).

Since the 1959 Mental Health Act, all mental disorders have been dealt with under the same code of practice and law although the features of mental illness and mental handicap are quite different.

Mental illness is essentially characterized by emotional instability. It occurs in many forms, at all ages, and in all types of individuals. It is as common in highly intelligent as in unintelligent persons.

Mental handicap is, by contrast, essentially a defect of development of the intellect in which the intelligence of the person is seriously retarded. It is usually present from birth (intelligence usually being determined by heredity) but occasionally may follow certain acute forms of brain disease in young children. Occasionally a person with mental handicap may also develop mental illness.

The recent DHSS documents on *Priorities in the Health and Social Services* have emphasized that the *development of more community based services for the mentally disordered is a top national priority*. The rate of growth advocated is high and it is hoped that joint financing (see p. 24) will enable such services to be developed even at a time of national economy.

MENTAL HEALTH ACT, 1959

The Mental Health Act, 1959, which followed a complete review by a Royal Commission 1954–7, entirely changed the law relating to mental disorders. These changes can be summarized by stating that the Act envisaged a shift from hospital care to community care. This Act introduced a more modern approach to mental problems and had seven main aims:

(1) to combine arrangements for mental illness and mental subnormality under one code of practice and law—both come within the term *mental disorder*; (2) to place the treatment of mental disorder and physical illness on the same basis; (3) to remove the stigma attached to mental disorder; (4) to encourage voluntary admission to hospital; (5) to simplify compulsory admission to hospital; (6) to develop widespread community services for those with mental disorder; (7) to introduce a new definition for mental subnormality (now called mental handicap).

1. *Mental disorder*

Until 1959, mental illness was treated quite separately from mental handicap. Separate hospitals and staffs dealt with both and the law was quite different. Now both mental illness and handicap are considered together. The justification for this lies in the fact that, in many instances, this is the most practical way of looking at the person's individual problem. For example, in the case of a moderate degree of mental handicap in which the intelligence of the client is retarded, the prognosis in terms of employment or training will depend on the emotional stability of the individual. If this is quite normal, there is a greater chance of successfully training that person to carry out an occupation and lead a reasonably normal life. If, on the other hand, there is a moderate degree of emotional instability this may prove quite impossible.

2. *Basis for treatment of mental illness*

There are certain important basic differences between the problems of treatment of physical illness and mental disorders. In physical illness, treatment is designed to carry out a full investigation, to correct various pathological processes discovered and, if possible, to restore the patient to full health or, if this is not possible, to arrest development of the disease and to control problems. Treatment and investigation may take place at home by the general practitioner, or the patient may be referred to hospital either as an outpatient or an inpatient. Once, however, treatment is completed, *the patient invariably returns home.* Even in a hopeless case (such as a malignant neoplasm or progressive neurological disorder) the patient is sent home and remains there as long as possible. *The treatment of mental disorders should be on a similar basis* but has the following additional problems.

a. The necessity of protecting either the patient or the community from the effects of mental illness, such as the danger of suicide or violent behaviour, means that special arrangements have to be made to admit and retain compulsorily a few patients in a mental hospital.

b. Much mental illness and handicap is a chronic problem. By comparison, the majority of physical illness is either acute or subacute and the disease lasts a relatively short time.

More long-term care is now undertaken in the community. Discharge from hospital of the chronic patient suffering from mental disorder has been made possible by newer and more effective treatments now available. Tranquillizer drugs have also assisted and better rehabilitation facilities within the community have helped. The present aim is to attempt to *use hospital admissions in mental disorder mainly for investigation and early treatment* and to *carry out chronic treatment and rehabilitation within the community.*

3. *Incidence of mental illness and stigma*

Mainly due to ignorance as to the nature and causation of mental disorder, many people feel ashamed or have feelings of guilt when a member of the family develops some form of mental illness. Study of the incidence of all forms of mental disorder shows that there is little logical basis for such a reaction. Only a tiny proportion of mental illness is hereditary. But mental illness is quite common—each year about 59 000 persons (127 per 100 000 population in England) who had not been previously treated are admitted to a mental hospital.

A survey carried out in 53 general practices (serving 300 000 people) in 1970–1 by OPCS showed that 1 in 14 males and 1 in 7 females consulted their general practitioner each year for some form of mental illness. This means that many families have some individual who has suffered from at least a minor degree of mental disorder. This does not, however, alter the fact that *there is still a serious stigma attached to this condition* because it is difficult to bring about a rapid change in public opinion towards mental illness. One of the ways it is hoped to combat this and to reduce prejudice is to replace treatment and investigation in an isolated mental hospital by care in a special mental health department of a district general hospital. The reason then for a patient's admission would not be so obvious or self-evident. It would create a better understanding between medical and nursing staff treating physical and mental disease.

4. *Informal admissions* of all patients suffering from mental illness are arranged wherever possible (in practice in 82% of cases). Only in serious cases, where the patient objects to admission which is obviously essential, is any formal procedure necessary.

5. *Compulsory admissions*

When compulsory admission is necessary, the procedure under the Mental Health Act, 1959, has been greatly simplified. The decision is now only a medical one and does not involve the intervention of a justice of the peace (see p. 471).

6. *Community mental health and social services* arrange for the treatment and rehabilitation of the patient or client to be undertaken while he is living at home—within the community. If the person has no suitable home, he may move to a special hostel and then into normal housing (see p. 478)—an arrangement which is preferable to a further stay in hospital. Community care is only possible if greatly extended treatment and rehabilitation facilities are made available in each area—hostels, training centres, special workshops, occupational therapy, job placement services and after-care services designed to help and support the client. Many of these are directly provided by social service departments, but there are also important duties to be undertaken by the primary health care team.

7. *Definitions*

The Mental Health Act defines two types of mental handicap as well as introducing an additional category of mental disorder, 'psychopathic personality'.

Severe subnormality means 'a state of arrested or incomplete development of the mind, which includes subnormality of intelligence and is of such a nature or degree that the patient is incapable of living an independent life or of guarding himself against serious exploitation, or will be so incapable when of an age to do so'. This includes all the very lowest grades of subnormality and most of these will need to be permanently cared for in special institutions. Mortality is highest in this group.

Subnormality means 'a state of arrested or incomplete development of the mind (not amounting to severe subnormality) which includes subnormality of intelligence and is of a nature or degree which requires or is susceptible to medical treatment or other special care or training of the patient'. This category contains the majority of mentally handicapped persons, including some low-grade patients only a little better than the 'severe subnormals' and all grades up to those who are borderline. Some of these are difficult to distinguish from normal persons with a somewhat limited intelligence. Unless there are additional serious emotional problems, it should always be possible to train and care for this group in the community.

Psychopathic disorder is defined as 'a persistent disorder or disability of mind (whether or not including subnormality of intelligence) which results in abnormally aggressive or seriously irresponsible conduct on the part of the patient, and requires or is susceptible to medical treatment'. Promiscuity or other immoral behaviour' is *not* considered sufficiently abnormal to constitute the legal definition of psychopathic personality. As 'psychopath' has come to carry considerable stigma, the term 'personality disorders with antisocial trends' is now often used in preference.

Review of the Mental Health Act

At present (1978) a review by the DHSS of the Mental Health Act is occurring as many indications are that progress towards the aims outlined above has been too slow. In addition the review will consider the recommendations of the Committee on Mentally Abnormal Offenders (the Butler Committee).

HEALTH AND SOCIAL SERVICES FOR THE MENTALLY ILL

Although it is convenient to describe various forms of medical, nursing and social services for the mentally ill, it is most important to emphasize that a *multidisciplinary approach* is essential. No one form of service can succeed without working very closely with the other services. The aim is to provide for each individual person the range of facilities (professional staff, day care, treatment or residential accommodation) which he needs.

Primary health care teams

These are responsible for the management and treatment of milder forms of mental illnesses. Specialist psychiatric advice may be needed and, in the elderly person, this is likely to involve the geriatric specialist. The primary health care team of general practitioner, health visitor, home nurse and social worker also has an important role to play in prevention—this involves early diagnosis and intervention to avoid the more serious episodes developing. The team also should be concerned *with the early recognition of mental stress and, particularly through the work of the health visitor*, be able to recognize stress in the young mother (often an accompanying factor of non-accident injury, see p. 434) and in young children.

Specialist services

These are mainly based within hospitals but, with the reorganization of the health services, the psychiatrist is increasingly concerned with helping with community care through day hospitals (often referred to as a psychiatric day activity area), outpatient care and domiciliary visiting with the primary health care team.

Hospital Care

In 1975, in England, 84 000 mental illness hospital beds were occupied daily and on average 196 000 patients attended as new outpatients in the year. The reduction in hospital beds and increase in outpatients (from 1959–70) is shown in Table 77.

TABLE 77 Hospital Psychiatric Services, England

<table>
<tr><th></th><th>1959</th><th>1968</th><th>1970</th><th>1973</th><th>1975</th></tr>
<tr><td>Average daily occupied beds</td><td></td><td></td><td></td><td></td><td></td></tr>
<tr><td>Mental illness</td><td>132 600</td><td>113 400</td><td>106 400</td><td>94 200</td><td>83 800</td></tr>
<tr><td>Mental handicap</td><td>53 900</td><td>55 600</td><td>54 500</td><td>51 700</td><td>48 800</td></tr>
<tr><td>New out-patients</td><td></td><td></td><td></td><td></td><td></td></tr>
<tr><td>Mental illness</td><td rowspan="2">151 000</td><td>213 300</td><td>215 300</td><td>208 600</td><td>195 900</td></tr>
<tr><td>Mental handicap</td><td>2400</td><td>2600</td><td>4000</td><td>4000</td></tr>
</table>

(From *Health and Personal Social Services Statistics*, 1977, DHSS)

The diagnosis of all admissions to mental hospitals is given in Table 23, p. 78.

The main *role of the hospital service in mental disorder is to provide investigation and treatment facilities*. Reference has already been made to the need to bring much of this work into district general hospitals in the future. At present, the majority still have to be admitted to mental hospitals. There is, however, a greater turnover of patients annually and the average length of stay of inpatients has diminished. Much follow-up and medical after-care is linked with outpatient facilities which have been extended in most district general hospitals.

Large psychiatric units providing 120–150 beds are being opened in many general hospitals and it is planned that such units should accept all types of mental illness except the special categories (drug addiction or alcoholism). The recommended scale of inpatient provision is 50 beds per 100 000 population—this means that for England and Wales there should be approximately 27 000 beds. Such a provision is based upon there being adequate day hospital places and community mental health services (see below).

Compulsory Hospital Admissions

About 18% of mentally ill patients enter hospital compulsorily. In many instances the reason for the admission is serious and acute. Under Part IV of the Mental Health Act, *compulsory admissions can only be applied to patients who cannot be persuaded to enter hospital informally and only then if such admission is essential.* An application for compulsory admission must be made either from the nearest relative or social worker and must normally be supported by recommendations of two medical practitioners. Admission may be arranged to any hospital willing to receive the patient. There are three types of compulsory admission used.

1. *Admission for observation in emergency* (S29) is the commonest form of compulsory admission arranged and is specially designed for the urgent acute case. Under S29 an emergency application can be made by any relative or the social worker. This application must state that the case is urgent and that ordinary procedure for admission for observation under S25 would involve undesirable delay. This must be verified *by one medical recommendation* given, if possible, by a doctor who has known the patient previously. Admission under S29 only lasts 72 hours, unless a second medical recommendation is made to the managers of the hospital, when the patient may be detained in hospital for 28 days in all, beginning with the day of admission.

2. *Admission for observation* (S25)—this is the second commonest form used. Application is made by nearest relative or by a social worker. *Recommendations of two doctors are necessary* one of whom must be approved by the AHA as having specialist knowledge of the type of mental disorder from which the patient is suffering. The other doctor is usually the patient's general practitioner. *Both must have personally examined the patient at the same time or within a period of seven days.* The medical recommendations must state: (*a*) that the patient is suffering from mental disorder of a nature or degree which warrants his detention in a hospital under observation for a limited period: and (*b*) that he ought to be so detained in the interests of his own health or safety or with a view to the protection of other persons; and (*c*) that informal admission is not appropriate. The patient may then be admitted to hospital with authority to detain him for a period not exceeding 28 days.

3. *Admission for treatment* (S26) is the least used method of compulsory admission. It can be used for: (i) patients of any age if suffering from mental illness or severe subnormality; (ii) for

patients under the age of 21 years if suffering from subnormality or psychopathic disorder.

The two medical recommendations must state: (*a*) that he ought to be so detained for treatment in the interests of his own health or safety or with a view to the protection of other persons; (*b*) give a clinical description of the patient's mental condition; (*c*) state the form of mental disorder from which he is suffering and that it is of a nature or degree which warrants detention in hospital for medical treatment; (*d*) indicate whether other methods of care or treatment are available and if so, why they are not appropriate and why informal admission is not suitable.

This means that *such admissions should only be recommended where there is no adequate alternative community care.*

Procedure

As soon as the patient refuses informal admission, the general practitioner should get into touch with the *social worker of the social services department* who then usually makes the application under the appropriate section already described and in the case of S25 or S26 admissions, arranges for a second medical examination. If all is in order, the social worker admits the patient and usually accompanies him to hospital. Social service departments have an emergency out of hours service to deal with emergency mental health admissions.

Mental Health Review Tribunals

To make certain that no patient is detained in hospital compulsorily unless essential, 15 Mental Health Review Tribunals have been set up, each operating in the area of the RHA. Each Tribunal consists of the following members appointed by the Lord Chancellor: (*a*) persons with legal experience, one of whom must be appointed as chairman; (*b*) medical practitioners, appointed after consultation with the Secretary of State; (*c*) persons appointed, also after consultation with the Secretary of State, who have experience in administration, knowledge of social services or other qualifications or experience considered suitable.

A tribunal for the hearing of applications is appointed by the

Chairman and must have at least one person from each of the above three categories.

Applications for discharge can be made by patients or relatives and are heard by the tribunal. In all cases, the patient or applicant is seen by the tribunal which also hears evidence from doctors and social workers. After hearing the application the tribunal may direct the patient's discharge. *It must direct the patient's discharge if they are satisfied:* (*a*) that he is not then suffering from mental illness, psychopathic disorder, subnormality or severe subnormality; or (*b*) that it is not necessary in the interests of the patient's health or safety or for the protection of other persons, that the patient should continue to be detained; or (*c*) in the case of a psychopathic or subnormal patient whose discharge at the age of 25 was barred or a patient whose discharge by his nearest relative was barred, that if released he would not be likely to act in a manner dangerous to others or himself.

In all cases, the decision of the tribunal must be communicated in writing to the applicant, the responsible authority and the patient within seven days. Each year approximately 750 applicants were determined by Mental Health Review Tribunals. Discharge of the patient was directed in approximately 100 cases.

Informal Admission

The general practitioner who has a patient acutely mentally ill needing admission to hospital can arrange informal admission in the same way as in physical illness by direct arrangement between himself and the hospital psychiatrist and this is the most usual method (in 82% of admissions).

Day Hospitals (Psychiatric Day Activity Area)

Day hospitals have been increasingly developed during the last 10 years in an attempt to bridge the gap between inpatient treatment and community rehabilitation. It is now more usual to refer to a *psychiatric day activity area* which is usually an integral part of any psychiatric unit within a general hospital. Such a unit has the dual function of providing day activity both for inpatients and for patients living in the community (rather more than half the places are used by in-patients). Industrial therapy, occupational therapy and forms of social rehabilitation play an important part in any psychiatric day activity area and there should be a close link between such units and the social service provision within the community. The recommended scale of psychiatric day activity places is 65 per 100 000 population.

Mental illness in the elderly

More mental illness occurs in the elderly than in any other section of the community. In 1975 in England 21·5% of all mental hospital admissions occurred in persons aged 65 years and over (the proportion of this age group in the population was 14%). In the elderly there is a special need for joint assessment by a psychiatrist and geriatric physician. *Short term admission to hospital, holiday relief, day hospitals, community nursing services* as well as domiciliary and support social services are often needed.

One of the special problems of mental illness is the care needed for *psychogeriatric cases* (previously referred to as senile dementia cases). There are two main requirements:

1. *Psychogeriatric assessment* involves admission of the patient to a *special assessment* unit. This should preferably be in a geriatric assessment ward (see Chapter 26) and there should be close cooperation between the geriatricians and psychiatrists. Approximately 10 to 20 beds are likely to be needed in each district management team area for this assessment.

2. *Provision of long stay beds for psychogeriatric cases.* The latest recommendation is that the care of the long term cases should be in *community hospitals* which will generally be smaller units (such as the former 'cottage' type of hospital).

A psychiatrist with special interest in the elderly would control the unit with assistance from the geriatrician and a general physician; day-to-day medical staffing would be provided by general practitioners as it is hoped that such an arrangement would enable stronger community links to be maintained with both the primary health care teams and the families. It is expected that the remedial professions (especially occupational therapy) would have a large contribution to make to such a unit.

It is estimated that approximately *25 to 30 long stay beds will be needed for every 10 000 elderly persons.* This means that approximately 10 000 beds would be required for England and Wales.

One very important feature planned for these community hospitals is that a *large day activity area* should always be provided (20 to 30 places per 10 000 elderly) as the maintenance of daily activities is most essential if the development of senile dementia is to be slowed down.

Psychiatric Community Nursing Services

There should be a full district psychiatric nursing service within the community which will be organized under the *district psychiatric nursing officer*. Such a service will provide the psychiatric nursing service needed in the community hospitals dealing with psychogeriatric patients, undertake nursing services in the outpatient and day patient parts of the psychiatric units as well as carry out a *domiciliary psychiatric nursing service*.

This will be developed in close conjunction with the primary health care teams and will deal with three main areas of work:

1. arrange pre-admission psychiatric nursing services
2. follow-up psychiatric nursing services after discharge from psychiatric units
3. assist local authority social service departments with psychiatric problems in their residential accommodation and in their day centres

Social Rehabilitation

Mental illness often affects the social adjustment of the individual, his personal friendship and family relationships. Many people recovering from mental illness are not immediately able to bear the full responsibility for organizing their life. Special strains are also imposed upon the family who may also require considerable support.

Most of the community supporting services for the mentally ill are organized by local authority social service departments. These mainly fall in three categories.

1. *Social work support* provided by social workers
2. *Day care facilities* to assist in the reintegration of the person

who has had mental illness. These include social rehabilitation facilities, occupational therapy, industrial therapy and workshops.

3. *Residential facilities* for those who have no satisfactory home to return to which could support them after their illness.

Social work support is provided by social workers (before the Local Authority Social Services Act, 1970, such officers were called mental welfare officers), many of whom have had special experience and training in dealing with the mentally ill. Much preventive and after-care work in the mental health field is concerned with the avoidance of further breakdown and with general rehabilitation. It is important to develop organized *community support systems by voluntary bodies and self-help groups*. The emphasis should be on measures to support the family and to improve social relationships as well as to increase the general awareness and understanding of mental health. In some instances follow-up care will be necessary for many years and this help will be provided in close cooperation with those working in the primary health care teams. After-care home visits by social workers are always best arranged after discussion with the general practitioner, psychiatrists and the nursing staff concerned with the community psychiatric nursing services. Unless social workers have very close working arrangements with all members of the primary health care teams, some clients and some doctors may resent the apparent interference of after-care and visiting may then be refused.

The effects of mental illness may appear to be hidden beneath other problems; in some instances, social problems within families may result mainly from mental illness of a member of that family. Early intervention in the social problem can very often prevent a much more serious crisis developing. The family may need much advice and help in a wide range of social problems including financial worries, housing and domestic difficulties, and upsets with children. In many instances employment is of very great importance.

Importance of Occupation

A correctly chosen occupation can do much either to prevent a person developing a mental illness or to avoid a relapse. Help in finding a job is one of the most important after-care services. Mental illness sometimes impairs an individual's ability to work in a constructive way, to keep regular hours, to deal with colleagues or staff or to maintain adequate output under pressure. In the rehabilitation, therefore, it is important that the rhythm and discipline of working are encouraged—hence the value of special workshops and industrial therapy units.

It is the duty of a Disablement Resettlement Officer (DRO) (see p. 443) to find employment for all handicapped people, including those with mental disorders. It is often difficult to find employment for clients who have had a mental illness because they may have lost their original job and there is usually a resistance among employers to re-employ them for fear they will again break down and perhaps disrupt their staff. It is important that the delay in obtaining a suitable post should not be allowed to depress the person. *Occupational therapy* at a special rehabilitation centre should be available, as this will not only help the client in training him in physical skills, but also restore his self-confidence. Most local authorities and AHAs provide such occupational therapy in their care and after-care services.

The social worker carrying out the after-care should cooperate very closely with the Disablement Resettlement Officer so that the former mental health patient can not only find suitable employment but be helped to settle down in the new job.

Day Care Facilities for the Mentally Ill

Day care facilities play an increasingly important role in the rehabilitation of many former mental hospital patients. Such centres should provide a wide opportunity for the individual to meet many different people and to improve his social rehabilitation. Many such people lack confidence and their self-respect has been shaken by their illness. They need to gain confidence by demonstrating that they can manage quite well on their own (when they are away from their families). Daily attendance at such centres which are reached by a bus or train journey helps them greatly to gain such self-confidence.

The functions of such centres often overlap those of day hospitals and sheltered employment. *Occupational therapy* should be available at day centres. As well as helping with the problems of readjusting to the demands of work, *cultural and educational activities* such as a study of art, music, drama or literature should also be provided at day centres. As regards the organization of such centres, the ex-mentally ill person himself should be encouraged to help in the running of the centre.

Residential Care

Many persons who are recovering from mental illness can return home from hospital. But those who have no satisfactory homes will need residential care on either a short-term or a long-term basis. Accommodation is provided by local authorities or voluntary bodies in (*a*) hostels; (*b*) staffed homes; (*c*) small unstaffed homes; (*d*) supervised lodgings; and (*e*) in ordinary housing. Hostels or homes should ideally cater for eight to ten persons and every person should attend a day centre initially. There should be a steady progression to normal independent living. However considerable support and rehabilitation will be needed with some persons who may require a short intensive programme of rehabilitation in a staffed hostel.

It is estimated that in England and Wales 30–48 long stay places will be needed for a population of 200 000 (at least 10–16 of these should be in staffed homes).

Voluntary help

Many persons recovering from a long mental illness will have difficulty in re-establishing social ties, particularly if they have no family support. Volunteers can be of great value in this respect and many of those in small unstaffed homes or housing rely to a large extent upon the help and support they receive from local voluntary bodies. It is therefore most important for social services departments when setting up unstaffed group homes to arrange for such support to be available.

ALCOHOLISM

Alcoholism can be defined as dependence upon alcohol to such a degree that the individual shows noticeable mental disturbance or an interference with bodily or mental health. In addition alcoholism is a medico-social problem in both its origins and manifestations for it interferes with interpersonal relations and with the normal economic and social functioning of the alcoholic and his family.

It is estimated that there are 300 000 to 400 000 alcoholics in England and Wales. There is some evidence that the incidence is increasing especially among women and young people.

Causes of alcoholism

There is no one cause of alcoholism. The greater the amount of alcohol drunk the more likely is alcoholism to occur. Social factors are always very important and there is a significantly higher proportion of alcoholism in persons who are single, widowed or divorced. The mean age for male alcoholics is the mid-forties while in women it is higher. The greatest incidence of alcoholism is in social classes I and V. Certain occupations have high risks—commercial travellers, business executives, publicans, seamen and doctors.

No particular type of personality is specially liable although both excessively shy people and the gregarious extravert show a higher incidence of alcoholism than normal.

Types of alcoholism

Two main types are described:

1. *Alcoholic addiction*—people who cannot go for long without drinking alcohol or who get withdrawal symptoms if they do so.

2. *Chronic alcoholism* in which serious physical and mental symptoms are the dominating feature. Loss of appetite and poor food intake encourage the development of cirrhosis of the liver or peripheral neuropathy (interference with peripheral nerves in the limbs). Severe memory loss is usual and dementia may occur. Withdrawal symptoms including delirium tremens may also occur.

Treatment

Early diagnosis and recognition is most important. Increasing absenteeism, decline in job efficiency, increasing marital disharmony and self-neglect are suggestive. Memory losses, misinterpretations and feelings of guilt and low self-esteem should also raise suspicions. It is also important to realize that ill effects may be presented by other members of the family especially wives.

Treatment is aimed at reversing the damage to the physical, mental and social life of the alcoholic and then to deal with the underlying addiction. There are 18 special alcoholism units; in addition most mental hospitals treat alcoholic patients. In a few areas where homeless, chronic alcoholics congregate and where the police are faced with large numbers of habitual drunken offenders, a few special experimental '*detoxification centres*' have been set up.

Rehabilitation and after-care

Once successful treatment has been completed, relapses are common unless a careful rehabilitation process is instituted. Doctors and social workers from social service departments and voluntary bodies all play very important parts in rehabilitation. It may be helpful to use special *hostels* and *day centres*. Many alcoholics have lost their job and retraining for a suitable job may be needed (it is sometimes important for treated alcoholics to change their job to ensure that they can work in drink-free conditions—e.g. publicans, waiters and barmen). The Disablement Resettlement Officer of the Department of Employment should be able to help with job placements and retraining.

Many voluntary bodies, such as various Councils for Alcoholism and Alcoholics Anonymous can give most useful support and help. In all instances it is most important that those helping in the rehabilitation—general practitioners, social workers and voluntary workers—ensure that their efforts are coordinated and that a team approach is adopted. Some relapses are likely and rehabilitation in many instances will therefore be a lengthy process.

DRUG ADDICTION

Many different drugs can be misused. There is a small illicit market in heroin and methadone in the UK, and probably about 2000 persons are involved (in 1974, 1885 addicts were known to the Home Office, of these approximately 175 are receiving heroin and 1250 methadone). Many of the addicts are young persons with a variety of problems and often a history of emotional deprivation; 39% of known addicts are under 25 years of age and 74% under 30. The majority of drug addicts are centred in large urban communities particularly in London.

The rehabilitation of drug addicts is a lengthy process involving medical and social services. Voluntary organizations play a very important part in providing *hostels* of various types, *day centres*, *counselling* and *information services*. It is most important that methods of communication are improved between the hospital and day dependence treatment units and the social service department.

An Advisory Council on the Misuse of Drugs was established in 1972. Its function is to advise the Home Secretary and Secretaries of State for Education and Social Services on health and social measures to deal with problems produced by the misuse of drugs. Recently the Council has set up a steering group of doctors to direct a campaign of education aimed at persuading doctors to reduce their prescribing of barbiturates.

SERVICES FOR THE MENTALLY HANDICAPPED

Incidence and Ascertainment

It is convenient to use intelligence quotient (IQ) (see p. 146) as a basis for determining mental handicap. This is not a precise measure of any person's ability because emotional factors are also relevant but the use of IQ has less subjective errors than any other criterion. In three recent surveys in Wessex and Newcastle hospital regions and in Camberwell in London, it is estimated that there were approximately *120 per 100 000 population with an IQ of 50 or less living at home* and *about 115 per 100 000 in hospitals or other* residential care. On this basis it would indicate that an approximate 66 000 severely mentally handicapped are living at home and 63 000 in hospitals and residential accommodation in England and Wales.

An important finding of these surveys was that, in many severely mentally handicapped children in hospitals, *there were also multiple physical handicaps present.* One in three such children suffered from epilepsy, one in five had defects of vision or hearing and 1 in 20 was blind. The incidence of multiple defects in adults was slightly less.

Most of these cases are discovered in early childhood and

reference has already been made to the role of health visitors, day nursery staff and nursery teachers as ascertained in Chapters 5 and 6.

Since April 1971 when the Education (Handicapped Children) Act, 1970 came into operation, mentally handicapped children are no longer segregated from the education services but receive their education and training in special schools for the mentally handicapped (see p. 148). These include some '*special care units*' for mentally handicapped children who also have severe physical handicaps or behaviour difficulties. Such children can often in this way remain at home rather than in hospital.

Social services for the mentally handicapped

The domiciliary or community services for the mentally handicapped are the responsibility of social services departments. There are three main types of service.

Day care

Many *special day care services* have been developed to help in their community care while the mentally handicapped person remains living at home. These include the following:

1. adult training centres
2. occupational therapy centres
3. sheltered workshops
4. industrial therapy and open industry

1. *Adult training centres* carry on the training of mentally handicapped young persons when they leave special school at 16 years. Many are mixed but a few cater only for one sex. Problems occasionally arise as puberty develops and it should always be carefully explained to parents that close supervision must be maintained on their activities at home. In particular, it is most important that every parent of a mentally handicapped girl realizes that her mental handicap will make her more vulnerable to the advances of unscrupulous men. Parental control that is too lax often results in their mentally handicapped daughter becoming pregnant.

Training in the adult training centre concentrates upon two main features: *social training* and the preparation of the young person to enter a *special sheltered workshop*. Girls concentrate their social training on housework and boys become more skilled in carpentry, woodwork and model making. In order to prepare the mentally handicapped young person to take his/her place in a sheltered workshop, it is necessary *to teach them how to work with other persons and to get used to longer hours*, as both are important for successful workshop placement. It is an advantage for the adult training centre to be sited beside the sheltered workshop so that those in the centre have a target to reach.

Often the mentally handicapped school leaver spends six to twelve months in the adult training centre before progressing to the sheltered workshop.

2. *Occupational therapy* centres are an important integral part of any day centre complex for the mentally handicapped. In them, the mentally handicapped young person is given an opportunity to become involved in many different activities—both individual handicraft, and in particular how to integrate into various group activities. It is not unusual for special recreational activities to be arranged in an *evening club* once a week. If possible, such clubs are run in such a way that the mentally handicapped young people themselves do much of the organization.

3. *Sheltered workshops*. Many very successful sheltered workshops for the mentally handicapped are now run by social service departments. The most successful undertake simple tasks which can best be done by hand or by some simple hand operated machine. Tasks include work contracted out from industry as well as the manufacture and marketing of simple products (i.e. toys) made within the workshop, which remains open for the whole of the year with the exception of a fortnight's holiday in the summer, planned to fit in with the local industrial holidays. The standard of work is usually high, for all is carefully supervised by the staff.

Although the sheltered workshop is a place of employment for the mentally handicapped, the training process started in the training centres still continues. This is often reflected in the system of payment adopted. One successful scheme is to base weekly payment upon a points system in which points represent part of the maximum wage and are added for good steady work and high standard of production, and deducted for bad behaviour, lateness or non-attendance. In this way, the mentally handicapped persons employed at the workshop quickly learn the importance of hard work and good behaviour. It is usual to arrange for the maximum wage to equal the amount each may earn without having any deduction made from his Supplementary Allowance from the DHSS. At present, this means each mentally handicapped person may earn up to £4 per week.

One of the most encouraging and remarkable changes, which has followed the introduction of workshops, has been the *great improvement in the behaviour and outlook of the mentally handicapped persons employed in them*, and they obviously feel they have taken a great step forward by showing that they can carry on a useful occupation. The speed and concentration of each person improves and after some months a few begin to approach the productive capability of an unskilled industrial worker.

There is no doubt that the introduction of workshops has done much to improve the opportunities and facilities for the adult mentally handicapped. By demonstrating the skills of the mentally handicapped to industry which subcontracts work, the workshop is helping to educate the general public and show that the potential of many such persons is considerable.

4. *Industrial therapy units and open industry*. The success of the sheltered workshops with the mentally handicapped has enabled the best workers to go into special industrial therapy units where they are trained to take their place eventually in normal industry (open industry). Industrial therapy units are organized in similar ways to sheltered workshops but conditions and hours approximate much more to those in normal factories. With these improved methods of training and better liaison with local industry, it is possible to employ more mentally handicapped in open industry. It must be stressed however that in only a minority of cases will this be possible and then only after very careful selection and training. Experience has shown that *10 to 15% of the mentally handicapped in sheltered workshops should be able to leave eventually and take their place in normal industry*.

Social Work Support

Social workers from social service departments provide continuous social work support. Such help should start while the mentally handicapped child is in school and continue into adult training centre, workshop and open industry. Support will also be needed for the family and, if possible, the social worker should be looked upon as the person who can help in the various crises to be faced. Some social workers specialize in such work while remaining essential members of a general social work team.

Residential Care

If possible, and provided it is satisfactory, it is always best for the mentally handicapped person to live at home. However, in a few instances the home conditions are quite unsuitable, and in the past many such mentally handicapped persons had to be admitted to hospitals. This is no longer necessary as social service departments have developed many types of small homes or hostels and even sheltered housing units.

Small homes or hostels should preferably take from eight to ten mentally handicapped. Such small units make it possible to produce more homelike conditions. Such homes should be scattered throughout the community and an excellent way to achieve this is the amalgamation of two adjacent council houses or similar types of dwellings. Residents in such hostels or homes should be as self-sufficient as possible and be encouraged to look after themselves with some constant overall supervision. About 8700 mentally handicapped persons are now looked after in such homes run by local authority social service departments in England.

It is most important that those mentally handicapped persons living in such hostels should be able to *attend day care facilities* and eventually attend either a *special sheltered workshop* or go to work in *ordinary industry*.

Different forms of *sheltered housing* in which one or two mentally handicapped persons look after themselves with minimum support from social workers or voluntary organizations are becoming popular. Such residential provision is best because the mentally handicapped person can eventually be helped in this way to become completely independent.

Short term Care

Many parents look after their mentally handicapped children devotedly at home but this involves a great deal of strain on them and other members of the family. It is most important for such parents to have a break from time to time to enable normal family holidays to be undertaken.

One of the best ways for social service departments to help is to provide short term care for the mentally handicapped child for a short period of two to four weeks to allow the parents and family to have a complete break. Such an arrangement helps such parents and enables them to return refreshed to the arduous task of looking after a mentally handicapped child.

Prevention of Mental Handicap

Most cases of mental handicap are caused by developmental abnormalities, by birth injuries or by chromosome abnormalities such as in 'Mongol' defectives (Down's syndrome) or rare metabolic conditions such as in phenylketonuria (see p. 113). Very occasionally mental handicap will follow a severe infection of the brain or meninges and for this reason, it is *essential that no delay ever occurs in diagnosing and treating such conditions.*

Methods of prevention can be summarized:

1. *Genetic counselling.* This is usually only possible after the birth of one affected child or where there is a history of possible familial tendency to transmit a hereditary disease which is likely to lead to mental handicap. With modern techniques, it is possible to predict the chances of parents who have already had one Mongol child of having another. In most instances these risks are low but in others risks rise (e.g. with an elderly mother) and then amniocentesis (see below) is of value. Genetic counselling is important so that intending parents can get expert advice and judge what risks are involved.

2. *Amniocentesis* is the removal of a small quantity of amniotic fluid and if this is done at 16 weeks, it is possible to detect mongolism (Down's syndrome) just in time to enable a termination of pregnancy to be safely carried out if the fetus is abnormal. This prevents the birth of a further child with mental handicap.

3. *Immunization of girls (aged 11 to 14 years) against rubella* (see p. 185) will prevent the danger of infection with rubella in the first three months of pregnancy and thus reduce the incidence of congenital abnormalities including mental subnormality.

4. *Immunization with anti-D immunoglobulin* and proper diagnosis and care of the child at risk of haemolytic disease of the

newborn will reduce the chance of kernicterus and of subsequent mental handicap (see p. 96).

5. *Expert midwifery* will reduce the risk of asphyxia in the newborn and brain damage to the child—approximately 45% of children with spastic diplegia have also some degree of mental handicap.

6. Intensive care for babies of low birth weight during the neonatal period.

7. Screening for phenylketonuria (see p. 113).

8. *Earlier completion of families* will reduce the risk of mental handicap. The relationship of age of the mother to the risks of developing a chromosome deficiency (Down's syndrome or mongolism) is dramatically shown by the chances of such a child being born to a normal mother:

The chance of a mongoloid birth to a mother aged 20 years is 1 in 260.

The chance of a mongoloid birth to a mother aged 30 years is 1 in 100.

The chance of a mongoloid birth to a mother aged 40 years is 1 in 40–50.

SPECIAL PROBLEMS WITH MENTALLY DISORDERED PERSONS

Criminal proceedings

Courts have power to authorize the admission and detention of a mentally disordered person found guilty of offences by the Courts. A Hospital Order may be made if the Court is satisfied that, on the written or oral evidence of two doctors (one of whom must be specially approved), the offender is suffering from mental illness, severe subnormality, subnormality or psychopathic disorder warranting hospital treatment. This order authorizes the removal of a patient to hospital within 28 days. The Court may, if necessary, make an order for the detention of the patient in a place of safety, which includes residential accommodation provided by a local authority, a hospital or mental nursing home, a residential home for mentally disordered persons, a police station or any other suitable place where the occupier is willing to receive the patient.

Alternatively the Court may make a Guardianship Order

instead of a Hospital Order if it is thought that the client should be cared for within the community. It is usual in such cases for local authorities to assume the office of Guardianship.

Protection and management of property and affairs

Once a person becomes mentally incapable of managing his own affairs, he cannot legally authorize anybody else to do so on his behalf. If power of attorney has been given to another person before the mental illness then such authority will probably become inoperable because of the illness.

In such cases, *the Court of Protection* exists to protect and manage the affairs and property of any person who is mentally incapable of doing so himself. The Court of Protection usually acts by appointing a receiver—usually a close relative (parent, brother or sister)—to administer the patient's affairs under the direction of the Court after considering medical evidence that the person is now fit to do this himself.

In all cases, application to the Court of Protection (at 25 Store Street, London, WC1) can be made by a close relative or by instructing a solicitor to make the approach.

26 Care of the Elderly

Proportion of elderly persons within the Community

The proportion of elderly persons within the population has been rising steadily since the start of the century. In 1900 less than 5% of persons were over the age of 65 years; today the figure is 14%. This represents 7·1 million people in England and Wales. But the *largest increases are in the older age groups.* By 1986, there will be approximately 24% more people aged 75 years and over. Yet the greatest increases are going to be seen in the very old age group—those aged 85 years and over. Now there are 1 in 104 persons in the country aged 85 years and over but *by 2001, this will be 1 in 65.*

There are many striking differences between the proportion of elderly men and women; 60% of all old persons are women but this proportion is much greater in very old age (see Table 1, p. 58). Falling birth rates during this century have accentuated the rising proportion of old persons but the *biggest reason is associated with the increased life expectancy of young persons today.* The life expectancy of a boy today is 70 years and a girl 76. In 1911 the figures were 49 years and 52 years. Yet the life expectancy of a man aged 65 is now 12 years and a woman 16 years (compared with 11 and 12 years in 1911). There has always been much speculation about the *longevity of women compared with men.* There are probably many reasons—the majority of women have an active job looking after their home and also seem better able to withstand the effects of chronic crippling diseases which so often occur in old age.

Distribution and conditions of the elderly

Figure 26 shows clearly who the elderly lived with in 1976. These figures come from a survey of the elderly undertaken in England in 1976. Note that *94% of all old persons live at home*; the remaining 6% live in hostels, hospitals, etc., 28% live alone and only 12% are living with children. In fact two-thirds of all

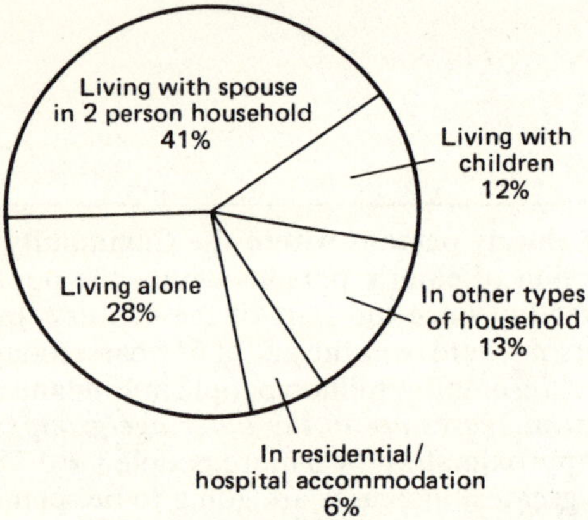

FIG. 26. Who the elderly live with, England, 1976. (From *A Happier Old Age*, 1978, DHSS)

elderly households contain no one under the age of 65 years and one-third of the elderly have never had children or their children have not survived—they have no near immediate next generation family.

Disability among the elderly

The incidence of physical and mental disability among the elderly is high. About 65% of all physically disabled persons are aged 65 years and over. There is also a higher rate of mental illness in the elderly than in any other age group. The OPCS survey showed that 4% of all persons aged 65 years and over were bedfast but *this figure rose to 20% of those aged 85 years and over.* Of those who are not bedfast, 2% have difficulty in seeing and 3%

in hearing. Reference has already been made to the fact that most blind persons are aged over 65 years of age (see p. 454). It will be clear that doctors and social workers meet many case problems in the elderly. Because so many old people live at home, *domiciliary services in both the medical and social fields are very important* if the likelihood of illness, accident or other problems is to be decreased.

Planning for old age—housing

Much can be done to ease the problems of the elderly by better planning for old age. Many serious mistakes are made by people about to retire; all too often they move to some unknown seaside resort for their retirement, are disappointed and find it difficult to settle down. It is not easy for an old person to readjust himself and make new friends and human companionship is often worth more in old age than living in some attractive place. It is important for an old person not to remain too long in a house which is too large and unmanageable, but to move to a smaller dwelling preferably before retirement. This means that, if possible, *an old person should be settled in his last home by the time he is 60 years of age.*

It is equally important that the old person lives in the right type of dwelling. This can be either a house, bungalow or flat, but it should have the following four essentials: (1) it should be sited on the level. So many of the traditional seaside towns to which people retire are too hilly; (2) it should have an entrance which can be directly approached by a car so that a vehicle can be driven up to the front door; (3) it should have a downstairs room which can be converted into a bedroom; (4) it should have a downstairs lavatory and washbasin (a downstairs bath is most helpful but is usually not possible).

These four points are connected with the inevitable fact that physical limitations will eventually develop as age increases. Another very desirable feature is that *the dwelling should be heated automatically* by oil, gas or electricity because most elderly people feel the cold acutely and need some heating for much of the year. A frail old person finds the problems of collecting fuel and stoking the fire increasingly difficult and both may be hazardous and result in falls.

Preparation for retirement

Short courses to help persons due to retire have become popular and many excellent examples are run by local authorities, local committees and other interested bodies. If possible, such *courses should be held for persons about four to five years before they are due to retire* so that plenty of time is available to put into practice the ideas introduced. This means that the best groups to aim at for these courses are those aged from 55–60 years.

All old people should cultivate some hobby or pastime, preferably one which involves routine and constant interest and gives the old person a real sense of purpose. It is always useful to encourage an elderly person to do some voluntary work helping other people, either the elderly, handicapped or children. Occasionally suitable part-time occupation is available and this is ideal. If the old person has physical limitations, routine activities should be continued for as long as possible, even if it is obvious that these are difficult. Thus, a woman should always be encouraged to look after the house even if she can only do a portion of the work.

Independence is very precious to the elderly. It is, therefore, important that relations do not take the old person permanently into their home, unless this is clearly inevitable, although many relatives are tempted to do this when difficulties arise. Children who precipitantly take their elderly parents into their homes may soon find it is a great mistake as the old person is not happy and more difficulties are caused. It is far better to arrange a temporary stay for a few weeks, so that the elderly person can retain her own home and independence.

HEALTH PROBLEMS IN THE ELDERLY

There are important differences between disease in elderly persons and other age groups. These can be summarized in the following five points:

1. *Social factors are far more important* with the elderly. To live in unsuitable surroundings is a disadvantage for any person but for an elderly person to do so may be quite disastrous. The cause of ill-health in many elderly persons is connected with poor living conditions which may also be the main reason why normal

treatment fails and relapses occur. For these reasons, *no one looking after an elderly person can afford to ignore social factors.*

2. *Multiple diseases* (the incidence at the same time of more than one disease in the same person) are common in the elderly but rare in all other age groups. An older person may present with heart failure but the cause of this may well be chronic bronchitis, ischaemic heart disease and anaemia or a combination of any two of these causes. This means that not only is diagnosis of the real cause made less easy, but treatment is more difficult, because one of the diseases may require a totally different type of treatment from the other, e.g. one may require rest and the other exercise.

4. *Rehabilitation is essential in the elderly.* In most younger persons there is considerable incentive for the individual to recover quickly so that he can get back to work or indulge in some favourite sport. Rehabilitation in younger people is relatively easy as the individual is keen to get back to normal. In elderly people, however, this motivation towards rehabilitation is often absent or not very marked, and it is most important that the doctor, nurse and social worker realize this so that special regimes can be introduced to ensure *active rehabilitation.*

4. In old persons, *the disability or limitation of function is often more important than the diagnosis.* It is essential to keep the old person as active as possible so that normal function about the house is maintained and the treatment of a number of serious conditions in old people is often modified because of these features. With young persons it is usual in most serious illness for the individual to go to bed. With many elderly persons it is much better to treat them in a chair in a warm room, as many serious complications (such as pneumonia) are much less likely if the old person can be kept up and more active in this way.

5. *Old people respond quite differently to many illnesses.* With infections, fever is often absent or very slight and its absence may give a false sense of security. However, *mental confusion* commonly presents as the main first sign of an infection or other acute illness in an old person. For this reason, the doctor, nurse or social worker should never ignore the sudden onset of mental confusion in an old person who previously had been quite normal, or assume that it is due to irreversible degenerative

causes. It is more likely to be caused by sudden acute illness which may respond quickly and completely to proper treatment.

The significance of these five differences is to make the care of the elderly a rather more complicated process than the care of younger persons. The recognition of this has been responsible in the last 20 years for the establishment of the speciality of *geriatrics*. Because of the extreme susceptibility of all elderly people to poor social conditions, a much closer link between the medical services and the social services in the community has been developed in geriatric practice.

One unusual condition mainly seen in old persons —*hypothermia*—illustrates many of these points and is now described.

Hypothermia

This is a serious condition in which the body loses heat and cannot maintain correct temperature control. It is extremely important that the methods of diagnosing and recognizing this condition are fully understood by doctors, nurses, health visitors and social workers, as hypothermia is a dangerous condition if not recognized and is particularly liable to occur in old people living alone at home in houses which are inadequately heated.

Hypothermia may also dangerously occur in elderly persons who have suddenly been taken ill (as in pneumonia) even though the elderly person is seated in a chair in a room which is not unduly cold. It can also occur after strokes, or after heart attacks in which the old person may sit quietly in a chair for hours on end.

Whatever the cause, it is most important that *the condition is recognized early* and that all staff dealing with the elderly know the early signs of hypothermia. The elderly person *does not usually look cold* and certainly does not shiver. The hands and face often appear warm and are red or reddish-purple in colour. The person often is drowsy and very inactive and his speech may become slow and slurred. Hands, feet, and face feel cold and the body temperature (as measured on a special low recording thermometer) is usually well below 35°C (95°F).

Once the condition is recognized, emergency treatment must be started which is often difficult and unsatisfactory. Rapid warming is very dangerous to old people with hypothermia and the aim should be to limit the warming up process to approximately 1°F per hour. The room should be kept warm and a few extra blankets should be used but *no direct heat* should be applied.

Prevention

The prevention of hypothermia involves three factors:

1. ensuring that, by good housing, elderly people are accommodated in warm conditions
2. encouraging old people to move around and not allow them to sit all day (even if they are in relatively warm conditions)
3. always being on the look out for hypothermia and realizing that it can develop slowly and unexpectedly, especially in elderly persons who are suffering from some illness

The full range of usual medical services from general practitioners is, of course, available to elderly persons living at home. In addition, there are: (1) special hospital services (geriatric services) (2) many nursing and preventive medical services provided by AHAs.

Special Geriatric Services

Old people use hospitals about twice as much as those under the age of 65 years. Although at any one time *only 2·5% of the elderly are in hospital, they occupy more than half of all the beds* and those over 75 nearly a third.

Although old people are often admitted to ordinary wards in acute hospitals, it is better if they are admitted to a geriatric unit. This may be a separate hospital or part of a general hospital. In such units, a complete medical and social investigation can take place as well as *special rehabilitation facilities* so necessary for successful treatment. The great difference between hospital care for the elderly and other age groups is that, with the elderly, there is often more than one system of the body diseased and producing symptoms. The investigation is, therefore, usually more involved and is further complicated by the fact that social circumstances of the patient do much to determine the outcome. There must therefore, be plenty of coordination between those working in the geriatric unit and the social services departments of neighbouring local authorities. The geriatric unit is concerned with initial diagnosis and treatment and rehabilitation; it therefore relies more on its physiotherapy section than other hospital units. Another essential stage is the *assessment of the more chronic cases* to decide whether they should be discharged: (*a*) home, often with special assistance such as attendance at a day hospital or day activity area within a hospital or if this is not available, at hospital outpatients for physiotherapy and occupational therapy; (*b*) to special residential accommodation (either hostels or sheltered housing); (*c*) to hospital chronic sick accommodation. Such units deal with two types of cases: firstly bedridden elderly persons suffering from a chronic illness in which there is no likelihood of marked improvement, and secondly severe psychogeriatric (senile dementia) patients.

Geriatric day hospitals (or day activity areas) help with the rehabilitation of elderly patients. They act as a half-way stage between hospital and home, patients being brought there by ambulance transport and returned home in the evening. Attendance may be daily or on a specified number of days per week, and physiotherapy and occupational therapy services are provided for old persons attending. There has been a dramatic increase in their use—attendances numbered 600 000 in 1971 but by 1976, had reached 1200 000.

The main value of day activity areas is: (1) they enable the elderly patient to be discharged home earlier, so encouraging independence; (2) they help with the rehabilitation of the patient; (3) they enable a better bridge to be maintained between the geriatric unit and the community services for the elderly.

It is valuable if *health visitors and social workers can visit the day hospital and geriatric units* periodically to assist in coordination between the two services. Recently community hospitals have been developed (see p. 166) and have been found very useful in dealing with elderly patients within the community.

Psychiatric services for the elderly

Reference has already been made in Chapter 25 to the increased incidence of mental illness in the elderly (over a quarter of all mental illness beds are now occupied by patients over the age of 75). Initial treatment usually takes place in the general hospital psychiatric unit and long term care in local or community hospitals. *There are increasing problems with the elderly mentally infirm.* The most severe cases ideally should be cared for in long stay hospital accommodation but there is a shortage of beds. Most mildly confused cases can be looked after at home if there is someone to care for her or alternatively she may settle in a hostel.

PRIMARY HEALTH CARE, COMMUNITY MEDICAL AND NURSING SERVICES

The appropriate health and nursing services provided to help elderly persons in the community are described in Chapters 7, 8 and 15 and include:

1. home nursing (see p. 164)
2. chiropody (see p. 167)
3. health education (see p. 159)
4. prevention of home accidents (see p. 265)
5. visual acuity (see p. 267)
6. nutrition of aged (see p. 268)

SOCIAL SERVICES AVAILABLE FOR THE ELDERLY

Prevention of mental deterioration

The mental state of the majority of old people living at home is good, for only about 11% show minor problems and 4% more serious symptoms. The prevention of mental deterioration in old age is closely connected with living in familiar surroundings and with having something useful to do. Human contact is also important and elderly persons living alone should be encouraged to visit clubs, luncheon centres, etc. for unless they have an opportunity to talk normally, their vocabulary will deteriorate and, with it, many mental processes. Recent research has shown that some form of *occupational therapy can do much to arrest the development of early senile dementia* by ensuring that the old person is given an opportunity to keep his mind active. Many problems and anxieties are due to the old person not properly understanding certain financial or legal problems and careful explanations and the sorting out of pension and legal difficulties such as rent, lease or will can often do much to help. Social workers spend much time in ensuring that elderly people understand the social services at present available.

It is always important to recognize promptly impending mental deterioration in the elderly at home, as it makes early treatment possible and may prevent a serious and perhaps final mental breakdown. Danger signs in such cases include:

1. *Change in outlook* of the old person—a change towards apathy or agitation.
2. *Eating habits may change*—the old person often becomes very fussy and will eat very little.
3. *Depression* becomes commoner. This may be associated with occasional outbreaks of verbal aggression making the old person difficult to live with.
4. *Memory*—a failure of memory is another sign or the old person may mislay things and accuse others of stealing them.
5. *Talk*—the usual tendency for old people to talk a lot disappears.
6. *Worries* become morbidly increased.
7. There is usually a marked loss in the ability of the old person to look after himself.

There may be quite marked swings in the behaviour pattern of elderly persons showing early mental deterioration. A visitor, such as a doctor or social worker, is very liable to see old persons at their best as they put on a special effort only to become just as abnormal within half an hour of the end of the visit.

Home help (see also Chapter 27)

In England in 1977, approximately 600 000 elderly persons were helped by the home help service. The main function of the home help is to assist the elderly in their homes, perhaps two or three times a week for 2–4 hours at a time. It has been estimated that approximately 10–15% of the elderly would benefit from such help. At each visit, the home help, usually a married woman, will do the housework, go out to collect essential shopping and prepare the old person a meal. They do not attempt to do all the housework, but rather tackle the jobs which the elderly person finds difficult because of her frailty. Thus the home help cleans the windows, gives the rooms a thorough cleaning, collects coal and does many of the heavier tasks. A charge is made for this service based on a sliding scale and this may mean that the elderly person with a reasonable income will pay full charge. But only a small minority can afford this and *elderly people living on a pension will be provided with free service.* The provision of home help services for the elderly is valuable and enables those to remain at home who otherwise would be too frail.

An important aspect of the home help's duties includes *observing the elderly at home in a sensible but inconspicuous way.* Someone visiting regularly in this way is in an excellent position to judge when the old person is becoming too frail to manage and adequate alternative arrangements can then be made.

Good neighbour schemes

In 1976, the Secretary of State for Social Services launched a national Good Neighbour Scheme designed to stimulate community support for the elderly; 8% of the bedfast or household elderly never receive visits from relatives and 47% never see friends. In addition to interesting themselves with the old person, Good Neighbours can help with shopping, minor household jobs, gardening, etc. and can completely alter the pattern of life of any frail elderly person living alone.

Meals-on-wheels

Meals-on-wheels is a service whereby a hot meal is taken to the old person at home. All social service departments provide meals-on-wheels either directly or with the assistance of the Woman's Royal Voluntary Service (WRVS). Such meals are cooked in large kitchens and are then put into special insulated containers and delivered by van. It is usual for one van and its team to collect and deliver in an urban community about 30–40 meals from 12 noon to 2 p.m., and again in the late afternoon deliver a light evening meal. A modest charge is made towards the cost of the meal, the content of which is specially planned to suit the elderly. Meals should ideally be supplied six days a week or at least three days a week (see Table 79, p. 512).

Luncheon clubs

Another excellent way in which social service departments help the elderly living at home is to provide lunch clubs to which old people can go for a meal say on three or four occasions a week. In many cases, the local branch of Age Concern provide helpers who serve the meals. These arrangements have *the added value that the old person is encouraged to leave her home*, get exercise and keep mobile, as well as benefiting from the social contacts at the centre. Some lunch clubs are held in specially built centres, but many are arranged in buildings such as church halls. A similar charge to that for meals-on-wheels is usually made.

Home care programmes

Recent surveys have shown that *one of the most critical times for many old people occurs when they are discharged home from hospital after an illness.* Elderly persons living on their own are particularly susceptible to rapid deterioration at such a time. New home care programmes are being experimented with to support old people at such times. One such programme aims at providing home help and meals services plus home nursing services for 20% of elderly persons discharged from hospital (selected to include those at greatest risk) for at least four weeks following discharge. A feature of such schemes is that consultants and hospital social workers select the cases to be helped and give *at least one week's notice of discharge* so that the home help and other services *can be waiting for the old person on discharge.* At the end of the four week period those in need of further help are assisted through the normal home help services enabling the special home care programme staff to care for new discharges.

Further experimental schemes are linked with special geriatric teams (of doctors and nurses) to treat an acutely ill person at home in the case of an acute illness in the hope that the elderly person can be rapidly improved within four to five days and thus prevent the need for admission to hospital (which in itself is very unsettling for many old people and the starting point of deterioration).

Clubs and handicraft centres

Many old people enjoy the social life at a club or rest centre, where they can enjoy the company of others. Some elderly people also attend a *handicraft centre at which they can carry out some recreational hobby*, and the value of this provision is the interest it creates. Recent research has emphasized the usefulness of handicrafts in arresting the development of early senile dementia. Clubs, rest centres and handicraft centres are provided both by social service departments and by many voluntary bodies. In many instances, there is a joint arrangement whereby the local authority provides the building and pays the running costs, while the voluntary staff run the centre.

Day centres

Many social service departments and voluntary bodies provide day centres which elderly people can visit during the day. Simple meals are often served at such centres and in some various handicrafts are also encouraged.

Day care centres

These provide an entirely different service and have often been referred to as 'hostels without beds' as they are intended to care for frail elderly people requiring the kind of care and attention which is often provided in hostels. *The old person is brought to the day care centre daily by transport* and is provided there with all meals and other services usually found in hostels. In the evening, transport takes the old person back again to their home.

This form of care is particularly useful where a frail old person is living with younger relatives who both go out to work during the day, and means that the elderly person can be looked after during the day without the need to be admitted permanently to a hostel. It also has been used to help old people living alone by taking them to a day care centre on two to three days a week so that they do not lose contact with the community outside. Problems do arise in some of these instances where the old person has to return to an empty and perhaps cold house in the evening. For this reason, it is best to link such arrangements with help from a good neighbour scheme.

Visiting

Regular visiting of old people living at home is an important function of social service departments. The numbers are so large that only those needing special attention can be visited regularly. Social workers concentrate upon those elderly people who urgently need special accommodation and determine the priority for admission to hostels and make adequate arrangements for those who cannot immediately be accommodated. This will include the arranging of home helps or meals-on-wheels. Health visitors are continuously visiting many families and will also be seeing many elderly persons living at home. Special arrangements are usually made for a link between geriatric hospitals, social workers, and health visitors to assist in the after-care of elderly persons recently discharged from hospital. They also visit those elderly persons being investigated in outpatient departments and those in need of after-care. *Voluntary visiting is also very important* and is increasingly arranged by community councils and other neighbourhood groups. In many instances, it is possible for a friendly visitor to be found who will call on the old person regularly.

Financial help

In many cases, *financial problems still arise, for many elderly persons worry excessively about money* and may stint themselves trying to economize, even when their financial circumstances are quite sound. This anxiety about money increases with age. The visitor must repeatedly explain pension entitlements, the true nature of Social Security and to what extra help the old person may be entitled (such as rent or rate rebates). Aid may be needed to complete pension and other forms.

Help with heating costs

Considerable concern has been expressed recently about the sharp increase in fuel prices which have affected the elderly more than any other group. Quarterly gas and electricity bills have caused difficulties and wherever possible pay-as-you-go schemes have been introduced to help the elderly on low budgets. Pensioners are now largely protected against disconnection of gas and electricity under the *Code of Practice* (introduced by the Government in 1977). Additional Supplementary Benefit can be paid to old persons in special need of extra fuel. Local authorities have started loft insulation schemes in their council houses and priority has been given to the elderly.

Outings and holidays

Most social service departments arrange special summer outings for old people and this is also supplemented by voluntary bodies. One important provision is for holidays for the elderly living alone or for those living with a family, as a separate holiday may be of value both to the old person and the family. Some local authorities own holiday homes while others may make block bookings at a seaside resort.

Rent rebates

Under the Housing Finance Act, 1972, local authority housing tenants can obtain a rent rebate when the gross income is below a certain level. Nearly 800 000 receive assistance in this way with their rents.

Rate rebates

There is a national scheme of special rate rebates which are available to all elderly persons over the age of 65. The scheme is based on a sliding scale by which elderly persons living on low incomes are excused a substantial part of their local rates (under the General Rate Act, 1967); 1·8 million pensioners benefit from rate rebates.

Bus passes or concessionary fares

Most local authorities have introduced special schemes by which elderly persons can obtain special free passes or concessionary fares on their buses. These schemes vary in different parts of the country and in an increasing number of authorities are available to women over 60 and men over 65 years of age who are in receipt of a pension. Most schemes enable the old person to travel free in non-peak periods of the day (9.30 a.m. to 4.30 p.m.). The value of these schemes is very great because they encourage independence in the elderly and remove any constraint on travelling to visit relatives and friends. Previously the high cost of bus fares prevented many elderly people from travelling and led to their isolation. British Rail also offers reduced fares for the elderly.

Accommodation

Houses, flats, bungalows or flatlets

All authorities provide special housing accommodation for the elderly. The type of dwelling varies with the district. In urban areas, small flats and flatlets are popular and these should be compactly planned with all accommodation on one floor and easily reached by lift. An ideal arrangement is bedsitting room with kitchenette and small bathroom. Heating should be automatic—either electric or central heating. In rural areas, bungalows are ideal.

Collective homes

There is an increasing need for a combination home to be provided along the pattern of the collective home so popular in Denmark, and local authorities have planned similar projects. Flatlets are provided in conjunction with a small old persons' home and large restaurant. The old people live in the flatlets and are provided with a regular midday meal in the attached restaurant, the charge for which is included in their rent. They stay in the flatlets for as long as possible but, if they become too frail to remain in them, they have priority to enter the old persons' home. This means that the old people need never leave the district and, when they become very frail, are cared for by the staff already known to them.

Sheltered housing

Many different types of 'sheltered housing' have been provided during the last five years. The essential feature of 'sheltered housing' is specially built or adapted accommodation often in a flatlet or flat for old people with a *resident warden in attendance* to ensure that the old person can get help in an emergency. The old people living in such accommodation are all capable of looking after themselves, but can remain safely in such accommodation much longer if there is a resident warden to help. The housing accommodation is provided by housing authorities (district councils in county areas or metropolitan districts or in accommodation built by housing trusts or voluntary bodies).

The Social Services Committee usually pays a varying sum annually to those providing sheltered accommodation dependent upon the facilities provided (from £50 to £130 per unit of sheltered housing), as a contribution towards the cost of providing the resident warden, the alarm system, telephone installations, or other communal facilities (midday meals, lifts, TV room, central heating, etc.). In this way, encouragement is given to the provision of extra facilities which will help to enable the old person to remain independent as long as possible.

Many social service departments are now concentrating on rapidly developing more different types of such sheltered accommodation rather than extending their hostel provision. This is because sheltered housing provides a better and more normal answer and is more popular with the elderly since it encourages independence. Sheltered housing is also cheaper to provide (an important feature at a time when new capital development is difficult). New schemes of community support (visiting, home helps, good neighbours, meals services, various care programmes) are being rapidly developed to enable frail old people to stay longer in such accommodation. In particular, it is important to concentrate upon times of great stress when the old person is at special risk, such as during illness or on returning home after a spell in hospital (see home care programme, p. 500).

Hostels for old people

Under the National Assistance Act, 1948, *every social services department has to provide hostels for elderly persons.* Most modern hostels are specially designed but a few have been converted from large houses. Each hostel usually contains from 35–50 old people as a larger one would not maintain the friendly atmosphere which is so important. The majority of bedrooms are single but some double rooms are provided. There are lounges of varying sizes on each floor and a lift is always provided so that all the accommodation is of the ground floor type eliminating the climbing of stairs. A resident matron is in charge and she and her staff look after minor illnesses, but more prolonged or serious cases are admitted to hospital, returning when fit. The residents receive medical attention from a general practitioner just as if they were living in their own home. The standard of care is very high and all needs, including clothing, are provided.

One important feature is that every resident contributes to the cost of their accommodation. Each hostel has a *standard charge* which represents the economic weekly cost of a resident and every old person entering a hostel is asked if they can afford to pay this. If they can, they do so. If not, each resident must pay a proportion of his/her old age pension leaving approximately £3.90 (1978) a week pocket money for personal spending. The local authority is then responsible for the additional cost. This financial arrangement ensures that every old person (even if his only income is an old age pension) contributes to the cost. The type and standard of accommodation are the same for all, regardless of the amount paid.

Every attempt is made to ensure that modern old people's homes have no institutional atmosphere. However, as the numbers of elderly persons rise in the country very frail old people are now being looked after in hostels. Quite a number of these are mildly confused and a few suffer from incontinence. Although everything is done by the staff of the hostel to encourage the residents to be active, increasing numbers seem unable to respond because of their frailty. The increasing numbers of elderly mentally infirm present particular problems in residential homes. Their presence can be very disturbing to others and make staffing difficult. Some homes now segregate the very confused from others and special homes for the elderly mentally infirm are now also being developed.

Hostels do not set out to provide accommodation for chronic sick old people; that is a responsibility of the Health Services. The dividing line between social services and health services is whether the old person needs constant nursing care—if so, he is the responsibility of the health services not social services. The frailest old people local authorities can care for in their hostels are those who can do all the following: (1) get up daily; (2) dress, even if only with assistance; (3) make their way across a room with help; (4) eat a meal without assistance.

Legislation

Emergency compulsory admission of old people

Under section 47 of the National Assistance Act, 1948, and the Amendment Act, 1951, power is given for the compulsory removal of aged and certain other persons to hospital or other institutions.

Those who can be compulsorily removed must be: (*a*) suffering from grave chronic disease or being aged, infirm or physically incapacitated, are living in insanitary conditions; *and* (*b*) are unable to devote to themselves, and are not receiving from other persons, proper care and attention.

The Area Specialist in Community Medicine (Environmental

Health) or District Community Physician and another doctor must certify that it is in the interests of the person to remove him from his dwelling. This being so, the local authority (through the social services department) applies to a magistrate (or court) for removal. If the magistrate (or court) is satisfied, then the order for removal to hospital or institution is made.

Few elderly people are removed in this way as the majority readily agree or can be persuaded, but occasionally action is necessary. Such cases are old people who have neglected themselves badly or who are very ill, such as those suffering from late neoplastic disease, and who are afraid to go into hospital. If a general practitioner meets with such a case and cannot persuade the patient, it is best to apply to the Director of Social Services who will arrange the necessary medical examinations and, if necessary, compulsory removal.

27 Other Community Social Services

Home Helps

Local authorities have a duty to provide home helps and all have developed these services. The Local Authority Social Services Act, 1970 transferred the control of the home help service from the health services to the Social Services Committee and to the Director of Social Services.

The object of the home help service is to provide assistance in the home where because of age, maternity, or acute or chronic illness (physical or mental), the housewife cannot look after the home. In 1976, 652 800 clients were helped in England in this way and it is interesting to note how these were made up (Table 78).

TABLE 78 Number of persons receiving home help, England, 1976

Old age (65 years and over)	570 400	(87·3%)
Chronic sickness and tuberculosis	43 200	(6·6%)
Other	29 100	(4·5%)
Maternity	5800	(0·9%)
Mentally disordered	4300	(0·7%)
Total	652 800	

(From *Health and Personal Social Services Statistics for England*, 1977, OPCS)

It will be noticed that elderly people make up by far the largest group of clients (87·3%) and the percentage of them is steadily increasing. This trend is not only due to the ever larger number of elderly persons living within the community, but also because most of them qualify for free service, being pensioners. There is a sliding scale of charges for home help service—the full charge now is about 98p per hour—but those on social security or those receiving old age pensions as their only income are given the service free.

In England in 1976, there were 88 065 home helps; the majority worked part-time and thus were equivalent to 42 141 whole time staff.

Duties of home helps

The duties of each home help include many of the usual tasks carried out by the housewife: cleaning rooms, preparing food and meals, cooking, shopping, lighting fires, and looking after the children (if any), etc.

Service can be provided for a client on a full-time or part-time basis and will vary from a few hours a week to full-time attendance. In the majority of instances, and especially in those receiving help over a long period of time (as with the elderly), home help service is provided for two to three sessions per week. In this way it is possible for the home help to provide service for more persons and, at the same time, encourage the elderly person to continue to do quite a lot of her housework herself and keep herself active for as long as possible. By sensible use of the home help service, together with the meals-on-wheels service, it is often possible to keep an elderly person living in her own at home for some years longer than would otherwise be the case.

For the acute and sudden illness in the housewife or in a maternity case, it is usual to provide full-time help for the period of the emergency or at least for two to four weeks until other arrangements can be made by the family. Of course, in many instances, such sudden emergencies can be looked after by other members of the family; the home help service is however, a most valuable safeguard for the family which has few adult relatives and is especially useful for those living in a large city or suburban area where neighbourly help is not so common as in country districts.

The home help soon gets to know very well the elderly person she is permanently visiting and learns a great deal about her personal problems. For this reason, it is important that home helps work in close contact with social workers, for the home help will act as a very useful source of information about elderly persons living alone. The majority of home helps are women aged 25 to 65 but recently a few men have been recruited in some areas. Male helpers generally undertake especially dirty or heavy work. They also have been used successfully to help difficult old men or people whose behaviour might be unacceptable to women. Occasionally specialized cleaning equipment is taken to the home in a specially equipped van to clean up very dirty houses in readiness for someone about to be discharged from hospital.

Organization of home help services

Most social service departments have a senior home help organizer directly responsible to an assistant director of social services (see Fig. 22, p. 392). Although the senior home help organizer is responsible for recruitment and training, the day to day control and deployment of staff is being linked in more and more authorities with the new area teams of social workers. In this way, the very closest links are maintained with social workers. In each area social work team, there is usually an assistant home help organizer to help with assessment of need, distribution of home help services and with the supervision of the home helps.

Referrals

Referrals for home help services still come mainly from the health service although social workers are increasingly requesting home help services for their clients.

An increase in demand for home helps has been noticed from primary health care teams especially from those with health visitor attachments. Hospital referrals still account for many new cases and the increase in hospital geriatric services has swelled the demand for more home help services. For the individual general practitioner (or hospital doctor, especially geriatrician) who wishes to arrange home help service for his patients, a request should be made locally first to the Director of Social Services who will give the address of the local supervisor of home helps.

Good neighbour schemes

There is usually a waiting list for those requiring home help services and a few authorities have experimented with an official good neighbour scheme in which a local volunteer is sought who will agree to carry out a number of the lighter duties of home helps—shopping, lighting a fire, cooking, etc. Such good neighbour schemes are different from the scheme the Secretary of State introduced in 1976 (see p. 499). Often an individual recruited as a good neighbour lives close by to the old person requiring assistance so that no travelling is involved. It is usual to pay the good neighbour an honorarium based on the number of tasks undertaken per week; for a full-time type of service involving some help on most or all days per week, the honorarium would be about £4–5 per week.

Meals Services

Brief reference has been made (p. 499) to the meals-on-wheels and luncheon club services provided by social service departments for the elderly.

This is a rapidly developing service which, although designed mainly to help the elderly, also assists many severely disabled persons living at home. In England approximately 41 million meals were provided in 1976, 60% being delivered to the client's home (meals-on-wheels) and 40% being served in various day centres and luncheon clubs. The growth of meals services has been most marked in London and the large provincial cities where much of the expansion has been provided by direct development by social service departments, and has been made possible by greater use of frozen foods and packing each meal in a foil disposable pack. In the rural and country areas and in smaller towns, the service still largely depends on the help of voluntary bodies such as the WRVS. In the large towns, special delivery vans are used and in many instances lunch and a light supper is provided to ensure that maximum use is made of the cooking and delivery services. In country areas many of the meals are still delivered by volunteers in private cars.

In the last few years a survey has been carried out each November to establish the number of meals which each recipient receives in that week. The figures for 1976 are given in Table 79.

TABLE 79 Main meals provided in recipients' homes, England, 1976

1 meal	7·6%	5 meals	18·5%
2 meals	43·6%	6 meals	1·7%
3 meals	17·7%	7 meals	2·9%
4 meals	8·0%		

(From *Health and Personal Social Services Statistics for England*, 1977, OPCS)

Comparison with earlier years shows that the proportion of persons receiving more meals per week is gradually rising but still the majority of meals-on-wheels are served twice a week to old people at home. In day centres, over half of the persons taking meals have them on at least five days per week.

Referral for meals

Referrals for meals come from the health services (especially geriatric hospitals and primary health care teams with health visitor attachment) and from area social service teams. Most social service departments arrange for meals to be prepared and distributed centrally but increasingly all referrals for new meals are being dealt with directly by area teams of social workers. Any doctor wishing to arrange for a meals service for his patients should contact the local Area Social Services Officer.

HOMELESSNESS

The Housing (Homeless Persons) Act, 1977

On 1 December 1977 a new Act—the Housing (Homeless Persons) Act, 1977—came into force in England and Wales. The main effect of this Act was to transfer the responsibility and duty for providing temporary accommodation for those who are in urgent need of help because they were homeless, from social services authorities to local housing authorities (metropolitan district councils and other district councils). *These local housing authorities now have a clear legal duty to assist those who are homeless* or who are threatened with homelessness. *Social services authorities are still required to cooperate with a housing authority* by giving reasonable assistance to them *by giving clients who are homeless or threatened with homelessness social work support and advice.*

The Act also requires all authorities, in carrying out their functions, to have regard to the *Code of Guidance* which has been issued by the Department of the Environment, the DHSS and the Welsh Office which should always be consulted by staff who wish to clarify some detailed point under the Act.

Definitions

A person is defined as homeless if he has no accommodation which he can occupy (together with any other person who normally resides with him as a member of his family or household). This would include a housekeeper or companion living with an elderly or disabled person. Details are given in the Code of Guidance of circumstances which may render a person homeless because he cannot use his accommodation, i.e. he cannot secure entry to it or he has a mobile home (caravan or boat) but has no place to put it.

A person is *'threatened with homelessness'* if he is likely to become homeless within 28 days. Authorities should, however, preferably advise and help people where the possibility of their becoming homeless is known more than 28 days in advance (rent arrears cases), i.e. they are encouraged to undertake prevention of homelessness.

Priority need

The Act introduces a new concept—it divides those who are homeless into priority cases and others. For all priority cases (unless they have become homeless intentionally), the *local housing authority has a clear legal responsibility to find them suitable permanent accommodation.* Others must be given temporary help and advice. There are four main categories of priority need:

1. A person who has one or more children living with them. The Code of Guidance notes that all those under 16 and others under the age of 19 who are either receiving full-time education or training or are otherwise unable to support themselves should be considered to come into the category of 'children'.

2. A person who has become homeless as the result of an emergency: fire, flood or other disaster.
3. A person has a priority need if his household includes *one or more persons who are vulnerable* for the following reasons:
   a. *Old age:* those above normal retirement age (65 for a man and 60 for a woman) and any others approaching normal retirement age who are particularly frail or in poor health or vulnerable for any other reason.
   b. *Mental illness* or *mental handicap* or *physical disability*.
   c. Special cases. The Code of Guidance particularly mentions battered women without children who are at risk of further pursuit or violence (if they were to return to the marital home) and *homeless young people who are at risk of sexual and financial exploitation*.
   d. *Pregnant women*, together with anyone who lives, or might reasonably be expected to live with them; this includes all pregnant women irrespective of the length of time they have been pregnant.

Intentional homelessness

The Act differentiates between whether the person has become homeless by chance or intentionally and this will be relevant to the obligations of the housing authority towards those who are homeless, even those who have a priority need. The Code of Guidance makes it clear that the numbers of those to be regarded as having become homeless intentionally are expected to be small. Generally for someone to have become homeless intentionally three features must be satisfied:

a. the person must have deliberately done, or failed to do, something in consequence of which he ceased to occupy accommodation which was at the time available, or if he is threatened with homelessness, something of which the likely result was that he would be forced to leave such accommodation
b. it must have been reasonable for him to continue to occupy the accommodation
c. he must have been aware of all the relevant facts (an act or omission in good faith on the part of someone unaware of any relevant facts is *not* to be regarded as deliberate)

The Code of Guidance gives examples. A person who chooses to sell his home, or who has lost it because of wilful and persistent refusal to pay rent, would in most cases be regarded as having become homeless intentionally. But if the person was obliged to sell because he could not keep up the mortgage repayments, or got into rent arrears, this would not be intentional because of real personal or financial difficulties, if he was incapable of managing his affairs on account of old age or mental illness or some physical disability, his act or omissions would *not* be regarded as deliberate and his homelessness would not have been intentional.

A battered woman who has fled the marital home *should never* be regarded as having become homeless intentionally.

A person who is unaware that they are entitled to rent allowances or rebates or other welfare benefits and therefore gets into rent arrears and may be evicted would not be classified as 'intentional homelessness'. In the same way, those who have left rented accommodation on receipt of notices to quit because they were unaware of their legal rights as tenants would not be intentionally homeless.

In all instances where the question of possible intentional homelessness arises, the Act makes it quite clear that it is for the housing authority to satisfy themselves whether someone who approaches them became homeless intentionally. The onus is *not* on the applicant to satisfy the authority that he did not do so. If the authority is not satisfied that he became homeless intentionally, the applicant is automatically entitled to full benefits of the Act.

Duties of Housing Authorities to Those Who are Homeless

For those with a priority need

Homelessness not intentional

The housing authority in this case *has a duty to provide permanent self-contained accommodation as soon as possible.* Usually this will mean local authority housing accommodation and this must be provided if there is no alternative. The accommodation offered must be reasonably convenient and avoid undue disruption of education or employment. Other types of housing may be arranged by the local housing authority such as accommodation in the privately rented sector with perhaps a rent allowance; another housing authority may be able to offer accommodation; new or expanding towns may offer opportunities for a new start in a different environment for those who want to move; housing associations or other voluntary bodies may be able to help. A mortgage may be arranged for those who may wish to consider house purchase.

In the case of persons under the age of 18 years a *social services department may underwrite a tenancy agreement where this would be appropriate.*

Where people are homeless because they have a caravan but no site, the housing authority are not obliged to make equivalent accommodation available. The authority may, however, arrange for the County Council to make available a site (note that County District Councils do *not* need to provide a gypsy caravan site). Or the District Council may provide some other form of permanent housing.

All accommodation provided *must enable the family* (or other members of the homeless household) *to live together.* The practice of splitting families is not acceptable even for short periods. *Under no circumstances should children be brought into care because their family are homeless* (this also applies to families whose homelessness is intentional).

Homeless persons with a priority need should not be obliged to spend a certain period of time in interim accommodation as a matter of policy. In rare cases, however, where it is the opinion of the social services authority that a person is in need of a greater degree of care and support than is available in any form of housing, they may offer that person a place in accommodation provided by them under section 21(1) (c) or 21(1) of the National Assistance Act 1948 and schedule S(1) of the National Health Service Act 1977. (In such cases the Housing Authority will have fulfilled their duty.)

Where it is not possible to arrange a permanent long term housing solution straight away, some *form of interim arrangements must be made for the household.* Such arrangements must enable members of the household to remain together and self-contained accommodation is needed, although for very short periods, reception centres or hostels can be used. For women who have been subject to violence, a woman's refuge in the area could be a sensible interim arrangement. As a last resort accommodation in lodgings, guest houses or bed and breakfast hotels may be used but these are generally considered unsatisfactory. Where families have to leave their rooms during the day (as in bed and breakfast arrangements), day centre provision should be provided.

The prevention of further homelessness should always be borne in mind. Where homeless families have been rehoused, it is important, particularly during the early weeks of the tenancy, to maintain contact to avoid circumstances developing which might lead to their becoming homeless again. In appropriate cases, social services departments should be able to help. It is most important that families who have become homeless due to financial difficulties should be given up-to-date relevant information or rent rebates and other financial assistance, and arrangements for direct payment of rent or rent guarantees.

Homeless is intentional

For those with a priority need but who have become homeless intentionally, the local housing authority is obliged:

1. to provide accommodation for the household on a temporary basis 'for such period as the authority consider will afford them a reasonable opportunity to secure accommodation'
2. to provide advice and assistance

In such cases, the legal responsibility for obtaining permanent accommodation rests with the homeless people themselves, but the Code of Guidance makes it quite clear that Housing Authorities should respond as helpfully and constructively as possible by giving widespread advice on financial aspects of accommodation, rent rebates and allowances and mortgages. Housing authorities are also asked to do all they can to ensure accommodation is secured. Such clients should be registered on the housing waiting list and section 6 (2) of the Housing (Homeless Persons) Act, 1977 amends section 113 (2) of the Housing Act, 1957 so that all persons who are homeless or threatened with homelessness, whether or not they have a priority need or become homeless intentionally are now added to the groups which a housing authority must give reasonable preference to in the selection of tenants.

As already mentioned, *children should never be received into care simply on the grounds of their parents' homelessness* and, in such cases, even though homelessness may have been intentional, local housing authorities should take all possible steps to ensure such families are not left without shelter.

For those who do not have a priority need (whether intentional or not)

For all such cases, the housing authority have a duty to give advice and assistance as they consider appropriate in any attempts the homeless person may make to obtain or retain accommodation for himself. That is the minimum statutory requirement, but the Code of Guidance indicates that authorities should do all they can to help, and that such assistance should always be positive and should include registration on the housing waiting list, help through a housing aid centre and the referral to housing associations or voluntary bodies. Lists of accommodation agencies, hostels, lodging and possible accommodation in the privately owned sector should be maintained and advice offered.

Local connections

If the housing authority considers that the homeless household has no local connection with their area but that there is such a connection with another area, section 5 of the Housing (Homeless Persons) Act 1977 provides that they may notify the other authority. *Providing there will be no risk of domestic violence, the duty may then transfer to the notified authority.* But in all such cases the original authority (to whom the homeless family first turned for help) must provide accommodation or advice. Their responsibility only passes to the notified authority when that authority accepts the position and, in all such cases, the homeless family or householder *must* be notified in writing.

Incidence of homelessness

The problem of homelessness has been growing steadily during the last 10 years but has now become fairly static. In 1976, in England, there were 33 680 applications made by homeless families to local authorities for help. The majority of these came from large urban connurbations (38% came from the Greater London area). The types of last accommodation and the reasons for becoming homeless are given in Table 80. As regards reasons for becoming homeless, disputes of various kinds made up the largest simple cause followed by repossession by landlords requiring the home, illegal letting and rent arrears.

TABLE 80 Homeless households: by type of last accommodation and by reason for loss of accommodation: application to local authorities England, 1976

	Percentage
Type of last accommodation	
Living with friends/relatives	28
Owner-occupied	14
Local or public authority	14
Rented	
private unfurnished	9
private furnished	11
Housing Association	1
Tied accommodation/rent-free	12
Squat	3
All other tenures	8
Reasons for loss of accommodation	
Dispute	39
husband, wife, cohabitee	13
other relatives	19
other	7
Rent arrears	8
Illegal letting/unauthorized occupancy	4
Landlord requires/repossessed	10
All other cases	39
Total number of applications	33 680

(From *Social Trends,* 1977, OPCS)

Prevention of homelessness

The prevention of homelessness is more important than its treatment and is a responsibility of all local government and especially of housing authorities and social service authorities. In London boroughs and metropolitan districts, the same local authority is responsible for housing and for social services. It should therefore be possible in all instances for a completely collaborative approach to be adopted. In non-metropolitan counties it is the local district council which is responsible for housing and the larger county council for social services. It is therefore necessary for the closest cooperation and collaboration to be developed between these two authorities if the problem of homelessness is to be prevented.

In the future, it is hoped to arrange for housing authorities to provide temporary and permanent accommodation for the homeless and for social service departments to provide the social work support services to help sort out and particularly to play *a more active role in the prevention of homelessness.* In particular, a very crucial period is that which immediately follows the rehousing of a family which has been homeless. Many families need support and help if they are to avoid further problems (especially financial ones) and thus be in danger of a further loss of home.

Methods of dealing with evictions and rent arrears

Some of those who are homeless have left when they get their first notice to quit and before a possession order has been obtained.

Rent arrears is a serious problem and the following is a list of a number of actions which housing and social service departments can undertake to deal with it without resorting to eviction (which will only create more difficult problems for many local authorities).

1. An early warning system after a few missed payments should be instituted to enable special arrangements for rent collection to be made, and for social service advice to be sought.
2. If rent arrears are still accumulating, housing authorities should check whether the tenants are eligible for rent and rate rebates.
3. There should be a vigorous pursuit of rent arrears and this should include selective visiting in certain cases to prevent the arrears becoming greater.
4. If there are serious family and social problems, it may be possible to assist by payments of rent arrears, using powers of Section 1 of the Children and Young Persons Act, 1963.

5. If the family are receiving supplementary benefit, then this will contain a sum equivalent to the rent (the rent element) and arrangements can be made in suitable cases for this to be paid directly to the local authority.
6. It may be appropriate for a civil action to be taken to recover the debt and subsequent deduction of earnings where a person is in regular employment. In such cases, a careful watch must be kept to ensure that the current rent is paid after the Court decision.
7. Transfer to cheaper accommodation to help reduce a tenant's financial difficulties. A difficulty with this action is that a concentration of families in social difficulties (a ghetto) could be created.

If all these measures fail and the tenant refuses to move without a court order for possession, an eviction notice might have to be issued followed by proceedings for possession. Such action should only be taken as a last resort and only if the authority is satisfied that other accommodation is available.

Where private landlords are concerned, similar arrangements should be taken to set up an adequate early warning system. The social services department should arrange for information about such cases to be sent to it early to enable effective preventive work to be undertaken. Such a link-up should include County Courts, Housing Associations, Probation Officers, Housing Aid Centres, Citizens' Advice Bureaux.

After-care of homeless families

As already stressed, it is essential that active rehabilitation work is carried out on many of the families rehoused in permanent housing accommodation. As might be expected, in a number of instances, the parents are immature and often inadequate and have drifted into debt or into serious family problems. Just rehousing them in council accommodation without any further help has often been shown to be of little use, for invariably further problems recur. Such families need continuous help from social workers especially in the early stages of their resettlement. Such help may need to be given periodically over two to three years.

Single homeless

There is a special difficult group of homeless persons who have been described as 'rootless'—they are without a settled way of life. Such a group contains a very wide range of persons: some are elderly lonely old people, others are young 'drop-outs' who have lost their family ties and seem to be drifting. They are often referred to as 'social inadequates'. There is a close connection within this group with persons who have a heavy drinking problem or suffer from mental ill-health or may have some physical handicap such as epilepsy. Others are addicted to drugs or gambling and seem to be unable to cope with modern life without continuing support and supervision. Some sleep rough and are seen to congregate in the inner city areas of large cities. Recently there has been far less of a tendency for such persons to travel continuously (like tramps of 40 years ago) and the problem is becoming increasingly local.

The care of the single homeless (some of whom do not strictly come within the priority groups defined in the Housing (Homeless Persons) Act 1977) is a very special problem, not only because of the diversity of the individuals who make up the group, but because many of them reject the attempts made by authorities and voluntary bodies to organize their lives on a more structured basis. The Supplementary Benefits Commission is responsible for approximately 20 directly administered reception centres (or reception and day centres) throughout the country, including eight in London. It also supports by grants many voluntary and church bodies who are active in caring for the single homeless. *CHAR (Campaign for Single Homeless People)* is the umbrella organization for voluntary bodies working in this field and regular meetings are held between the Supplementary Benefits Commission and CHAR to improve services.

Research into the problems of the single homeless is supported by DHSS—currently there is an Action Research Project of the St Mungo Community and this has included a study of comparison between the St Mungo Community and the Camberwell and Battersea Reception Centres. The Institute of Psychiatry is also conducting further research into the social and medical characteristics of men who are admitted to London reception centres other than Camberwell and to assess the short term resettlement functions of these centres.

Because of the concentration of social problems among the single homeless, some social services departments (especially in large connurbations) have a specialized small section of social workers whose main task is to help the single homeless. Other local authorities give grants to various voluntary and church bodies who have set up various services for this group.

28 Hospital Social Workers

Medical training and practice are concerned with the recognition and understanding of various physical signs and symptoms which result from pathological changes in the human body. In many instances, successful diagnosis follows the correct linking together of physical signs and symptoms and the many complicated biochemical, radiological and other tests carried out. There is however a further factor which must always be considered—*the individual reaction of the patient to the various social circumstances in his life (his environment)*. These play some part in the production of most illness but in some they are predominant and are then often spoken of as '*psychosomatic*'.

In the treatment and management of all illness the reaction of the patient to the various social factors which he faces (his family, his job, etc.) are often quite crucial. Where the illness is largely produced by the psychological reaction of the patient (the psychosomatic diseases), successful diagnosis and treatment is dependent upon the ability to understand, change or influence for the better the patient's reaction and adjustment to these social aspects.

This is particularly so in any longstanding or permanent illness such as a congenital abnormality, or a disabling condition such as rheumatoid arthritis, multiple sclerosis or hemiplegia or a sudden serious accident. Also the reaction of the patient and family is often most important in a terminal illness (leading to the death of the patient) and this is especially so in some incurable cancers which come on suddenly in middle age.

Doctors are taught to appreciate the importance of social

factors in diagnosis and treatment but, especially in hospitals, the unravelling of many of the more complicated social features in disease is undertaken at the request of the consultant by a trained social worker—the *hospital social worker.* Her work in all its aspects forms part of a team approach and assists and complements that of the consultant and his medical team.

The numbers of hospital social workers has steadily increased in the last 30 years and their tasks have altered considerably since their predecessors were appointed as 'almoners', who were among the earliest social workers and were functioning in some hospitals at the end of the last century.

At present there are approximately 2250 hospital social workers. Most of these work in district general hospitals or in geriatric and paediatric units. Those who work in psychiatric hospitals and are specially qualified are called *psychiatric social workers.*

These are four main areas of work for hospital social workers.

1. *Medical casework* concerned with the adjustment of the patient and his/her family to their disease. This is the largest and most important aspect of hospital social work. It mainly involves working with the patient in hospital (including in-patient and out-patient work) but may also necessitate the hospital social worker visiting the patient's home.
2. *Environmental help*—arranging how the patient's home can be assisted to help cope with the illness. This may involve complete rehousing of the patient or the adaptation of the home either structurally or by the introduction of certain aids.
3. Arrangements of *immediate assistance to the patient* or his relatives. This includes financial help, convalescent arrangements, provision of escorts and accommodation for relatives.
4. *Liaison with various other social work agencies* to enable long term care and assistance to be provided for the patient.

The nature of hospital social work, its value and its limitations can best be illustrated by a series of examples now given which are classified under the four main general headings.

MEDICAL CASEWORK

Casework by hospital social workers is undertaken for most types of patients and for most ages. There is however a greater need in certain age groups who are potentially more vulnerable. Hence more work is done with children, elderly persons, and certain groups who obviously are going to face more social problems—unmarried mothers, patients who show signs of maladjustment (anxiety states, suicides, alcoholics), the homeless and any other patient who obviously has an acute difficult personal problem—marital difficulties would be an obvious example.

Another important group to the hospital social worker is the longstanding or chronic patient especially if he/she has a disability. After the acute treatment of any such patient has been carried out, the next stage—successful rehabilitation back into the patient's own home and normal life (back to employment) may depend on solving as many social problems as medical ones. For instance *mobility is of paramount importance for anyone who is going to return successfully to work.* The hospital social worker is expected to know how these can be best dealt with and has the responsibility to arrange all the various solutions—special transport, industrial training, special housing, etc. (see below).

Hospital Social Work with Children

A particular problem seen in paediatric work is connected with congenital disabilities of all kinds. Their recognition, diagnosis and treatment is obviously a task for health visitors and midwives, paediatricians and all their specialized teams which will include hospital social workers. Many parents find it very difficult to accept and adjust to the realization that their young baby is seriously disabled and may always be so. *There is a natural tendency for all such parents to disbelieve the paediatrician* and not to accept the true position. Very often the parent will rationalize this natural disbelief by suggesting that the doctor is wrong or that there must be some treatment which will help. Any tendency on the part of the medical team to become impatient with such an attitude can quickly result in the parent seeking other medical help—perhaps privately in another part of this country or even abroad. They may even, in extreme cases, spend large sums of money which they cannot afford (and which they will need later) in a futile attempt to find someone who will 'cure their child'.

Much of this fruitless effort can be avoided if the medical team recognize that most parents always find it very difficult to accept at once reality and that many need the support over a long period of time before they will finally come to terms with the true situation. But the immediate problem can be helped by a sympathetic hospital social worker who can quietly assist the parents by discussion, listening and practical advice and by arranging the special aid such parents need—how to help their child to develop more normally. *Many such children suffer from the disadvantage of isolation* (because the child is unable to mix in normal ways) and this can be overcome by attending a special day nursery or playgroup. If the hospital social worker sees the parents and child regularly and arranges for health visitors, teachers or social workers to meet the parents and child too, slowly the parents begin to accept the diagnosis and will be better able to face the various difficulties. Similar problems are often seen with the parents of mentally handicapped children. In all these cases, it is often *very helpful if the parents can meet other parents who have older children who are disabled in the same way*. It is for this reason that many local associations for many congenital disabilities have developed and hospital social workers in paediatric hospitals often can introduce the parents to such a group. Many parents, in a curious way, feel guilty or ashamed about their congenitally disabled child (although many would never admit it) and may be stubbornly resentful of meeting similar parents. Patient persuasion can overcome this and can make so much difference to the eventual acceptance of the problem and its solution.

Home accidents are a serious problem in paediatric work (see p. 122). In many instances, the question may arise whether the accident could not have been prevented if only some precaution had been taken. Studies of children with burns show in some cases that this is the second case in the same family or even in the same child. This may be coincidental but usually there is a reason for this—the home circumstances may be not very satisfactory and young children may be left on their own for long periods at home or in the care of an older child. Occasionally the question of serious neglect may arise and the accident may be the only means of bringing this to light. For these reasons, hospital social workers often undertake further investigations for the paediatrician to see whether the home cannot be made safer and therefore reduce the chance of further accidents. In most instances, the hospital social worker would discuss the case with the health visitor who is visiting the home.

In some instances, the question arises whether the injury which the child has suffered is the result of an accident at all or whether it may not be a case of *non-accidental injury*. Suspicion in such cases usually starts with the doctor seeing the child recognizing that the injuries are not consistent with the parents' story, the type of injury or the attitude of the parent (see p. 434). As soon as reasonable suspicion occurs, the hospital social worker will help arrange a '*case conference*' with the doctors and local social service department officers (see p. 435). The hospital social worker will also help follow up the consequent treatment of such cases and, in this respect, work very closely with social workers, health visitors and voluntary bodies in the community.

It is known that non-accidental injury is more likely to be found in certain groups of parents—very young teenage parents or those who, in the past, have had a mental illness. Teenage parents often do represent an 'at risk' group for they are not only less tolerant of difficult children (and especially of babies who cry persistently) but are also relatively immature and, to make things much worse, are often living in poor housing conditions (sharing accommodation or living with in-laws). Apart from any possibility of non-accidental injury in children of very young parents, it means that when normal illness occurs in such children their parents will probably need more help and advice. Very often the paediatrician arranges for the hospital social worker to pay special attention to such cases. Close links must be maintained by the hospital social worker with health visitors and social workers from the local area office of the social services department so that all the support and help needed can be given at home—when the child has been discharged from hospital.

Hospital Social Work with the Elderly

The elderly are a very important section of the community in whom any serious illness may often be accompanied by many social problems (see Chapter 26). It therefore follows that any serious illness in an old person necessitating admission of that old person to hospital should be followed by inquiry into the home circumstances to see whether the old person when medically fit for discharge can safely go home, i.e. whether there is suitable supportive help at home. In most old people living in a family, home discharge is quite safe provided that nursing and medical care is available. A substantial proportion of the elderly live alone and home discharge in such cases calls for special arrangements—the provision of a home help, or a meal being delivered or arrangements made for some friend or relative to come and help temporarily to bridge the immediate period following discharge, until the old person is completely fit again to look after herself. Most geriatricians, physicians and surgeons treating elderly patients in hospital will usually refer those who live on their own to the hospital social worker so that she can ensure that the care of the old person will be satisfactory on discharge home. Some progressive local authorities have set up special *home care programmes* to help such cases but all can arrange for a home help to be available. A further problem which hospital social workers will have to consider is that some elderly people although in urgent need of such help may refuse to accept it. In many instances *the real reason for refusal is financial*—the old person feels he/she cannot afford such help. Careful explanation may help—no charge is made for home help services to the elderly whose only income is their old age pension but there can still be a difficulty in those few cases, who, although able to afford to pay for the home help, are so conscious of rising costs that they still refuse. Such elderly patients usually rationalize their refusal by firmly stating they do not need such help. Careful cooperation between the doctor and social worker will help and particularly if the old person clearly realizes, *before admission* if possible, that this form of support is all part of the necessary treatment.

Terminal Cases

Obviously many problems will have to be faced in terminal illnesses and these will depend on the age of the patient, his or her family responsibilities and the likely length of the terminal illness (short terminal illnesses usually provide fewer social problems than illnesses which last many months).

Carcinoma cases of all kinds especially in younger persons or in adults with family commitments often call for a considerable amount of medical casework. An infinite variety of problems occur. First there is the *initial treatment and the support, reassurance and anxieties of the patient to be faced.* Any adult in this situation with a family to support—such as a mother with a family still at school with say, a carcinoma of the breast or ovary—has a greater chance of success with her treatment if her natural anxieties about how the family are going to cope in her absence are reduced by sympathetic and effective practical help. In all instances, the problems faced by the family immediately will depend on the attitude of her husband and other adult relatives and on the age of the children. In many instances, the family may be able to cope but, in a number, help will be needed at once or may become necessary as the family perhaps, later, begins to show signs of strain or of being unable to manage. Many types of assistance are possible—social service departments will be able to do much to enable the family to stay together by providing a home help. In other instances it is best to arrange for a young child to go into a day nursery so that the father can leave the child there on his way to work and collect him on his way home knowing that the child will be properly looked after. In some cases, such arrangements would not be satisfactory and it may be necessary for the children to be taken voluntarily into temporary care in a children's home until the mother has had her treatment and is fit enough again to look after them. In some cases a mixture of such arrangements may be appropriate—one or two children coming into care and one (or two) staying with the father.

The hospital social worker will need to work very closely with other social workers in the community and also with health visitors who may already be well known to the family in the course of their ordinary home visiting of young children. The hospital social worker must be able to see the patient in hospital and to discuss with the doctors, nurses and other staff the prognosis and assess the assistance required.

In some terminal cases, other types of problems will have to be faced. In many elderly patients with a fatal illness, the type of home they live in and the health of their spouse may be crucial in deciding whether to discharge the patient home at all and what further supportive services will be required. Within the hospital, the consultant medical and nursing staff usually will refer such cases to the hospital social worker to investigate the home circumstances. Most hospital social workers will not carry out a home visit in such instances but will depend on the views of the primary health care team (general medical practitioner, health visitor, home nurse) and the local social worker.

In some cases, the solution is unlikely to be permanent—the patient may return home for a period and then may suddenly deteriorate and need either readmission to hospital or admission into a nursing home dealing with such cases. Obviously the closest coordination is necessary between the hospital social worker and the primary health care team. In many instances admission may finally be arranged into one of the many excellent nursing homes or hospices run by dedicated religious bodies and hospital social workers will have a local list available and help choose the one most suitable and which will also enable relatives to visit.

Single Parent Families

In single parent families, any illness in that parent will usually produce many social problems. Single parent families represent 1 in 10 of all families with dependant children; about 660 000 single parents look after 1 million children, most of these are women including 190 000 deserted or separated, 120 000 divorced, 120 000 widowed and 90 000 unmarried mothers. Obviously the care of the children will depend upon their age but in many instances unless the family can help, the younger children will need to come into the care of the local social services department. If the illness is long and protracted, such children may need to be fostered with foster parents (see p. 420) and the hospital social worker will be expected to initiate the arrangements.

Unmarried mothers represent about 9% of all mothers and, although today there is a much more liberal view held towards illegitimacy, any such birth always presents some extra problems which will usually fall to the hospital social worker to solve. Many mothers will wish to keep their child and fortunately there are many excellent schemes to help with housing accommodation (the local social services department should be able to help find places). In some instances, the mother may wish to have her baby adopted and, if the mother decides early enough, the hospital social worker arranges for this to be undertaken by either the local social services department or by a voluntary adoption agency (see p. 431).

Gynaecological Cases

In gynaecology departments, many special social problems have to be sorted out. Many women have deep-rooted fears about gynaecological conditions which need careful explanation. Much of this is carried out by the consultant and his medical staff but the multidisciplinary team approach is being increasingly used in such hospital departments and the hospital social worker in that team is expected to deal with those problems. A variety of marital difficulties may have to be tackled by the hospital social worker especially in the rehabilitation of hysterectomy patients. Some of the troublesome symptoms may be connected with marital or sex difficulties and such hospital social workers need special training and must work very closely with the medical team in the hospital and the primary health care team in the community.

Many such departments now have to deal with questions such as *abortions* and the hospital social workers must know all the alternative arrangements which are available if an abortion is either refused or cannot take place in hospital because of the shortage of beds.

Accident Cases

In accident cases involving adults, many social problems occur. Some of these are due to the suddenness of the injury and to the period of doubt which follows concerning the outcome if the seriously injured patient remains unconscious. There may still be a very difficult period for the family and patient to face until it is clear that there is no permanent brain damage. Not only is it necessary for the hospital social worker to help support the family but *she will also need to help with rehabilitation*—with possible employment problems and perhaps with industrial retraining. In most of these instances, the hospital social worker acts as the coordinator between the doctors in the hospital and with those responsible for industrial retraining including the Disablement Resettlement Officers of the Employment Service Division.

In accident cases which result in permanent paralysis (such as *paraplegia*), there may still be a period of doubt about the outcome for it may be weeks before it becomes certain whether the paralysis is permanent due to a division of the spinal cord or whether it is temporary due to severe bruising. If the case turns out to be one of *permanent paraplegia*, then a *great deal of social work needs to be undertaken by the hospital social worker in conjunction with social workers in the community*, and with occupational therapists to ensure that the home will be suitable for the patient. He will be in a wheelchair on his discharge. Many adaptations and modifications will probably be necessary but these will take a long time to arrange and therefore it is most important that the hospital social worker starts such arrangements (which will necessarily involve many outside agencies) early in the stay of the patient in hospital. It is for this reason, that many regional hospitals looking after paraplegia patients arrange for their hospital social workers to discuss each patient's home conditions in detail with a social worker from the local social services department *shortly after the admission of the patient.*

Rheumatoid Arthritis and Similar Chronic Disabling Diseases

Many serious disabling conditions which develop suddenly in adult life (but which are not fatal) such as *rheumatoid arthritis always provide a range of social problems.* Some of these may be obvious, like the care of young children if the mother is affected and has to be admitted to hospital for a long period. But others may be related to the difficulty of adjustment which many patients find. If a normal active young adult suddenly develops a crippling and painful condition such as rheumatoid arthritis, the initial reaction is usually one of incredulity. Much patience is needed by the doctors and nurses to overcome this, and the hospital social worker backed up by other social workers and health visitors in the community can play a major part by casework and counselling (by sympathetic listening, explanation and encouragement) to enable the patient finally to accept the immediate limitations of the illness and therefore to help the rehabilitation process.

In other diseases such as *multiple sclerosis* and *muscular dystrophy*, there is usually a general slow deterioration and progression although there will be periods of remission and relapses and, in some cases, the disease will suddenly abort. Crises are bound to occur in some of these cases as the effects of the disease produce their social problems. Many of these have to be dealt with by those working outside hospital such as social workers, primary health care teams but, in many instances, hospital admission becomes inevitable and the hospital social worker has to help solve the difficulty. This will vary from complete family breakdown as when a married partner leaves the home, to more minor problems connected with various aids and adaptations which need to be fitted to help the partially paralysed patient.

Mental Disability

Social workers employed in mental hospitals form an important part of the team under the psychiatrist. The successful discharge of many patients depends upon not only the correct psychiatric treatment but on being able to find out the home conditions. All psychiatric patients are particularly influenced adversely by unsatisfactory living conditions. In fact the 'extrinsic' conditions are always one of the most important predisposing factors in sudden deterioration or breakdown in mental illness. It therefore follows that the success or failure in many such patients will depend on the social conditions surrounding the patient on discharge—his home, his family, the availability of suitable employment.

Follow-up of all discharged mentally ill patients is also most important and the hospital social worker should help the psychiatrist to assess how the patient is managing after discharge. This can only be satisfactorily undertaken by the hospital social worker if she has excellent links with the primary health care team and the social worker undertaking the after care. The provision of day care facilities in the community are also important (see p. 477) and reports should always be available from such units. In the past, many psychiatric social workers in hospital undertaking such after care work did many visits themselves. With the larger number of discharges being arranged from psychiatric hospitals, this is now rarely possible and arrangements have been made for the social workers in the area teams in the community to visit the hospital regularly, to attend weekly conferences on patients about to be discharged and to act as the visiting after-care force for the hospital treatment team.

In the case of the *mentally handicapped, a great deal of social problems occur.* Reference has already been made to the difficulties many parents have in accepting the diagnosis (see p. 137). Apart from this, a great deal of advice needs to be given to such parents (see Chapter 6). In many instances, hospital social workers will not be involved as most of these persons live at home. But in some cases, the mentally handicapped patient is also disabled in some other respect (about 48% of those with spastic diplegia are also mentally handicapped) and the hospital social worker may be involved in helping and advising during a stay in hospital or on attendance at outpatient or assessment clinic.

General Medical, Surgical and Orthopaedic Cases

In small proportion of such cases, the hospital social worker will be brought into the diagnostic and treatment team in hospital by the consultant because of *special difficulties connected with social problems of the patient at home or at work.* Any illness which may become longstanding is more likely to produce social problems. For this reason *diabetes*, *epilepsy*, *chronic bronchitis* and *ischaemic heart disease (coronary thrombosis)*, *hemiplegia*, *tuberculosis* and many other diseases often involve the hospital social worker either during the initial illness or during a relapse. The uncertainty of outcome (prognosis) adds to the various social problems to be faced by such patients and their families.

ENVIRONMENTAL HELP

Housing always plays an important part in the development of disease and in its treatment and rehabilitation (see p. 292). In the paraplegic or the serious disabled mentioned above, the house may need to be adapted in various ways (see p. 448) or new specially designed accommodation may be necessary. It is *most important that the inevitable problems are considered early enough to enable a satisfactory solution to be worked out by the time the patient is ready for discharge.* This virtually means shortly after admission of the patient and not, as is done in many cases, shortly before discharge. Six months will probably be required to carry out any major structural adaptations and if new accommodation must be built a longer time will be needed. Smaller adaptations take a shorter time but even these will require three months. It should be possible to supply small handrails more quickly but it is surprising how many small snags can arise to delay the job. Therefore the hospital social worker should anticipate such difficulties by arranging with the corresponding local authority social services department to order the necessary structural work or aid required as soon as possible after the need has become firmly established.

ARRANGEMENTS OF IMMEDIATE ASSISTANCE

A further function of hospital social workers could be classified *as arranging features which facilitate medical care.* It includes a wide range of functions many of which might be described as routine or superficial services for patients and their relatives which do not involve social casework. They include financial help, convalescent arrangements, provision of escorts and accommodation for relatives.

Financial help

Many patients will need advice about their '*welfare rights*'—what financial help they are entitled to—sickness benefit, invalidity benefit and the various industrial injury benefits. Many of these are extremely complicated and are constantly changing and most patients find them confusing. In the case of accidental injuries, the hospital social worker must explain that compensation may be available through civil action in the courts and stress the importance of the patient and his relatives seeing a solicitor at the earliest possible moment, to ensure that he receives the proper advice. If the patient belongs to a professional organization or trade union, that body usually will be most helpful in such cases.

There are also special financial grants available through the local Social Security office to assist with the visiting of children and others who are patients in hospital. The hospital social work department has to undertake this type of work.

Convalescent arrangements

Convalescent arrangements of various kinds are made by hospital social workers. These include a range of such facilities within the health service, i.e. by transfer to special convalescent hospitals and with the convalescent type of holiday formerly arranged by local authority health departments and now transferred to the reorganized health services. In addition there is a wide variety of other convalescent homes available which are run by industrial concerns, nationalized bodies and trades unions which assist with convalescence for those working in the corresponding industry. There are also many voluntary organizations which before 1948 used to help with the payment of hospital provision for its contributors which have bought or built convalescent homes (e.g. the Merseyside Health Benefits Council). The hospital social worker therefore has a wide range of convalescent facilities to choose from in helping any individual patient.

Provision of escorts

In some instances, an *escort has to be arranged to travel with a child or elderly person leaving hospital* and the hospital social worker is responsible for arranging this. She usually uses a panel of voluntary helpers or a local voluntary organization.

Accommodation for relatives

In some cases, the patient has been admitted to a hospital which is a long way from home and close relatives may find it very difficult or impossible to visit unless they can arrange to stay for a short time near the hospital. The hospital social worker usually has a list of suitable addresses—covering a range of accommodation and price—and will assist relatives to find suitable accommodation. This is particularly important if the patient is dangerously ill or is due to have an operation and the relatives wish to be close at hand.

LIAISON WITH VARIOUS COMMUNITY AGENCIES

Another function of hospital social workers is the necessary *liaison work* between the team in the hospital treating the patient; doctor, nurse, physiotherapist, occupational therapist; and the various other statutory and voluntary agencies working in the community. Most of this liaison is with the social services department of the corresponding local authority for every such department should act as a necessary link between the hospital services and the community social services. Many of the facilities required by patients either in the form of services, aids and adaptations, telephones—are initiated by the hospital social worker contacting the social services department who then provides the service required. To ensure that continuity of care can occur, social workers in the local area social service teams are encouraged to visit hospitals periodically to discuss with the hospital social worker which patients will require further help. Eventually it is hoped that hospital social workers will be alerted when anyone well known to the local social services department has to be admitted to hospital so that the doctors and treatment team can be given the fullest facts.

Hospital social workers also work closely with local health visitors so that after care services can be more fully mobilized. Health visitors can be most valuable when children are admitted to hospital, or with unmarried mothers, or with any family known to have been under constant observation by the health visitor. In many districts, the health visitors are very active in undertaking after-care of elderly persons at risk.

In any case in which possible adoption is raised, the local social services department should be contacted; in many instances, voluntary adoption agencies may be used.

Employment opportunities with disabled patients can be a most important and crucial feature in the rehabilitation of many handicapped persons. The hospital social worker should work closely in such cases with the Disablement Resettlement Officer of the Employment Service Division. Usually the DRO will visit the patient in hospital. Occasionally medical staff have to complete various registration forms in respect of their disabled patients and it is usually the Hospital Social Worker who obtains the form and arranges for the doctor to complete it and then returns it.

Organization

Hospital social workers are now members of the social services department but they are still based within hospitals (see p. 393).

Index

Abatement notice, 293
Abortion Act, 1967, 271
  introduction, 357
Accidents
  children, 122–3
  elderly, 266
  prevention in primary health care, 265–6
Active immunity, 180
Adaptations for the disabled, 448
Admission unit, 422
Adoption, 429–33
Adult training centres
  and school leavers, 143
  main functions, 482–3
Advisory Council on the Misuse of Drugs, 481
Aetiology, 171
Age Concern, 385
Agglutination test, 175
  in typhoid diagnosis, 207–8
Agricultural revolution, 335
Aids for the disabled, 448
Aid centres, 449
Albuminuria in pregnancy, 99
Alcoholism, 478–80
Aliens Order, 1953, 329
Alkali, etc., Works Regulation Act, 1906, 298
Allocation Committee, 30
Ambulance services, 169–70
Amenity beds, 34
Antenatal care, 98–100
Anthrax
  epidemiology and control, 222–3
  immunization, 185
Approved schools, 423
Area Chemists Contractors Committee, 31
Area comparability factor, 63–4
Area Health Authorities, 9–10
  structure and functions, 14–15
  main duties, 17–18
Area Medical Officer, 19
Area Nursing Officer, 20
Area Nurse (Child Health Services), 20
  main functions, 127–8
Area Review Committee, 435–6
Area Team of Officers, 18
Artificial Limb and Appliance Centre, 380
Ascaris lumbricoides, 318
Ascorbic acid, 281
Association of Directors of Social Services, 385
Asthma, schoolchildren, 145
Attendance allowance, 452
Attendance Order, 426
Augmentation of wages, 455–6
Autism, 150

Bacteriological investigations, 174–5
Barnardo, Thomas, 342
Barnardos children's homes, 420

Basic practice allowance, 35
Battered baby syndrome, *see* Non-accidental injury
BCG immunization, 184
Benzidine derivatives and bladder cancer, 249
Benzyl benzoate, 135
Beri-beri, 280
Beveridge, William, 350
Birth rate, 59–63
Black Death, *see* Plague
Blindness
  children, 144
  sheltered employment, 455
  social services, 453–8
  WHO work with, 328–9
Blood culture, 174–5
  in typhoid, 207
Blood group in antenatal care, 95
Blood transfusion
  and RHA, 16
  in pregnancy, 103, 349
Boarding out, 420
  regulations, 421
Boards of Guardians, 338
Borstal training, 427
  establishment, 346
Botulism, 213
Braille, 456
Bread, 282
Breast feeding, 115
  and cancer of breast, 246
British Association of Social Workers, 385
Bronchiectasis, schoolchildren, 145
Bronchitis, epidemiology, 252–4
Brucellosis, epidemiology and control, 223–5
Budd, William, 341
Bus passes, 503

Calcium, 279
Calorie requirements in diet, 281–2
Campaign for Single Homeless People, 522
Cancer
  education, 268
Cancer (*cont.*)
  epidemiology of, 239–49
  bladder, 249
  breast, 245–6
  cervix, 247
  lung, 243–5
  stomach, 246–7
  registration, 83
Canicola fever, 226
Carbohydrates, 278
Careers guidance, 142–3
Care order, 418
  procedure, 424–5
Carriers, 175–6
  convalescent, 175
  symptomless, 175
  typhoid and paratyphoid, 208–9
Case conferences
  problem families, 429
  Non-accidental injury, 435
Census, 57
Central Midwives Board, 92
Cervix cytology, 168–9
Chadwick, Edwin, 340
Cheese, 285
Chemical closets, 306
Cheshire Foundation Homes, 452
Chief Environmental Health Officer, 290
Chief Medical Officer, Annual Report, 53
Child abuse, *see* Non-accidental injury
Child guidance clinics, 149
Child health clinic, 116
Child minder, 415
Children Act, 1948, 350
  care proceedings under, 416–19
Children Act, 1975, 417–18
  custodianship, 421
  future changes in adoption, 431–3
Children and Young Persons Act, 1963, 416
Children and Young Persons Act, 1969
  observation and assessment under, 419
  and criminal proceedings, 425–6
Chiropody, 167
  development, 352

Chlorination, *see* Water
Cholecystectomy in typhoid carriers, 209
Cholera
  epidemiology and control of, 216–17
  and WHO, 324–5
Cholesterol, and ischaemic heart disease, 252
Chronically Sick and Disabled Persons Act, 1970, 441–2
  introduction, 357
Cigarette smoking
  and cancer of the lung, 245
  and ischaemic heart disease, 251
Cirrhosis of the liver, epidemiology, 257–8
Citizens Advice Bureaux, 384
Clean Air Acts, 1956 and 1968, 298–9
  introduction, 354
Clearance areas, 294
Clients, 393
Closing orders, 294
Clostridium perfringens food poisoning, 212–13
Clubs
  for disabled, 448
  for elderly, 500–1
Cockroaches, 315
Commonwealth Immigrants Act, 1962, 329–30
Communicable diseases
  statistics, 83
  control in primary health care, 264–5
  local control, 27
  in schools, 133
  virulence, 177
Community Health Councils
  and consumer protection, 25–7
  functions, 50–1
Community homes
  assisted, 424
  controlled, 424
  types of, 420–1
  with education on the premises (CHEs), 423–4
Community hospitals, 166
Community Relations Council, 356
Community development, 357
Compulsory purchase order, 295
Concessionary fares, *see* Elderly
Congenital dislocation of the hip, 113–14
Congenital malformations, 111–13
  study of, 357
Contact tracing
  in poliomyelitis, 219
  in sexually transmitted diseases, 231
  in tuberculosis, 195
Convalescence, arrangements made by hospital social workers, 537
Cooperation card in pregnancy, 101
Corporate management, 378–80
Coronary thrombosis, *see* Ischaemic heart disease
Cot deaths, 120–1
Court of Protection, 488
Court Report, 106, 123–5
Custodianship, 421–2
Cyanocobalamin, 280

Dark Smoke (Permitted Periods) Regulations, 1958, 298
Day centres
  disabled, 447
  elderly, 501
  mentally ill, 477
Day hospitals
  geriatrics, 166
  mental illness, 473–4
Day nurseries
  functions, 413–14
  in non-accidental injury, 438
Day surgery, 166–7
Deaf and dumb, social services for, 458
Deafness
  children, 144
  hard of hearing, 458–9
  hearing aids in children, 131
  high frequency, 131
  partial, in children, 144
Death rates
  crude, 63

Death rates (*cont.*)
  standardization, 63–4
Dental care
  in pregnancy, 99
  in schoolchildren, 151–2
Dental Services Committee, 31
Department of Health and Social Security
  control methods in health, 5, 6
  control methods in social services, 385–7
Depression in elderly, 498
Deratting Exemption Certificate, 331
Designated area, 29
Detention centres, 427
Detoxification centres, 480
Diabetes
  and ischaemic heart disease, 251
  epidemiology, 254–7
  in schoolchildren, 145
Diet in pregnancy, 98
Diphtheria
  epidemiology, 192
  immunization, 183
Director of Social Services
  and disabled persons, 444
  functions, 389–95
Disabled Living Foundation, 444, 449
Disabled Persons (Employment) Acts, 1944 and 1958, 440
Disablement Resettlement Officer
  and cerebral palsy, 461
  and corporate management, 380
  and disabled persons, 443–4
  and handicapped schoolchildren, 142
  and hospital social workers, 538
Discharges and deaths of hospital patients, 79–80
Disease prevention
  primary, 262
  secondary, 262
District Community Physician, 22
  and hospital infections, 192
  and immunizations in local outbreaks, 32
  and notification of communicable diseases, 176
District Handicap Teams
  functions, 124–5
  and multidisciplinary teams, 46
District Management Team, 21
District nursing, *see* Home nursing
District Nursing Officer, 21
Divorce, 405–7
Down's syndrome, 147
Droplet infection, 171–2
Drug addiction, 480–1
Dysentery, epidemiology, 209–10
Dyslexia, 150

Education
  problems in handicapped children, 139
  psychologist, 132
  and social problems, 409–10
Education (Handicapped Children) Act, 1971, 482
Educational Subnormality (Mild), ESN(M), 145–6
Educational Subnormality (Severe), ESN(S), 147–8
Elderly
  and hospital social workers, 529
  concessionary fares, 503
  disability in, 490–1
  health problems in, 492–4
  proportions of population, 58, 489–90
  sheltered housing, 504–5
  social services for, 497–503
Electron microscopy, 175
Employment Rehabilitation Centres, 443
Employment Service Division and disabled persons, 442–4
Endemic, 171
Environmental Health Officer and communicable diseases, 27
Epidemic, 171
Epidemiology of non-communicable diseases, 238–9
Epilepsy
  in schoolchildren, 149–50
  and social services, 461–2
Ergosterol, 280

Erythrogenic toxin, 189
European Health Committee of Council of Europe, 321
European Economic Community, 322

Family Allowances, 350
Family size, 399–401
Family Expenditure Survey, 54
Family planning provisions, 168
Family Planning Information Service, 156
Family Practitioner Committee, 20
  main functions, 28–31
Family Service Units, 383
Faecal-borne infections, 172
  culture in typhoid diagnosis, 207
Farr, William, 339
Fats, 278
Finance
  help for elderly, 502
  help for patients, 536–7
  DHSS control methods, 5
  payments to general practitioners, 34–7
Flies, control, 313–14
Fleas, control, 310–11
Fluoridation, *see* Water
Flying squad, 102–3
Food Hygiene (Docks, Carriers, etc.) Regulations, 1960, 289
Food Hygiene (General) Regulations, 1970, 287–8
Food
  contamination, 287
  and typhoid, 206
  port inspection, 330–1
  preservation, 286–7
  poisoning, 210–15
Foster parents, 420

Gamma benzene hexachloride, 316
Gamma radiation of food supplies, 215
Geriatrics
  day hospitals, 496
  services, 495
General Board of Health, 340
General Household Survey, 53
General Improvement Area, 296–7
General Medical Council, 34
General practitioner
  conditions of service, 31–4
  and health education, 159
  remuneration, 34–7
  size of practice, 30
Genetic counselling
  after congenital malformed birth, 111
  in mental handicap, 486
Gonorrhoea, epidemiology and control, 229
Good neighbour schemes, 499, 511
Group health education, 159
Guardian ad litem, 431
Guardianship Order, 487–8
Guide dogs for the blind, 457
Guthrie test, 102

Haemolytic disease of the newborn, 108
Handicapped children, 136–7
  overprotection, 145
  parents, 137–8
  special schools, 139
Handicraft centres
  for elderly, 500–1
  general provisions, 447
Health Advisory Service, 370
Health Bulletin, 54
Health care planning teams, 22–3
  and multidisciplinary teams, 46
Health centres, 162–3
  development, 352
Health education, 153–61
  in pregnancy, 97–8
  in schools, 134
Health Education Council, 155–6
  functions, 158
Health education officer, 154–5
Health Insurance, first schemes, 347
Health Service Commissioner, 37–8
Health Services and Public Health Act, 1968, 165

Health Trends, 55
Health visitor
  and health education, 155
  estimation of need of, 373
  roles, 115–18
Heating, 302
  for elderly, 502
Heat stagnation, 300
Hemiplegia, 459–60
Holder process, 283
Holidays
  for blind, 457
  for disabled, 449–50
  for elderly, 502
Home accidents
  children, 122–3
  elderly, 266
Home care programmes, 500
Home helps
  and disabled, 508–11
  and elderly, 447
  estimation of need of, 498–9
Homelessness, 512–23
  intentional, 517–18
  priority needs, 513–14
  single persons, 522–3
Home nursing, 163–7
Home workers schemes, 456
Hortvet test, 283
Hospital In-patient Enquiry, 54
Hospital Management Committees, 351
Hospital
  care in mental illness, 469–70
  confinements, 91
  community, 166
  Infection Control Officer, 192
  infections, 191–2
  statistics, 77–80
Hospital Order, 486
Hospital social worker
  estimation of need, 373–4
  main duties, 525–37
Hostels
  for blind, 457
  for elderly, 505–6
  for mentally handicapped, 485
  for mentally ill, 478
Houghton Committee, 432
Houses
  improvement, 296
  multiple occupation, 295–6
Household, projections, 402
Housing
  and disabled persons, 448–9
  and health, 273
  and illness, 292
  in Industrial Revolution, 337
  and social problems in, 407–8
  and the elderly, 491
  substandard, 293–7
  in tuberculosis, 196
Housing (Homeless Persons) Act, 1977, 512–13
Humidity
  in incubators, 109
  ventilation, 300
Hygiene in schools, 134–5
Hyperkeratosis, 279
Hypertension
  and ischaemic heart disease, 251
  in pregnancy, 98
Hypothermia
  primary health care, 267
  elderly, 494–5

Immunization, 180
  advances after 1942, 349–50
  against tuberculosis,198–9
  BCG, 184
  passive, 180, 187–8
  in primary health care, 264
  in schools, 133
  of travellers, 32
  schedules for in infants, 182
  triple, 183
  whooping cough, 182–3
Incubation periods, 173–4
Incubator care, 109
Industrial Revolution, 336–7
Industrial therapy units, 484
Infantile gastroenteritis, 217–18
Infant mortality rate, 66–70
Infectious diseases, *see* Communicable diseases
Infective hepatitis
  epidemiology and control, 220

Infective hepatitis (*cont.*)
passive immunization, 188
Influenza, 199–200
and WHO, 327
Inner Area Partnership, 357, 388
Insect-borne diseases, 235–7
Integration of handicapped children in schools, 140–1
Intelligence Quotient, 146–7
Interdepartmental Committee on Physical Deterioration, 344–5
Interim care order, 418
Intermediate area, 29
Intermediate treatment, 426
International Statistical Classification of Disease, Injuries and Causes of Death, 85
Insecticides, 316
Iodine, 279
Iron, 279
Ischaemic heart disease
epidemiology, 249–52
genetic factors, 251
rehabilitation, 262–3
and social class, 88
Issue analysis, 361, 368–70

Jenner, Edward, 335
Joint Care Planning Teams, 22–3
Joint Committee for children, 125
Joint Consultative Committee, 23–4
and corporate management, 380
Joint Financing, 24
Joseph Rowntree Memorial Trust, 461
Juvenile delinquency, 147

Kahn test, 95
Keratomalacia, 279
Key sector finance, 386
Keystone machine, 131
Koch, 335

Lassa fever, epidemiology and control, 232–5
Laundry service, 164
Leprosy, and WHO, 326
Leptospirosis
and rats, 309
epidemiology and control, 255–6
Leukaemia, epidemiology and control, 247–8
Lice, control, 311–12
Life tables, 64
Life expectancy, 64–5
Lighting, 303
Liquid Egg (Pasteurization) Regulations, 1963, 215, 331
Lister, 343
Local Authority Associations, 385
Local Authority Social Services Act, 1970, 389–93
introduction, 355
Local Executive Councils, 351
Local Government Board, 341
Local Government Act, 1929, 348
Locally determined schemes, 386
Local Medical Committee, 30–1
Low birth weight babies, 109–11
Luncheon clubs, 499–500

Maladjustment, children, 148–9
Malaria
epidemiology and control, 235–6
eradication schemes, 323–4
Management consultants, 369
Management
input and output measurements, 361–4
objectives, 361
priority determination, 375–8
Manpower Services Commission
and disabled persons, 442–4
Manpower shortages, 377–8
Margarine, 284–5
Mass media health education, 159
Mass miniature radiography, 198–9
campaigns, 353
Maternal mortality rate, 73–6
in 1930s, 349
confidential enquiry, 100
primary avoidable factor, 349
Meals on wheels
and elderly, 499

Meals on wheels (*cont.*)
development of, 352
for disabled, 447
organization of, 511–12
Measles
active immunization, 184
epidemiology, 200
passive immunization, 187
Meat inspection, 285
Medical Officer of Health, 342
Medical Practices Committee, 29
Medical Services Committee, 33–4
Meningitis, 193
Mental confusion in elderly, 493
Mental handicap, 464
hospital social worker, 534–5
in phenylketonuria, 113
in primary health care, 269
prevention of, 486–7
sheltered housing, 483–4
social services for, 482–6
Mental Health Act, 1959, 465–8
introduction, 355
Mental Health Enquiry, 54
Mental Health Review Tribunals, 472–3
Mental illness
and hospital social worker, 534–5
compulsory admissions, 470–2
epidemiology, 258–60
informal admissions, 467
intrinsic factors, 259
in primary health care, 270
statistics, 78
types, 464
Mental subnormality, *see* Mental handicap
Midwives Acts, 92
1902, 346
Milk and Dairies (General) Regulations, 1959, 283
Milk
composition, 282–3
pasteurization, 283–4
sterilization, 284
Mineral salts, 278–9
Minister for the Disabled, 357
Ministry of Health, creation of, 348
Mobility allowance, 450–1
Mongolism, *see* Down's syndrome
Monitoring of health services, 43–4
examples, 364–8
Morbidity, 76
factors connected with, 238–9
Morris, Alfred, 357
Mortality rates, 85–6
Mosquitoes
malaria, 235–6
control, 312–13
Mothercraft clinics, 94
Multidisciplinary team developments, 45–6
Multiple sclerosis
and hospital social workers, 534
social services for, 459–60
Muscular dystrophy, 459–60, 534
Myelomeningocele, 111

Named Person
in infants, 122
in schoolchildren, 138
National Children's Homes, 343, 420
National Development Group for Mentally Handicapped, 6
publications, 54
National Food Survey, 54
National Health Service, policy and planning, 6
National Health Service Act, 1946, 350
National Health Service (Family Planning) Act, 1967, 357
Needs, calculation of, 371–5
Neonatal cold injury, 108
Neonatal mortality rate, 70–1
Neonatal paediatrics, 108
Newsholme, Sir Arthur, 345
Nicotinic acid, 280
Night blindness, 279
Non-accidental injury
and hospital social workers, 528
diagnosis, and treatment, 433–9
in primary health care, 264
registers, 437
Northern Ireland, health and social services, 40
Notification of births, 56, 107, 345

NSPCC, 343
Nuisance order, 293
Nursery schools, 128–9
Nutrition, 276–82
  in 1930s, 349
  in primary health care, 267–8
Nursery schools and classes, 415

Observation and assessment
  children, 419
  units, 422–3
Obesity
  in diabetes, 256
  in ischaemic heart disease, 251
Obstetric list, 93
Occupancy
  in day nurseries, 368
  in hospitals, 366–7
  in old persons' homes, 367
Occupational mortality, 88–9
Occupational therapy
  and disabled, 446–7
  and elderly, 497
  centres for mentally handicapped, 483
  domiciliary, 352
Oedema in pregnancy, 99
Office of Population Censuses and Surveys, 3–4
Offices, Shops and Railway Premises Act, 1963, 302
  introduction of, 354
Open areas, 29
Open industry, 445
  for blind, 455
Optical Committee, 31
Orthodontic treatment, 152
Orthoptic treatment, 131
Osteomalacia, 280
Oxyuris vermicularis, 318

Paediatrics, developmental, 359
Paraplegia
  and hospital social worker, 533
  social services, 459–60
Parasitology, 317–19
Parental rights, cessation of, 419
Pandemic, 171
Paratyphoid fever, 205–8
Pasteurization
  ice cream, 284
  milk, 283–4
  milk and food poisoning, 216
  typhoid epidemics, 207
Patient Operated Selector Mechanism, 460
Pemphigus neonatorum, 191
Pensions, introduction of, 347
Peptic ulcer, epidemiology, 254–5
Perinatal mortality rate, 71–2
Personal Social Services Council, 385
Phage type, in typhoid, 208
Phenylketonuria, 113
Phosphorus, 279
Place of safety order, 435, 438
Plague
  and rats, 309
  epidemiology and control, 236–7
Playgroups, 414
  in non-accidental injury, 438
Plenum system, *see* Ventilation
Poliomyelitis
  epidemiology and control, 218–20
  immunization, 183
Pollution, atmospheric, 297–9
Population explosion, 357
Population
  projections, 401–4
  trends, 53
Poor Law Amendment Act, 1834, 338
Port medical work, 329–30
Postnatal care, 103
Posters in health education, 160
Precipitation test, 175
Preschool initial medical examination, 129
Premature babies, *see* Low birth weight babies
Preventive social work with children, 429
Primary health care
  and home nursing, 165
  and mental illness, 469
  preventive medicine in, 262–75
Prior approval, 298

Problem families, 119–20
  and social problems, 428–9
Proper Officer
  and communicable diseases, 290
  and environmental health, 27
  and unfit houses, 294
Proteins, 278
Psychiatric services
  community nursing, 475
  day activity area, 473–4
  for the elderly, 496–7
  and social worker, 525
Psychopathic disorders, 468
Public Health Act, 1848, 340
Public Health Laboratory Service, 28
  development, 353
Puerperal pelvic infection, 190
Pure tone audiometer, 131
Pyrethrum, 316

Q fever, 228

Rabies Act, 1974, 227
Rabies, epidemiology and control, 226–8
  immunization against, 185
Ragged Schools Movement, 342
Ramps
  in houses, 448
  in schools, 139
Rate rebates, 503
Rate support grant, 386–7
Rats
  description and control, 308–10
  disease spread, 309
  and plague, 236–7
Reform Bill, 1832, 337
Refuse collection and disposal, 307–8
Regional Health Authority
  functions, 15–17
  full list, 14–15
  structure, 8–9
Regional Hospital Boards, 351
Regional Planning Committee
  and children, 426
  functions, 428
Regional Plan
  for children, 423–4
  details, 428
Regional Team of Officers, 17
Registration
  of births, 55–6
  of cancers, 83–4
  of deaths, 56
  of disabled, 446
  of stillbirths, 56
Rehabilitation
  centres, 447
  in elderly, 493
  in mental illness, 475–6
Remand homes, 423
Renal dialysis units, dangers of infection, 232
Rent rebates, 503
Residential nursery, 422
Repiratory diseases in neonatal period, 120
Restricted area, 29
Retirement, preparation for, 492
Rhesus factor
  in antenatal care, 95
  prevention of incompatibility, 96–7
Rheumatic heart disease in children, 145
Rheumatoid arthritis
  and social services, 459–60
  social problems, 533–4
Riboflavin, 280
Rickets, 280
Royal Association for Disability and Rehabilitation, 383
Royal National Institute for the Blind, 456–7
Royal Society for the Prevention of Accidents, 156
Rubella
  active immunization, 185
  epidemiology, 200–1
  passive immunization, 187

Salmonellosis, 213–16
Scabies mite, 315–16
  in schools, 135

Scarlet fever, 189
School health service
  and medical examinations, 126–7
  organization, 126–51
  establishment, 334–5
Scotland, health services, 38–9
Screening tests
  development, 358
  in infants, 113–14
  in women, 268
Secretary of State for Social Services
  and appeals, 30, 33, 34
  functions in health, 3–5
  functions in social services, 384–7
  Parliamentary control, 7
Secretary of State for Wales, 39
Selective medical examinations in schools, 129
Senile dementia, 497–8
Seniority payments, 36
Septic tanks, 181
Serum sickness, 181
Serum hepatitis, 231–2
Sewage disposal, 306–7
Sex education, 270–1
Sex ratios and age, 399
Sexually transmitted diseases
  and WHO control, 326
  epidemiology and control, 228–31
  incubation periods, 174
Shaftesbury, Lord, 339
Shaftesbury Society, 343
Shellfish and typhoid fever, 285
Sheltered workshops, 445
  for mentally handicapped, 483–4
Ships, fumigation, 310, 331
Short-term care, 485
Sickness Benefit returns, 81–3
Simon, Sir John, 341
Single parent families
  and hospital social workers, 531–2
  day nursery provisions, 413–14
Slum clearance, 293–4
Smallpox
  consultants, 203
  epidemiology and control, 201–4
  eradication programmes, 324
Smog, 297
Smoke control areas, 299
Snow, Sir John, 340–1
Social class
  and age of mother at time of birth, 401
  and births, 61
  and cancers, 242
  and cirrhosis of the liver, 257
  and diabetes, 256
  and leukaemia, 248
  and mental illness, 259
  statistics, 57–9
Social educational teams, 151
Social factors in diseases, 239
Social indicators
  objective, 398–410
  subjective, 411–12
Social Security, 350
Social Service Department, 392
Social Trends, 53
Social Worker
  and health education, 155
  estimation of need of, 374
  in schools, 139
  non-accidental injury, 436
  training, 388–9
Social Work Service, 370, 386
Southwood Smith, Dr, 340
Spastic diplegia
  in children, 150
  social services in, 460–1
Spastics Society, 444
Special education advisory service, 138
Specialist Careers Officer, 142
Specialist in Community Medicine (Child Health), 20
  and school health services, 128
Specialist in Community Medicine (Environmental Health), 19
  and hospital infections, 192
  and immunization on local outbreaks, 32
  and notification of communicable diseases, 176
Specialist in Community Medicine (Social Services), 19, 394
Speech development, 118–19
Speech therapists, 150
Sphincter control in infants, 119
Spina bifida, 111

Sputum tests, 174–5
  disposal of in tuberculosis, 196
Standard capitation fee, 35
Standardized Mortality Ratio
  cancer, 241
  suicide, 261
  tuberculosis, 194
Staphylococcal infections
  food poisoning, 211–12
  pemphigus neonatorum, 191
Statutory nuisance, 293
Steatorrhoea, 281
Sterilization
  of air in premature baby units, 110
  of water supplies, 305–6
Stigma in mental illness, 466
Stillbirth rate, 73
Subnormality, 468
Suicide, 260–1
Sunshine Homes, 144
Supervision orders, 426
Supplementary practice allowance, 35
Surveillance
  in children, 114
  in poliomyelitis, 219–20
  in smallpox, 204
  in viral haemorrhagic diseases, 233–5
Sweep test, 131
Syphilis
  epidemiology and control, 229–31
  prevention in pregnancy, 95

Taenia
  echinococcus, 317
  saginata or *solium*, 317
Teachers
  and health education, 155
  and tuberculosis, 196
Telephones for the disabled, 451
Tetanus immunization, 182–3, 185
Thiamine, 280
Trichiniasis, 221
  and rats, 309
Throat swabs and washings, 174–5
Tonsillectomy in poliomyelitis outbreaks, 218
TOPS courses and disabled persons, 443
Toxaemia of pregnancy and maternal mortality, 75–6
Toxoid, 181
Toxoplasmosis, 220–1
Trachoma, 327
Training function of social service departments, 391–2
Training Services Division and disabled persons, 443–4
Transport for the disabled, 450
Tribunal, 33
Trichinella spiralis, 318
Trilene analgesia in labour, 101–2
Tuberculosis
  WHO control schemes, 325–6
  epidemiology and control of, 193–9
  BCG immunization, 184
  in schoolchildren, 145
  reduction of, 353
Typhoid fever
  epidemiology and control of, 205–9
  threshold infection, 205–6
Typhus fever, epidemiology and control of, 237–8

Unit costs, 366
Unmarried mothers, 104–5
Urban Aid, 357, 388
Urinary carriers, 208–9
  cultures, in typhoid, 207

Vaccine, 181
Vandalism, 356
Vehicle excise duty, exemption of in disabled persons, 451
Venereal diseases, *see* Sexually transmitted diseases
Ventilation, 300
  Plenum system, 301–2
Viral haemorrhagic diseases, 232–5
Virological investigations, 174–5

Virulence of communicable diseases, 177
Vitamins, 279–81
Vocalization in infants, 118

Wales, health services, 39–40
Warfarin, 310
Warnock Committee, 122
  and CHEs, 423
  recommendations, 135–43
Wassermann test, 95
Welsh Health Services Organization, 39
Water
  chlorination, 305
  fluorindation of, 306
  infection in typhoid, 206
  filtration, 305
  purification, 304–6
  supplies, 303
  wells, 303–4
Webb, Beatrice and Sidney, 347
Welfare food rationing schemes (1939–1945), 349
Weils disease, *see* Leptospirosis
Wireless for the blind, 457
Whooping cough immunization, 182–3
Women's Royal Voluntary Services, 383
World Health Organization
  development, 353
  functions, 320–9
Wright, Almroth, 343–4

Xerophthalmia, 27

Youth Treatment Centres, 427

Zermatt typhoid epidemic, 209